**PLATINUM COORDINATION COMPLEXES
IN CANCER CHEMOTHERAPY**

Other books in this series:

F.J. Cleton and J.W.I.M. Simons, eds., Genetic Origins of Tumor Cells
ISBN   90-247-2272-1

J. Aisner and P. Chang, eds., Cancer Treatment Research
ISBN   90-247-2358-2

B.W. Ongerboer de Visser, D.A. Bosch and W.M.H. van Woerkom-Eykenboom, eds., Neuro-
Oncology: Clinical and Experimental Aspects
ISBN   90-247-2421-X

K. Hellmann, P. Hilgard and S. Eccles, eds., Metastasis: Clinical and Experimental Aspects
ISBN   90-247-2424-4

H.F. Seigler, ed., Clinical Management of Melanoma
ISBN   90-247-2584-4

P. Correa and W. Haenszel, eds., Epidemiology of Cancer of the Digestive Tract
ISBN   90-247-2601-8

L.A. Liotta and J.R. Hart, eds., Tumor Invasion and Metastasis
ISBN   90-247-2611-5

J. Banoczy, ed., Oral Leukoplakia
ISBN   90-247-2655-7

C. Tijssen, M. Halprin and L. Endtz, eds., Familial Brain Tumours
ISBN   90-247-2691-3

E.M. Muggia, C.W. Young and S.K. Carter, eds., Anthracycline Antibiotics in Cancer
ISBN   90-247-2711-1

B.W. Hancock, ed., Assessment of Tumour Response
ISBN   90-247-2712-X

D.E. Petersen and S.T. Sonis, eds., Oral Complications of Cancer Chemotherapy
ISBN   90-247-2786-3

R. Mastrangelo, D.G. Poplack, and R. Riccardi, eds., Central Nervous System Leukemia:
Prevention and Treatment
ISBN   0-89838-570-9

A. Polliack, ed., Human Leukemias: Cytochemical and Ultrastructural Techniques in
Diagnosis and Research
ISBN   0-89838-585-7

W. Davis, C. Maltoni, and S. Tanneberger, eds., The Control of Tumour Growth and its
Biological Bases
ISBN   0-89838-603-9

A.P.M. Heintz, C.T. Griffiths, and J.B. Trimbos, eds., Surgery in Gynecological Oncology
ISBN   0-89838-604-7

PLATINUM COORDINATION COMPLEXES IN CANCER CHEMOTHERAPY

Proceedings of the Fourth International Symposium on
Platinum Coordination Complexes in Cancer Chemotherapy
convened in Burlington, Vermont by the Vermont Regional
Cancer Center and the Norris Cotton Cancer Center, June 22-24, 1983.

edited by

Miles P. Hacker
Evan B. Douple
Irwin H. Krakoff

Martinus Nijhoff Publishing
A member of the Kluwer Academic Publishers Group
Boston/The Hague/Dordrecht/Lancaster

Distributors for North America:
Kluwer Academic Publishers
190 Old Derby Street
Hingham, MA 02043

Distributors outside North America:
Kluwer Academic Publishers Group
Distribution Centre
P.O. Box 322
3300 AH Dordrecht
The Netherlands

Library of Congress Cataloging in Publication Data

International Symposium on Platinum Coordination
   Complexes in Cancer Chemotherapy (4th : 1983 : Burlington, Vt.)
   Platinum coordination complexes in cancer chemotherapy.

   (Developments in oncology)
   Sponsored by Bristol-Myers Company and others.
   Includes indexes.
   1. Cisplatin—Congresses. 2. Cancer—Chemotherapy—Congresses.
3. Platinum compounds—Therapeutic use—Testing—Congresses.
4. Coordination compounds—Therapeutic use—Testing—Congresses.
5. Complex compounds—Therapeutic use—Testing—Congresses.
I. Hacker, Miles P. II. Douple, Evan B. III. Krakoff, Irwin H. IV. Vermont
Regional Cancer Center. V. Norris Cotton Cancer Center. VI. Bristol-
Myers Company. VII. Title. VIII. Series.
RC271.C55I58 1983   616.99'4061   83-23722
ISBN-13: 978-1-4612-9792-5   e-ISBN-13: 978-1-4613-2837-7
DOI: 10.1007/978-1-4613-2837-7

DEDICATION

DAVID B. BROWN
1943-1983
Professor of Chemistry, University of Vermont
Member, Vermont Regional Cancer Center

This volume is dedicated to David Brown. He was one of the leaders in conceiving and planning the Fourth International Platinum Symposium. In his research, Dave exemplified the spirit of the symposium and was an example of the intense involvement of a laboratory scientist in clinical problems leading to new insights and more rapid progress. Unfortunately, the field of cancer therapy had not advanced rapidly enough for Dave to be able to benefit directly from the effort in which he had taken such an active part. And if he would have lived to attend the symposium, we hope that he would have been proud of this volume and its intent to advance the application of metal coordination complexes in cancer therapy.

SYMPOSIUM COMMITTEES

ORGANIZING
Joseph H. Burchenal
Michael J. Cleare
Thomas A. Connors
Evan B. Douple, *Co-Chairman*
Miles P. Hacker
Irwin H. Krakoff, *Co-Chairman*
Jean-Pierre Macquet
Barnett Rosenberg

PROGRAM
David B. Brown
Joseph H. Burchenal
Michael J. Cleare
Miles P. Hacker, *Chairman*
Karin Lindquist
Stephen J. Lippard
Charles L. Litterst
Robert A. Newman
Robert C. Richmond

ARRANGEMENTS
David B. Brown
Joan MacKenzie, *Chairman*
John J. McCormack

SPONSORS

BRISTOL-MYERS COMPANY

E.I. du PONT de NEMOURS & COMPANY

ENGELHARD CORPORATION

JOHNSON MATTHEY, INC.

NORRIS COTTON CANCER CENTER

A.H. ROBINS COMPANY

SMITH KLINE & FRENCH LABORATORIES

STUART PHARMACEUTICALS

VERMONT REGIONAL CANCER CENTER

WARNER-LAMBERT

The symposium was supported in part by Grant #CA 34679 from the National Cancer Institute.

CONTRIBUTORS

DONALD L. BODENNER, Department of Pharmacology and University of Rochester Cancer Center, University of Rochester, Rochester, New York, 14642, U.S.A.

RICHARD F. BORCH, Department of Pharmacology and University of Rochester Cancer Center, University of Rochester, Rochester, New York, 14642, U.S.A.

FRANCES E. BOXALL, Department of Biochemical Pharmacology, Institute of Cancer Research, Belmont, Sutton, Surrey, England.

WILLIAM T. BRADNER, Pharmaceutical Research and Development Division, Bristol-Myers Company, Syracuse, New York, 13221-4755, U.S.A.

JOSEPH BURCHENAL, Memorial Sloan-Kettering Cancer Center, New York, New York, 10021, U.S.A.

JEAN-LUC BUTOUR, Laboratoire de Pharmacologie et de Toxicologie Fondamentales du CNRS, 31400, Toulouse, France.

A. HILARY CALVERT, Department of Biochemical Pharmacology, Institute of Cancer Research, Belmont, Sutton, Surrey, England.

JOHN P. CARADONNA, Department of Chemistry, Massachusetts Institute of Technology, Cambridge, Massachusetts, 02139, U.S.A.

STEPHEN K. CARTER, Pharmaceutical Research and Development Division, Bristol-Myers Company, New York, New York, 10154, U.S.A.

MICHAEL J. CLEARE, Johnson Matthey Research Center, Blunt's Court, Sonning Common, Reading RG4-9N4 England

JERRY COLLINS, Clinical Pharmacology Branch, Division of Cancer Treatment, National Cancer Institute, Bethesda, Maryland, 20205, U.S.A.

BRIAN J. CORDEN, Clinical Pharmacology Branch, Division of Cancer Treatment, National Cancer Institute, Bethesda, Maryland, 20205, U.S.A.

J. WAYNE COWENS, Department of Clinical Pharmacology and Therapeutics and Department of Experimental Therapeutics, Roswell Park Memorial Institute, Buffalo, New York, 14263, U.S.A.

PATRICK J. CREAVEN, Department of Clinical Pharmacology and Therapeutics, Roswell Park Memorial Institute, Buffalo, New York, 14263, U.S.A.

JEROEN H. DEN HARTOG, Department of Chemistry, State University Leiden, 2300 RA Leiden, The Netherlands.

LEIGH A. FERREN, Environmental Sciences, Oak Ridge National Laboratory, Oak Ridge, Tennessee, 37830, U.S.A.

ANNE MARIE J. FICHTINGER-SCHEPMAN, Department of Chemistry, State University Leiden, 2300 RA Leiden, The Netherlands.

ALEXANDER P. FLORCZYK, Pharmaceutical Research and Development Division, Bristol-Myers Company, Syracuse, New York, 13221-4755, U.S.A.

DEVINDER S. GILL, Department of Biological Sciences, Carnegie-Mellon University, Pittsburgh, Pennsylvania, 15213, U.S.A.

MILES P. HACKER, Vermont Regional Cancer Center and Department of Pharmacology, University of Vermont, Burlington, Vermont, 05401, U.S.A.

STEPHEN J. HARLAND, Department of Biochemical Pharmacology, Institute of Cancer Research, Belmont, Sutton, Surrey, England.

KENNETH R. HARRAP, Department of Biochemical Pharmacology, Institute of Cancer Research, Belmont, Sutton, Surrey, England.

K. J. HIMMELSTEIN, Inter Research Corporation, Lawrence, Kansas, 66044, U.S.A.

JAMES D. HOESCHELE, Warner-Lambert/Parke-Davis Pharmaceutical Research Division, Ann Arbor, Michigan, 48105, U.S.A.

WILLIAM J. M. HRUSHESKY, Department of Medicine, University of Minnesota, Minneapolis, Minnesota, 55455, U.S.A.

PAUL C. HYDES, Johnson Matthey Research Centre, Sonning Common, Reading RG4 9NH, England.

NEIL P. JOHNSON, Laboratoire de Pharmacologie et de Toxicologie Fondamentales du CNRS, 31400, Toulouse, France.

MERVYN JONES, Department of Biochemical Pharmacology, Institute of Cancer Research, Belmont, Sutton, Surrey, England.

JANET C. KATZ, Department of Pharmacology and University of Rochester Cancer Center, University of Rochester, Rochester, New York, 14642, U.S.A.

DAVID P. KELSEN, Memorial Sloan-Kettering Cancer Center, New York, New York, 10021, U.S.A.

HARTMUT KÖPF, Institute für Anorganische and Analytische der Technischen Universität Berlin, D-1000 Berlin 12, West Germany.

PETRA KÖPF-MAIER, Institute für Anatomie der Freien Universität Berlin, D-1000 Berlin 33, West Germany.

STEPHEN J. LIPPARD, Department of Chemistry, Massachusetts Institute of Technology, Cambridge, Massachusetts, 02139, U.S.A.

CHARLES L. LITTERST, Laboratory of Medicinal Chemistry and Pharmacology, Division of Cancer Treatment, National Cancer Institute, Bethesda, Maryland, 20205, U.S.A.

PHUONG VAN T. LUC, Vincent T. Lombardi Cancer Research Center, Georgetown University Medical Center, Washington, D.C., 20007, U.S.A.

JEAN-PIERRE MACQUET, Laboratoire de Pharmacologie et de Toxicologie Fondamentales du CNRS, 31400, Toulouse, France.

STEFAN MADAJEWICZ, Department of Clinical Pharmacology and Therapeutics, Roswell Park Memorial Institute, Buffalo, New York, 14263, U.S.A.

ANTONIUS T. M. MARCELIS, Department of Chemistry, State University Leiden, 2300 RA Leiden, The Netherlands.

KEVIN G. MC GHEE, Department of Biochemical Pharmacology, Institute of Cancer Research, Belmont, Sutton, Surrey, England.

J. GORDON MC VIE, Department of Oncology, Netherlands Cancer Institute and Free University Hospital, 1007 MB Amsterdam, The Netherlands.

VEN L. NARAYANAN, Drug Synthesis and Chemistry Branch, Division of Cancer Treatment, National Cancer Institute, Bethesda, Maryland, 20205, U.S.A.

MOHAMED NASR, Starks C.P., Inc., Silver Spring, Maryland, 20910, U.S.A.

DAVID R. NEWELL, Department of Biochemical Pharmacology, Institute of Cancer Research, Belmont, Sutton, Surrey, England.

ROBERT F. OZOLS, Medicine Branch, Division of Cancer Treatment, National Cancer Institute, Bethesda, Maryland, 20205, U.S.A.

T. F. PATTON, Department of Pharmaceutical Chemistry, University of Kansas, Lawrence, Kansas, 66045, U.S.A.

LAKSHMI PENDYALA, Department of Clinical Pharmacology and Therapeutics, Roswell Park Memorial Institute, Buffalo, New York, 14263, U.S.A.

HERBERT M. PINEDO, Department of Oncology, Free University Hospital, 1007 MB Amsterdam, The Netherlands.

VICTOR M. PRIEGO, Vincent T. Lombardi Cancer Research Center, Georgetown University Medical Center, Washington, D.C., 20007, U.S.A.

AQUILUR RAHMAN, Vincent T. Lombardi Cancer Research Center, Georgetown University Medical Center, Washington, D.C., 20007, U.S.A.

HONORAT RAZAKA, Laboratoire de Pharmacologie et de Toxicologie Fondamentales du CNRS, 31400, Toulouse, France.

JAN REEDIJK, Department of Chemistry, State University Leiden, 2300 RA Leiden, The Netherlands.

A. J. REPTA, Department of Pharmaceutical Chemistry, University of Kansas, Lawrence, Kansas, 66045, U.S.A.

JOHN A. ROBERTS, Health and Safety Research Division, Oak Ridge National Laboratory, Oak Ridge, Tennessee, 37830, U.S.A.

WILLIAM C. ROSE, Pharmaceutical Research and Development Division, Bristol-Myers Company, Syracuse, New York, 13221-4755, U.S.A.

BARNETT ROSENBERG, Barros Research Institute, Holt, Michigan, U.S.A.

PETER J. SADLER, Department of Chemistry, Birkbeck College, University of London, London, WCIE 7HX England.

BERNARD SALLES, Laboratoire de Pharmacologie et de Toxicologie Fondamentales du CNRS, 31400, Toulouse, France.

PHILIP S. SCHEIN, Vincent T. Lombardi Cancer Research Center, Georgetown University Medical Center, Washington, D.C., 20007, U.S.A.

HOWARD I. SCHER, Memorial Sloan-Kettering Cancer Center, New York, New York, 10021, U.S.A.

JOHN E. SCHURIG, Pharmaceutical Research and Development Division, Bristol-Myers Company, Syracuse, New York, 13221-4755, U.S.A.

H. SHIH, Department of Pharmaceutical Chemistry, University of Kansas, Lawrence, Kansas, 66045, U.S.A.

ZAHID H. SIDDIK, Department of Biochemical Pharmacology, Institute of Cancer Research, Belmont, Sutton, Surrey, England.

IAN E. SMITH, Department of Biochemical Pharmacology, Institute of Cancer Research, Belmont, Sutton, Surrey, England.

LARRY A. STERNSON, Department of Pharmaceutical Chemistry, University of Kansas, Lawrence, Kansas, 66045, U.S.A.

W. W. TEN BOKKEL HUININK, Department of Oncology, Netherlands Cancer Institute and Free University Hospital, 1007 MB Amsterdam, The Netherlands.

W.J.F. VAN DER VIJGH, Department of Oncology, Netherlands Cancer Institute and Free University Hospital, 1007 MB Amsterdam, The Netherlands.

J.B. VERMORKEN, Department of Oncology, Netherlands Cancer Institute and Free University Hospital, 1007 MB Amsterdam, The Netherlands.

CLAUDE VIEUSSENS, Laboratoire de Pharmacologie et de Toxicologie Fondamentales du CNRS, 31400, Toulouse, France.

L. R. WHITFIELD, Warner-Lambert/Parke-Davis Pharmaceutical Research Division, Ann Arbor, Michigan, 48105, U.S.A.

EVE WILTSHAW, Department of Biochemical Pharmacology, Institute of Cancer Research, Belmont, Sutton, Surrey, England.

PAUL V. WOOLLEY, Vincent T. Lombardi Cancer Research Center, Georgetown University Medical Center, Washington, D.C., 20007, U.S.A.

MICHEL WRIGHT, Laboratoire de Pharmacologie et de Toxicologie Fondamentales du CNRS, 1400, Toulouse, France.

ROBERT C. YOUNG, Medicine Branch, Division of Cancer Treatment, National Cancer Institute, Bethesda, Maryland, 20205, U.S.A.

PREFACE

The idea for convening a Fourth International Symposium on Platinum Coordination Complexes in Cancer Chemotherapy was born in an assembly of researchers from the Vermont Regional Cancer Center and the Norris Cotton Cancer Center who shared a common interest in metal complexes. It was agreed by those assembled that sufficient time had passed since the Third International Symposium on Platinum Coordination Complexes in Cancer Chemotherapy held in 1976 at the Wadley Institutes of Molecular Medicine in Dallas, Texas, during which several advances in the chemistry, biochemistry, pharmacology and clinical use of platinum complexes had occurred, to warrant a fourth symposium. Furthermore, intensive investigations in progress were bringing sophisticated methodologies to bear on the problems in the field, clinical trials were yielding interesting results, and unique approaches to cancer therapy were being designed. Therefore, an organizing committee was formed and planning culminated in the symposium which was held in Burlington, Vermont, June 22-24, 1983.

This volume includes the manuscripts of the invited speakers from each of the six sessions representing key aspects relevant to the use of platinum and other metals as chemotherapeutic agents. These speakers and session leaders were charged to review recent developments and to highlight some of the new areas of focus and promise. The abstracts of the scientific posters which were presented appear in their respective sections. In order to keep the size of the proceedings to one volume the authors were unfortunately limited. The questions and discussions generated by active participation by the attendees are not transcribed and it is therefore impossible to capture the excitement and cross-disciplinary interaction which was present among the 180 participants throughout the symposium.

The editors wish to thank the contributors for delivering the manuscripts on schedule, and the session leaders for their assistance with the editing and refereeing of the manuscripts. Financial assistance in support of the symposium was provided by several sources as acknowledged elsewhere in this volume, and this support is gratefully appreciated. We also thank the other members of the organizing committee. The program committee deserves the credit for assembling speakers and special thanks is reserved for Joan MacKenzie, who along with staff of the Vermont Regional Cancer Center, provided the local arrangements which contributed to the effective exchange of ideas and the success of the symposium.

Miles P. Hacker, Evan B. Douple and Irwin H. Krakoff
August, 1983

TABLE OF CONTENTS

Nomenclature

Section I: Biochemistry of Platinum Coordination Complexes in Cancer Chemotherapy

Section II: Pharmacology and Pharmacodynamics of Platinum Coordination Complexes in Cancer Chemotherapy

xiii

David B. Brown Memorial Lecture

NOMENCLATURE

Nomenclature for Platinum Antitumor Compounds
J. Reedijk

1. INTRODUCTION

Throughout this symposium book and also in the literature a
variety of (often trivial) names and abbreviations have been used
to describe or indicate platinum compounds. To allow proper regis-
tration and classification of such compounds, and also to avoid
confusion or misunderstanding in referring to these compounds, it
is required to have and use a clear and concise nomenclature. Both
IUB (International Union of Biochemistry) and IUPAC (International
Union of Pure and Applied Chemistry) have nomenclature commissions
that deal with this subject. This paper will briefly summarize the
rules that lead to IUPAC-recommended names, and will also list
most of the trivial names and abbreviations that have been used so
far for a variety of platinum anti-tumor compounds.

2. NAMES AND FORMULAE OF PLATINUM COORDINATION COMPOUNDS

All platinum anti-tumor compounds belong to the group of
coordination compounds and should, therefore, be named as indicated by the rules of the IUPAC commission for Inorganic Chemistry
Nomenclature (1). These rules show how to derive <u>formulae</u> and
systematic <u>names</u>.

In <u>formulae</u> cations are always listed before anions. Within the
complex entity, the central metal ion is mentioned first, followed
by the anionic ligands and - thereafter - the neutral ligands.
Complicated ligand formulae may be abbreviated by <u>lower</u> <u>case</u>
letter symbols, such as en, py, dien, dach, ox. Square brackets
are often used to indicate the coordination entity, whereas a
geometric descriptor may be added - only when needed - in front
of the formula, separated by a hyphen.

Examples: K_2PtCl_4, $K[PtCl_3(C_2H_4)]$, cis-$[PtCl_2(NH_3)_2]$,$[PtCl_2(en)]$, $[PtCl(dien)]Cl$, $trans$-$[PtBr_2(py)_2]$, $[Pt(ox)(NH_3)_2]$.

The names for such compounds are easily deduced by applying the following simple rules (abstracted from the IUPAC (1) rules).

a. Cationic species are mentioned before anionic species (e.g. dipotassium tetrachloroplatinate; sodium chloride);

b. In a coordination entity (such as $PtCl_2(NH_3)_2$) the metal is always mentioned last. In front of the metal all the coordinated ligands (both ionic and neutral) are listed in alphabetical order of their names. The name is written as a single word, without spaces and with hyphens used only to separate structural prefixes (such as 1,2..., cis, α, μ, β). The valence state of the metal may be added when useful.

Example: amminebromochloropyridineplatinum(II)

c. When more than one ligand of a certain kind is present, numerical prefixes must be used, such as in tribromochloroplatinum(IV).

d. Certain coordinated ligands have special names, i.e.

NH_3 (ammine; NOT ammonia) OH^- (hydroxo; NOT hydroxy)

H_2O (aqua; NOT aquo) Cl^- (chloro; NOT chloride)

These ligands are used in combination with the numerical prefixes di, tri, tetra, etc. All other ligands are used in combination with bis, tris, tetrakis, etc. and application of parentheses. Anionic ligands usually end in -o; (e.g. -ato, -ido,-ito).

Examples: diaquabis(pyridine)platinum(II)-ion; diammine-oxalatoplatinum(II); diamminebis(nitrato)platinum(II).

e. When the coordination entity is negatively charged, the name should end in: ate; (NOT ite, ato, etc.), such as in disodium-tetrachloroplatinate(II).

f. Geometrical or structural indicators may be added in italics when needed, such as in cis-diamminedibromoplatinum(II). In many cases this is not needed, such as in $Pt(en)Cl_2$.

g. Ligands bridging between two metals are indicated by μ, such as in di-μ-hydroxo-bis[cis-diammineplatinum(II)] dinitrate.

h. Organic ligands are named according to the Organic Rules (2). Often used abbreviations are: en (ethylenediamine), py (pyridine), ox (oxalato dianion), dach (diaminocyclohexane), mal (malonato dianion).

3. USE OF NOMENCLATURE

To help the reader of this book and to contribute to a proper use of nomenclature in future work by investigations in this field, a Table has been set up. This Table shows the line formulae, structural formulae, IUPAC-recommended names, recommended abbreviations (only when agreement exists) and several other used abbreviations for most (but not all) compounds mentioned in the Proceedings.

Names for other, related platinum compounds should be derived accordingly. In case of doubt, however, the original IUPAC publications should be consulted (1,2).

It is recommended that in all future papers on platinum antitumor compounds, the authors at least mention:
i) the line formulae (or the structural formulae, when known)
ii) the systematic IUPAC-recommended names.

Used abbreviations (for instance in Tables, Figures, Schemes) should be clearly explained within the paper. Abbreviations should preferably be in capitals (where needed preceeded by *cis-*) to avoid confusion with ligand abbreviations.

4. ACKNOWLEDGEMENTS

The author is indebted to Drs. Miles P. Hacker, Charles L. Litterst, Ven L. Narayanan, Alessandro Pasini and Peter J. Sadler for helpful discussions during the symposium.

5. REFERENCES
1. Nomenclature of Inorganic Chemistry, Definitive Rules 1970. 2nd Edition, Butterworths, London, 1971. Also published in Pure and Appl. Chem. <u>28</u>. (1971) 1.
2. Nomenclature of Organic Chemistry, Sections A,B,C,D,E, F,H. Pergamon Press, Oxford, 1979.

TABLE. Formulae, names and abbreviations of Platinum coordination compounds

Line formula	Structure formula	Systematic IUPAC name[a]	USA-accepted abbreviation	Abbreviations still in use[d]
cis-[PtCl$_2$(NH$_3$)$_2$]	(structure)	cis-diamminedichloroplatinum(II)	Cisplatin	cis-DDP, CDDP, neoplatin, CP, PDD, cis-Pt, cis-platinum, NSC-119875
trans-[PtCl$_2$(NH$_3$)$_2$]	(structure)	trans-diamminidichloroplatinum(II)	–	trans-DDP, trans-platin, trans-Pt, TDDP, NSC-131558
cis-[Pt(NH$_3$)$_2$(H$_2$O)$_2$]$^{2+}$	(structure)	cis-diamminediaquaplatinum(II)-ion	–	–
cis-[Pt(OH)(NH$_3$)$_2$(H$_2$O)]$^{+}$	(structure)	cis-diammineaquahydroxoplatinum(II)-ion	–	–
[PtCl(dien)]Cl	(structure)	chloro(diethylenetriamine)-platinum(II) chloride	–	Pt-dien, No NSC number
[PtCl$_2$(en)]	(structure)	dichloro(ethylenediamine)-platinum(II)	–	cis-DEP, NSC-125181

TABLE (continued)

Systematic IUPAC name [a]	USA-accepted abbreviation	Abbreviations still in use[d]	Formula
diammine(1,1-cyclobutanedicarboxylato)platinum(II)	Carboplatin	CBDCA, JM-8, NSC-241240	$[Pt(C_6H_6O_4)(NH_3)_2]$
aqua(1,1-bis(aminomethyl)cyclohexane)sulfatoplatinum(II) (see footnote b)	Spiroplatin	TNO-6 NSC-311056	$[Pt(SO_4)(H_2O)(C_8H_{18}N_2)]$
cis-dichloro-trans-dihydroxo-cis-bis(isopropylamine)platinum(IV) (see footnote c)	Iproplatin	CHIP, JM-9, NSC-256927	$[PtCl_2(OH)_2(C_3H_9N)_2]$
diammine(2-ethylmalonato)-platinum(II)	–	JM-10, NSC-154849	$[Pt(C_5H_6O_4)(NH_3)_2]$
ethylenediaminemalonatoplatinum(II)	–	JM-40 NSC-146068	$[Pt(C_3H_2O_4)(en)]$ $[Pt(mal)(en)]$
aqua(1,2-diaminocyclohexane)-sulfatoplatinum(II) (see footnote b)	–	JM-20 NSC-250427	$[Pt(SO_4)(C_6H_{14}N_2)(H_2O)]$ $[Pt(SO_4)(dach)(H_2O)]$

TABLE (continued)

		Systematic IUPAC name [a]	Abbreviations still in use [d]
[Pt(C₃H₂O₄)(C₆H₁₄N₂)] [Pt(mal)(dach)]		(1,2-diaminocyclohexane)malonatoplatinum(II)	—	JM-74 NSC-224964
[Pt(C₉H₄O₆)(C₆H₁₄N₂)] [Pt(C₉H₄O₆)(dach)]		(4-carboxyphthalato)(1,2-diaminocyclohexane)platinum(II) (see footnote b)	—	JM-82, DACH-Pt DACCP, NSC-271674
[Pt(C₆H₆O₇)(dach)]		(1,2-diaminocyclohexane)-(isocitrato)platinum(II) (see footnote b)	—	PHIC NSC-350602
[Pt(C₃H₃O₃)₂(dach)]		(1,2-diaminocyclohexane)bis(pyruvato)platinum(II) (see footnote b)	—	PYP, NSC-268253
[Pt(ox)(dach)]		(1,2-diaminocyclohexane)-oxalatoplatinum(II)	—	l-OHP, NSC-271670

Footnotes

a) In many cases several alternatives are possible for the names of the organic ligands(2); the most commonly used name has been used in this Table.

b) The structure of the compound is not precisely known, and may be different in the solid state, compared to the aqueous solution.

c) Simplified name; the systematic name is more complex(1).

d) For use in Tables, Figures, etc. abbreviations using capital letters are preferred, to avoid confusion with ligand abbreviations (lower case letters).

SECTION I

BIOCHEMISTRY OF PLATINUM COORDINATION COMPLEXES IN CANCER CHEMOTHERAPY

Chaired by S.J. Lippard

Overview
S.J. Lippard

Considerable agreement about the major structure of cis-diamminedichloroplatinum (II) (cis-DDP or cisplatin) bound to DNA emerged from this
session. Enzymatic digestion of DNA that had been allowed to react with
cisplatin in vitro revealed binding in regions rich in oligo(dG)
sequences. Two general approaches were presented. In the first, an
exonuclease or a sequence specific restriction enzyme (endonuclease) was
used to digest platinated DNA. Electrophoretic analysis of the partially
digested DNA using Maxam-Gilbert sequencing gels permitted location of
the nuclease sensitive platinum binding sites. Practitioners of the second
approach used several enzymes to overdigest platinated DNA down to the mononucleotide or short oligonucleotide level. The resulting fragments were then
separated by high performance liquid chromatography (HPLC) and analyzed. The
results of both methods pointed to a cis-DDP intrastrand d(GpG) crosslink as
being the major bifunctional binding mode, followed by d(GpXpG), X = C,A,
d(ApG), and interstrand crosslinking. Using high resolution NMR spectroscopy,
the structure of the cis-$[Pt(NH_3)_2-(DGpG)]$ adduct with several synthetic oligonucleotides was shown to involve coordination of the N7 atoms of two
adjacent guanine bases to platinum. This chelate has been clearly established
for the cis-DDP reaction products with three self-complementary hexanucleoside
pentaphosphates, d(ApGpGpCpCpT), d(TpGpGpCpCpA), and d(CpCpApTpGpG) and with
the decanucleotide d(TpCpTpCpGpGpTpCpTpC).

Several laboratories are attempting to extract platinated DNA from tissue
cultures or whole animals treated with cis-DDP, digest the platinated DNA to
the mononucleotide or short oligonucleotide level, and identify the platinum
binding sites by HPLC. In a lively discussion that took place during an
unscheduled evening workshop on this topic, it was apparent that similar
results are emerging from the different groups and that the intrastrand
d(GpG) crosslink will be a major structural determinant. Strong evidence

that this structure forms in vivo was supplied by antibody recognition
studies of DNA extracted from the ascites fluid of mice bearing the L1210
leukemia tumor that had been treated with a chemotherapeutic dose of cisplatin.
These same antibodies showed good recognition for poly (dG)·poly (dC) modified
with cis-DDP but not for platinated poly d(GC) or DNA allowed to react with
the chemotherapeutically inactive trans isomer.

Although some consensus has been reached on the stereochemistry of the
cis-DDP/DNA adduct formed in vitro or in vivo, it has not been established
that this lesion is responsible for the antitumor activity of cisplatin. Is
DNA the real target of antitumor platinum compounds? This question was addressed through studies of the inhibition of DNA synthesis in L1210 leukemia
cells in culture by cis-DDP, trans-DDP, and [Pt(dien)Cl]Cl. At very low
levels of bound platinum the antineoplastic effects of cis-DDP did not
correlate with the inhibition of DNA synthesis. Subsequent discussion of
this result emphasized, however, that DNA synthesis had been monitored only
at short times (1-2h) following platinum treatment and that controls for
platinum binding to the cell membrane had not been run. Nevertheless, this
study served as an important reminder that future work should continue to
question whether the important cytotoxic lesion of cis-DDP involves the DNA
or some other component of the tumor cell.

Assuming that DNA is the target of cisplatin, why does the drug kill
tumor cells before destroying healthy tissue? And what is the basis for the
resistance developed by cells following prolonged treatment with the drug?
These questions were addressed through studies of the DNA repair characteristics of the sensitive and resistant cell lines. Although a clear answer has
not yet emerged, attention has focused on the possible formation of crosslinks
in regions of chromatin associated with the regulation of DNA replication
or cell division. Ancillary work of interest in this regard was presented on
several posters, including studies of platinum binding to nucleosomes,
chromatin, and minichromosomes. Experiments that revealed the extent of cis-
DDP crosslinking of DNA to be influenced by the presence of intercalators
such as ethidium bromide were also described.

Powerful physical methods have been employed to elucidate the structures
and dynamic properties of cis-DDP adducts with DNA and its constituents.
Results were presented of studies using ^{195}Pt and ^{15}N NMR spectroscopy,
EXAFS, and both Tb^{3+} and nucleotide luminescence to probe aspects of platinum
binding. Among other results was the find that ligands attached to platinum

can be fluxional, suggesting possibly that once the drug is attached to one or two binding sites on a biopolymer there might be subsequent, slow ligand migration reactions to produce a more stable and possibly more lethal binding mode. Further insight into this matter was provided by studies with nucleobases in which certain adducts were found, surprisingly, to be stable even to prolonged treatment with cyanide ion, which is usually quite effective in removing platinum from DNA. Perhaps these discoveries will be linked one day to the biochemical processes responsible for repair in tumor cells.

Chemical and Biological Studies of cis-Diamminedichloroplatinum (II) Binding to DNA
J.P. Caradonna and S.J. Lippard

INTRODUCTION

Over a decade has passed since the initial observation that neutral platinum amine coordination compounds with cis configuration of labile groups were effective chemotherapeutic agents.[1] Subsequent studies built a strong case that DNA is the relevant biological target of these complexes.[2,3] Substantial effort has therefore been directed towards defining and characterizing the interactions of cis-Pt(NH$_3$)$_2$Cl$_2$ (cis-DDP) and the inactive trans-Pt(NH$_3$)$_2$Cl$_2$ (trans-DDP),[4] the structures of which are shown in Figure 1, with DNA at the molecular level.

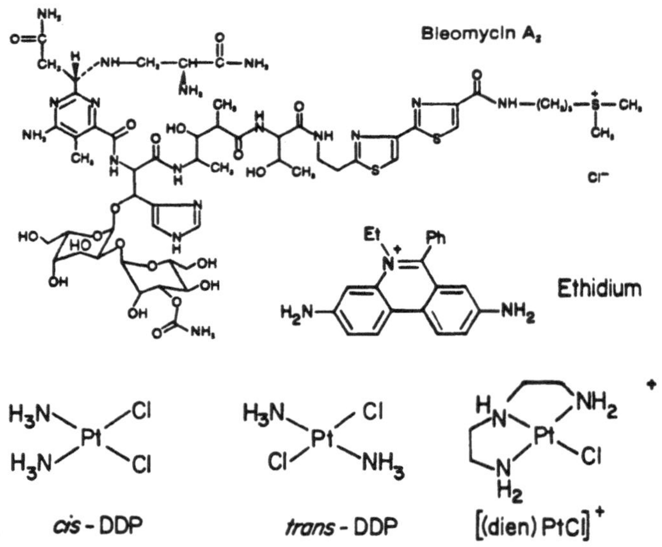

FIGURE 1. Chemical structures of bleomycin A$_2$, ethidium, cis–diamminedichloroplatinum(II), trans–diamminedichloroplatinum(II) and chlorodiethylenetriamineplatinum(II).

Currently, two major binding modes are believed to be important. Each involves the covalent[5] bifunctional coordination of platinum to heterocyclic nitrogen atoms of DNA bases in (1) two different strands (interstrand crosslink)[6,7,8] or (2) the same strand (intrastrand crosslink)[9] of the double helix. Although recent investigations have shown a correlation between interstrand crosslink formation and cell kill,[10,11] studies of Walker carcinoma cells[2] and mouse leukemia L1210 lines resistant to cis-DDP[10,12] demonstrate that the relationship between interstrand crosslink formation and cytotoxicity is not necessarily simple. Furthermore, studies on the inactivation of T7 bacteriophage[13] and phage λ[14] indicate the relative unimportance of the interstrand link compared with the intrastrand crosslink.

Results obtained by our group[15,16,17] and others[18,19] suggest that intrastrand d(GpG) crosslinking is the major event in the bifunctional interaction of cis-DDP with DNA. In this paper, we summarize recent experiments performed in our laboratory including (1) the use of enzymes to probe the base sequence specificity of cis-DDP for DNA;[16,17] (2) the characterization of the reaction product of cis-DDP with the self-complementary deoxyribohexanucleoside pentaphosphate [d(ApGpGpCpCpT)]$_2$;[20] (3) the mutual effects of intercalators and cis-DDP on their DNA binding properties;[21,22] and (4) the development of an enzyme-linked immunosorbent assay (ELISA) for cis-Pt(NH$_3$)$_2$-DNA, using a rabbit antiserum elicited against platinated calf thymus DNA modified to 4.4%.[23,24]

NUCLEASES AS PROBES OF PLATINUM BINDING TO DNA

The conformational changes produced by the binding of platinum complexes to double stranded circular supercoiled DNA are well documented.[25] Both cis- and trans-DDP are known to unwind double helical DNA (22° per bound platinum)[21] and to remove negative supercoils from plasmid DNAs.[26,27] Using agarose gel electrophoresis it was observed for either isomer that a bound drug to nucleotide (D/N) ratio of 0.050 ± 0.005[21] caused comigration of closed circular (Form I) with relaxed circular (nicked, Form II) DNA. Further positive winding of supercoiled DNA was detected by an increase in gel mobility of the DNA at higher values of bound platinum. Accompanying the dramatic changes in the electrophoretic mobility of Form I DNA was an increase in the migration of the relaxed form with increasing amounts of bound platinum.[21] This

effect was attributed to DNA shortening resulting from the formation of
intermediate to long range platinum-induced crosslinks. A significant
decrease in the contour length of platinated Form II DNA,[26] and the
observation that the intercalator ethidium bromide (EtdBr, Fig. 1)
minimizes this shortening as measured by electron microscopy, were taken
as evidence to support this conclusion.[21]

There is increasing evidence that the activity of DNA processing
enzymes depends on the local structure of DNA.[28] The observation that
bound platinum induces conformational changes in DNA suggested an assay
for determining the base sequence specificity of cis-DDP. In one such
study,[16] we examined how the normal activity of the restriction endonuclease PstI with the plasmid pSM1 was modified by the presence of bound
platinum. The plasmid has four necessarily identical cleavage sites and
the fragments (A through D) are easily separated by gel electrophoresis.
At low levels of platinum binding (D/N = 0.004) enzyme cutting at one of
these sites (D-B junction) was selectively inhibited as monitored by the
unique appearance of the D-B fragment in electrophoresis gels. Higher
platinum binding levels were required to suppress the remaining cleavage
sites. Comparison of the base sequences adjacent to the four restriction sites showed only the D-B junction to be flanked by oligo d(G)·
oligo d(C) sequences, specifically $d(G)_2 \cdot d(C)_2$, and $d(G)_4 \cdot d(C)_4$. These
and similar results suggested that cis-$Pt(NH_3)_2Cl_2$ binds to oligo
d(G)·oligo d(C) sites causing structural changes that selectively
inhibit restriction enzyme activity. At comparable binding levels the
trans isomer failed to produce these effects.

A more direct method for determining platinum binding to specific
sequences of DNA was developed simultaneously by our group[17] and that of
Haseltine.[29] The enzyme exonuclease III was used to digest platinated
duplex DNA exonucleolytically from the 3' end. A 165 bp piece of DNA
containing several oligo d(G)·oligo d(C) regions was isolated from
pBR322 and labeled with ^{32}P at the 5' end of one of the strands. The
platinated DNA was then treated with exonuclease III and the distribution
of fragments separated by size on a DNA sequencing gel. The enzyme
stopping points were determined by comparing the size of the exonuclease
III generated fragments with the length of DNA fragments produced by Maxam-
Gilbert sequencing reactions. It was observed that cis-DDP, but not
trans-DDP or [(dien)PtCl]Cl (Fig. 1), bound to oligo d(G)·oligo d(C)

sequences was efficient in stopping exonuclease III. Enzyme activity was not observed to stop at single G sites or other base sequences. This result suggests that either there is preferential binding of cis-[Pt(NH$_3$)$_2$Cl$_2$] to oligo d(G)·oligo d(C) regions at the exclusion of other sites, or that the resulting cis-Pt(NH$_3$)$_2$-oligo d(G)·oligo d(C) structure is singularly able to inhibit exonuclease III digestion.

NMR EVIDENCE FOR THE INTRASTRAND GpG CROSSLINK

The nuclease work described above showed that cis-DDP binds to (dG)$_n$·(dC)$_n$, n ≥ 2, sequences of DNA, a result consistent with the formation of intrastrand crosslinks between adjacent guanine or cytosine bases. It was therefore of interest to obtain a detailed spectroscopic characterization of cis-Pt(NH$_3$)$_2$Cl$_2$ adducts of G·C rich oligodeoxyribonucleotides. The evidence accumulated previously for cis-diammineplatinum(II) coordinated to mono-[30,31] and dinucleotides[32] revealed the heterocyclic nitrogen atoms of the purine and pyrimidine bases to be the most favored DNA binding sites. The ability of the cis-Pt(NH$_3$)$_2^{2+}$ moiety to form an intrastrand crosslink between two adjacent guanine residues has been supported by ^{1}H NMR studies of di-[32] and tetranucleotides[33] containing such sequences. Recently, we[20] examined the reaction of cis-DDP with the self-complementary deoxyribohexanucleoside pentaphosphate [d(ApGpGpCpCpT)]$_2$ and determined that the only detectable product was an intrastrand cis-diammineplatinum(II)-d(GpG) crosslink. The binding site of the covalently bound platinum was determined by comparing the chemical shifts (δ) of the non-exchangeable base protons as a function of pH* of the unplatinated and platinated oligonucleotides. The only significant difference observed upon platinum binding was a decrease of ~ 2 pH units in the guanosine H-8 chemical shifts vs pH* curves corresponding to the deprotonation at N1 of each guanine base in the platinated sample. The pK$_a$ of guanine N1 was found to be 9.8 and 8.0 for the unplatinated and platinated oligonucleotides, respectively. Such a decrease in the pK$_a$ of N1 is characteristic of guanine complexes in which cis-Pt(NH$_3$)$_2^{2+}$ is bound at the N7 position.[32,33] Coupled with the observation of the expected 0.3-0.9 ppm[32,33] downfield shift of guanine H8 induced by Pt(II) binding to N7, we concluded that an

intrastrand GpG crosslink had formed (Figure 2). The ^{1}H NMR spectrum of
the platinum adduct resembled spectra of the unmodified oligonucleotide
taken at high temperature (T > 80°C) or low pH* (pH* 3.2), conditions
under which the duplex structure and base stacking are largely
eliminated. This NMR spectral evidence demonstrates that significant
base unstacking accompanies the binding of cis-DDP to oligonucleotides,
confirming the earlier conclusions made on the basis of experiments with
plasmid DNAs.

cis - diammineplatinum(II) - d(GpG) intrastrand crosslink

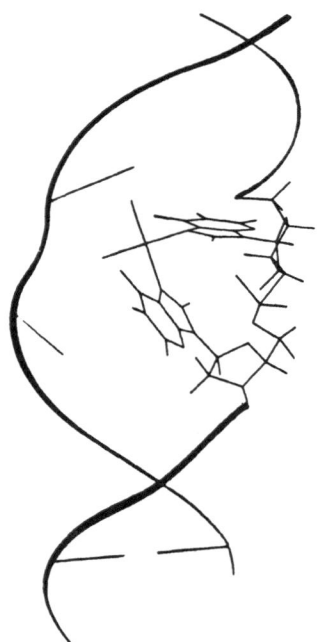

FIGURE 2. Intrastrand d(GpG) crosslink promoted by binding of the cis-
diammineplatinum(II) fragment to DNA. Conformational angles
used in the computer drawn portion of the diagram were kindly
supplied by Dr. J. Reedijk.

MUTUAL INFLUENCE OF cis-DDP AND INTERCALATING DRUGS ON DNA

Several of the drugs clinically used in combination chemotherapy to improve the efficacy of cis-DDP are intercalators,[4] a class of compounds known to alter the secondary and tertiary structure of DNA. It was therefore of interest to study the influence of intercalators on the binding of cis-DDP to DNA. As our initial compound we chose the simple intercalating agent ethidium bromide (EtdBr, Fig. 1).[34] We recently demonstrated that the binding kinetics of cis-DDP and its ability to unwind duplex DNA were unaltered when EtdBr was present during platination. However, EtdBr dramatically changed the exonuclease III detectable binding sites of cis-DDP.[22] In the absence of the intercalator, the enzyme stopped at $(dG)_n$ n = 2,3,5, sites which had been platinated.[17] Curiously, a $5'-(dG)_6-dC-(dG)_2-3'$ sequence 29 bases from the 3' end of the labeled strand of the 165 bp DNA, expected to be a prime site for platination and therefore a major enzyme stopping point, was only faintly observed on the electrophoresis gel. This result suggested that perhaps little or no platination had occurred at this site. When EtdBr was present in the platination reaction mixture, however, the $d-G_6-C-G_2$ site became the major band in the autoradiographic pattern. Even more interesting was the fact that, during an EtdBr titration experiment, low levels of intercalator showed the $3'-(dG)_2$ site to be the major stopping point with little or no detectable platinum on the $(dG)_6$ site. As the concentration of EtdBr increased, the $(dG)_6$ site became the major stopping point with a sharp decrease in intensity of the $(dG)_2$ site (Figure 3). Two possible explanations were proposed: (1) the $d-G_6-C-G_2$ site normally has a conformation unsuitable for cis-DDP binding which is modified in the presence of EtdBr to allow platinum binding to occur; or (2) platinum binds to the dG_6-C-G_2 region to the same extent whether or not EtdBr is present but, the enzyme is insensitive to bound platinum unless platination is carried out in the presence of EtdBr. In either case, these results demonstrate that local structure must play an important role in the binding of cis-DDP to DNA and that intercalators can modulate this interaction.

Recently, we have extended these studies through a series of collaborative experiments with Y. Sugiura designed to elucidate the interactions of the iron-containing antibiotic bleomycin (BLM, Fig. 1)

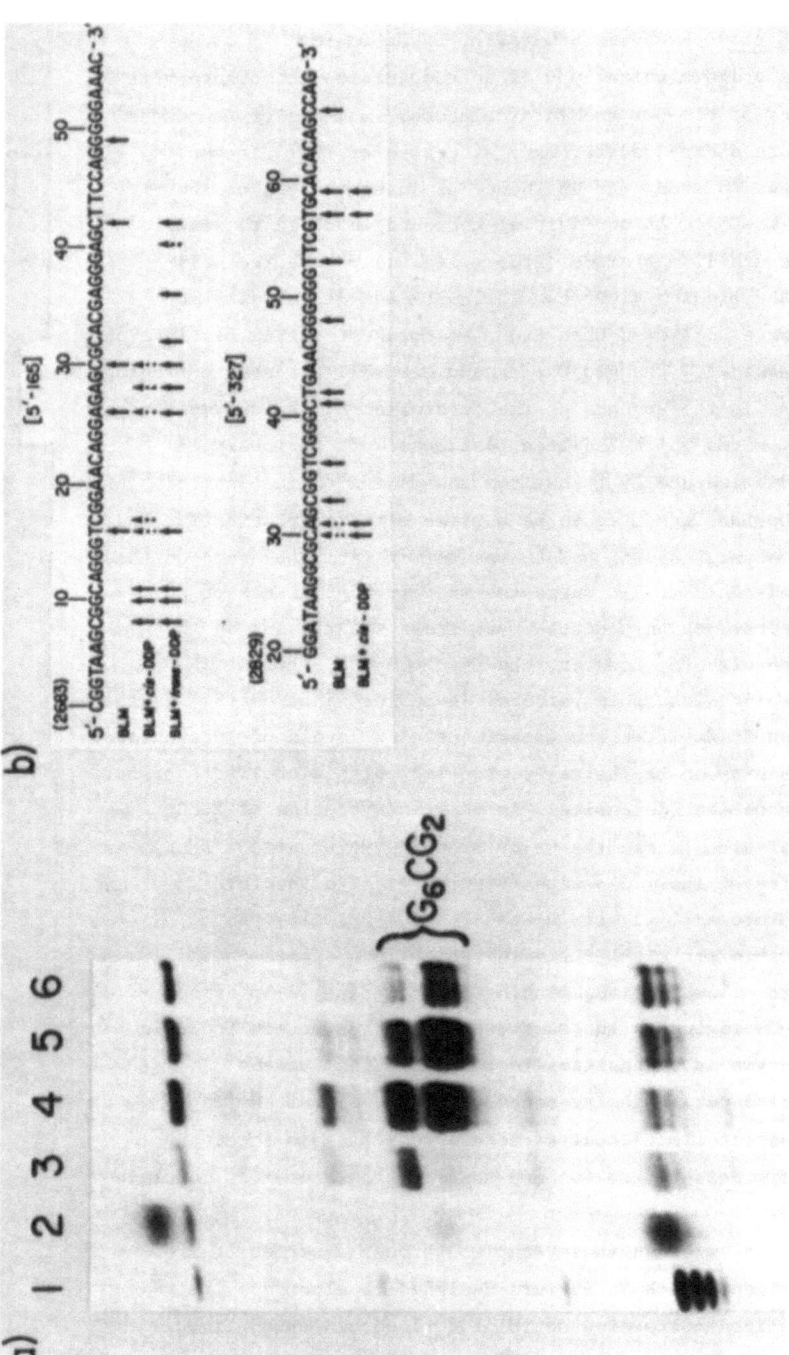

FIGURE 3. (a) Autoradiograph of an electrophoresis gel demonstrating the ethidium bromide induced change in the exonuclease III detectable cis-DDP binding sites of a 165 base pair DNA molecule (see ref. 22). Key: cis-DDP D/N: lanes 2-6, 0.05. EtdBr D/N: lane 2, 0,; lane 3, 0.012; lane 4, 0.057; lane 5, 0.12; and lane 6, 0.23. Lane 1 contains the exonuclease III digestion products of unplatinated ^{32}P-5'-labeled 165 base pair DNA. (b) Partial sequences of 165 base pair and 327 base pair restriction fragments obtained from pBR322 depicting the cleavage sites for bleomycin (BLM) in the absence and presence of cis- or trans-DDP. Strong cleavage sites are denoted as solid arrows while weaker sites are indicated by broken arrows. Full details are given in ref. 35.

with platinated DNA.[35] This glycopeptide antibiotic,[36] with its inter-
calative dithiazole moiety, is often used in combination chemotherapy
with cis-DDP to treat cancer. It cleaves double stranded DNA specifically at G–C and G–T (5' → 3') sequences.[37] In light of the exonuclease
III–EtdBr–cis-DDP results discussed above, it was of interest to
determine whether the synergism displayed by cis-DDP/BLM combination
chemotherapy could result from changes in the normal BLM activity due to
cis-DDP-DNA binding. Experiments were performed using 165 bp and 327 bp
restriction fragments, obtained from pBR322, labeled at the 5' end with
^{32}P. Cleavage sites were determined by separating the BLM produced
products on electrophoresis gels and comparing their lengths with those
obtained from Maxam–Gilbert sequencing reactions. Preliminary results
showed a significant increase in the overall ability of BLM to cleave
DNA treated with either cis– or trans-DDP. These platinum compounds
also brought about profound changes in the sequence specific BLM
cleavage products. For example, in a control experiment with
unplatinated DNA, BLM unexpectedly cut at internal GpG sequences of
oligo d(G) regions. These were completely blocked upon treating the DNA
with small amounts (D/N ~ 0.01) of either platinum isomer. Closer
inspection revealed differences in the BLM cleavage patterns obtained
following reactions of cis– and trans-DDP, with cis-DDP being more
effective at masking preferred bleomycin cutting sites in the vicinity
of oligo (dG) sequences. A summary of the BLM cleavage pattern changes
induced by platination of DNA is given in Figure 3 and analyzed in
detail elsewhere.[35]

USE OF ANTIBODIES TO PROBE THE BINDING OF PLATINUM COMPLEXES TO DNA IN
VIVO AND IN VITRO

The work presented thus far has focused on cis-DDP-DNA adducts
prepared in vitro. Until recently,[23] a sensitive and accurate assay for
probing this reaction in vivo was lacking. With the isolation of a
rabbit antiserum elicited against cis-DDP modified calf thymus DNA (D/N =
0.044) and its utilization in a competitive enzyme–linked immunosorbent
assay (ELISA), we have been able to identify cis-DDP-DNA adducts (lower
limit of detectability 0.2–0.3 fmol Pt/µg DNA) formed in vivo in a
variety of systems. The antiserum exhibits no reactivity towards cis-DDP
or DNA alone. When leukemia L1210 cells were subjected to a high dose of

cis-DDP (500 μM) the competive ELISA profiles revealed that DNA isolated from cells collected immediately after 1 hour treatment bound more antibody than DNA from cells allowed to incubate in fresh media for an additional 4 hours (Figure 4). It is known that cis-DDP induced interstrand crosslinking increases with time (up to 12 hours),[38] a fact confirmed in our study by alkaline elution profiles. Thus interstrand crosslinks are not readily detected by the antibody, a conclusion further supported by the lack of recognition of DNA treated with trans-DDP or L-phenylalanine mustard in the competitive ELISA. In both cases, the presence of interstrand crosslinks was proven by parallel alkaline elution studies. DNA obtained from malignant ascites cells of L1210 tumor bearing mice treated intraperitoneally (10 mg/kg) with cis-DDP bound to antibody (Fig. 4), demonstrating that a population of platinum-DNA adducts formed in the cancer cell is structurally highly congruent with calf thymus DNA platinated in vitro.

Studies were subsequently undertaken to define the nature of the bound platinum on the original immunogen calf thymus DNA.[24] Several platinum compounds having cis stereochemistry, $[Pt(en)Cl_2]$, cis-$[Pt(NH_2-CH_3)_2Cl_2]$, cis-$[Pt(NH_2-i-C_3H_7)_2Cl_2]$, $[Pt(CP)(DACH)]$ and cis-diammine-platinum-α-pyridone blue, were allowed to react with calf thymus DNA. All were able to bind antibody competitively. No antibody specificity was observed for DNA incubated with trans-DDP, trans-$[Pt(NH_2CH_3)_2Cl_2]$ or $[(dien)PtCl]Cl$. The most significant observation made, however, was the excellent immunoreactivity of the antiserum for cis-DDP bound to poly d(G)·poly d(C), with practically no recognition of platinated poly d(GC)·poly d(CC) (Fig. 4). These results strongly support the conclusion that cis-DDP forms a nearest neighbor intrastrand crosslink between adjacent deoxyguanosine residues (Fig. 2) as its major structural determinant. The documented specificity of the antibody for DNA from cultured cells and mouse acites fluid treated with cis-$[Pt(NH_3)_2Cl_2]$ strongly implies that this adduct is also formed in vivo. The observation that the ELISA profile of in vivo DNA samples show less efficient antibody binding than for immunogen DNA suggests a more heterogeneous in vivo adduct population.

cis-DDP-DNA COMPETITIVE ELISA

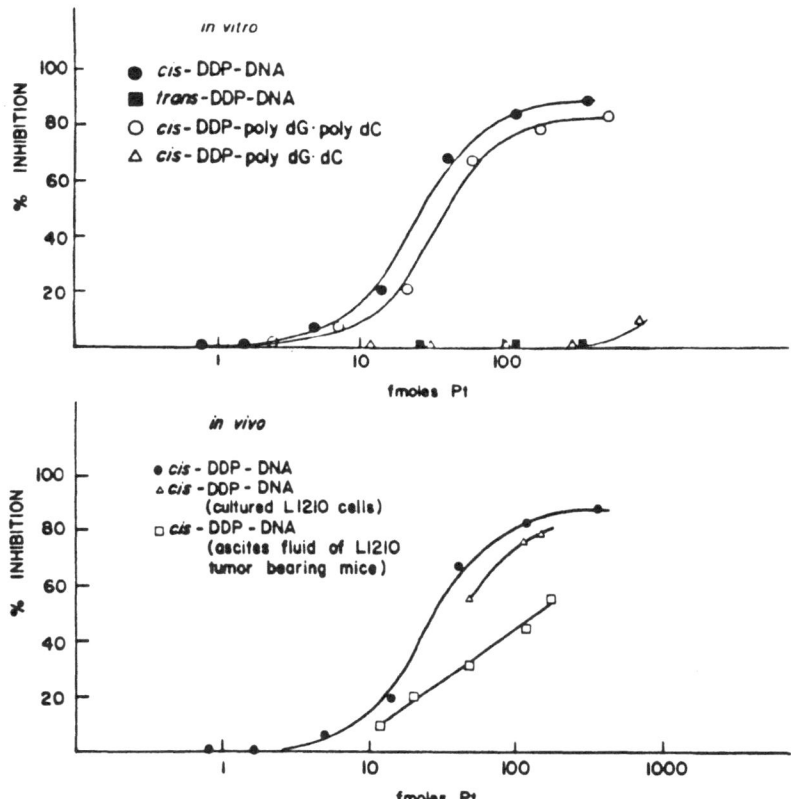

FIGURE 4. (top) Competitive ELISA with cis- (●, D/N = 0.062, control) and
trans- (■, D/N = 0.038) DDP modified calf thymus DNA, with cis-
DDP modified poly (dG)•poly (dC) (O, D/N = 0.042) and poly d(GC)•
poly d(GC) (△, D/N = 0.049). The abscissa corresponds to
increasing concentrations of competitor. (bottom) Profiles in
competitive ELISA with cis-DDP modified calf thymus DNA (●, D/N =
0.062, control), DNA isolated from suspension culture of murine
L1210 cells exposed to cis-DDP (500 µM) for 1 hour (△) and DNA
from ascites fluid of L1210 tumor bearing mice injected intraperitoneally (10 mg/kg) 5 hours prior to cell harvest (□).

CONCLUSIONS

The difference in activity between cis- and trans-$[Pt(NH_3)_2Cl_2]$ is
likely to be a direct result of the different stereochemistries of their
adducts with DNA. Sequence specific binding studies conducted with
exo- and endonucleases demonstrate that cis-DDP inhibits enzymatic

activity near $(dG)_n \cdot (dC)_n$, $n \geqslant 2$, regions while the trans isomer is less
effective. This interaction can be modified by intercalators, compounds
known to alter DNA structure, as demonstrated by the exonuclease III
assay of DNA platinated in the presence of EtdBr. This effect may help
explain the altered activity and specificity observed for the antitumor
antibiotic bleomycin with platinated DNA. A possible binding mode
specific to the cis isomer is a nearest neighbor intrastrand crosslink
between N7 positions of adjacent deoxyguanosine bases. This interaction
was the only one observed in the reaction of cis-DDP with
$[d(ApGpGpCpCpT)]_2$. Antibodies raised against calf thymus DNA modified to
4.4% with cis-DDP show excellent selectivity towards DNA isolated from
L1210 mouse leukemia cell cultures and tumor bearing mice treated with
chemotherapeutically relevant doses of the platinum compound. The
antiserum is specific for cis-Pt-DNA adducts with no activity towards
trans-Pt adducts or platinum induced interstrand crosslinked structures.
Furthermore, high activity was demonstrated towards platinated poly
d(G)·poly d(C), but not poly d(GC)·poly d(GC). We therefore conclude
that cis-diammineplatinum(II)-d(GpG) intrastrand crosslinks are formed
both in vitro and in vivo and that they are an important, if not the most
important, kind of cis-Pt(NH$_3$)$_2$-DNA interaction. Whether this lesion is
the major one responsible for the ability of cis-Pt(NH$_3$)$_2$Cl$_2$ to kill
cancer cells remains to be determined.

REFERENCES
1. Rosenberg, B.; Van Camp, L.; Trosko, J.E.; Mansour, V.H. Nature
   (London) 222 (1969), 385-386.
2. Roberts, J.J. Advances in Inorganic Biochemistry, Ed., Eichhorn, G.L.;
   Marzilli, L.G. Elsevier, 1981, p. 273-332.
3. Roberts, J.J.; Pera, Jr., M.F. Platinum, Gold and Other Metal
   Chemotherapeutic Agents, ACS Symposium Series #209, Ed., Lippard, S.J.
   p. 3-25.
4. Prestayko, A.W.; Crooke, S.K.; Carter, S.H. Cisplatin, Current
   Status and New Developments; Eds., Prestayko, A.W.; Crooke, S.T.;
   Carter, S.K., Academic Press, 1980.
5. Howe-Grant, M.; Wu, K.C.; Bauer, W.R.; Lippard, S.J. Biochemistry
   15 (1976), 4339-4346.
6. Pascoe, J.M.; Roberts, J.J. Biochem. Pharmacol. 23 (1974),
   1345-1357.
7. Roberts, J.J.; Friedlos, F. Biochim. Biophys. Acta 655 (1981),
   146-51.

8. Pera, M.F.; Rawlings, C.J.; Shackleton, J.; Roberts, J.J. Biochim. Biophys. Acta 655 (1981), 152-156.
9. Stone, P.J.; Kelman, A.D.; Sinex, F.M. J. Mol. Biol. 104 (1976), 793-801.
10. Zwelling, L.A.; Michaels, S.; Schwartz, H.; Dobson, P.P.; Kohn, K.W. Cancer Res. 41 (1981), 640-649.
11. Laurent, G.; Erickson, L.C.; Sharkey, N.A.; Kohn, K.W. Cancer Res. 41 (1981), 3347-3351.
12. Strandberg, M.C. Proc. Amer. Assoc. Cancer Res. 22 (1981), 202, A799.
13. Shooter, K.V.; Howse, R.; Merrifield, R.K.; Robbins, A.B. Chem.-Biol. Interact. 5 (1972), 289-307.
14. Filipski, J.; Kohn, K.W.; Bonner, W.M. Chem.-Biol. Interact. 32 (1980), 321-330.
15. Ushay, H.M.; Tullius, T.D.; Lippard, S.J. Biochemistry 20 (1981), 3744-3748.
16. Cohen, G.L.; Ledner, J.A.; Bauer, W.R.; Ushay, H.M.; Caravana, C.; Lippard, S.J. J. Am. Chem. Soc. 102 (1980), 2487-2488.
17. Tullius, T.D.; Lippard, S.J. J. Am. Chem. Soc. 103 (1981), 4620-4622.
18. Kelman, A.D.; Buchbinder, M. Biochimie 60 (1978), 893-899.
19. Brouwer, J.; van de Putte, P.; Fichtinger-Schepman, A.M.J.; Reedijk, J. Proc. Natl. Acad. Sci. USA 78 (1981), 7010-7014.
20. Caradonna, J.P.; Lippard, S.J.; Singh, M.; Gait, M. J. Am. Chem. Soc. 104 (1982), 5793-5795.
21. Tullius, T.D.; Ushay, H.M.; Merkel, C.M.; Caradonna, J.P.; Lippard, S.J. Platinum, Gold and Other Metal Chemotherapeutic Agents, Ed., Lippard, S.J. ACS Symposium Series #209, p. 51-71.
22. Tullius, T.D.; Lippard, S.J. Proc. Natl. Acad. Sci. USA 79 (1982), 3489-3492.
23. Poirier, M.C.; Lippard, S.J.; Zwelling, L.A.; Ushay, H.M.; Kerrigan, D.; Thill, C.C.; Santella, R.M.; Grunberger, D.; Yuspa, S.H. Proc. Natl. Acad. Sci. USA 79 (1982), 6443-6447.
24. Lippard, S.J.; Ushay, H.M.; Merkel, C.M.; Poirier, M.C., Biochemistry (in press).
25. Lippard, S.J. Accounts Chem. Res. 11 (1978), 211-217.
26. Cohen, G.L.; Bauer, W.R.; Barton, J.K.; Lippard, S.J. Science 203 (1979), 1014-1016.
27. Mong, S.; Prestayko, A.W.; Crooke, S.T. in Cisplatin, Current Status and New Developments; Eds., Prestayko, A.W.; Crooke, S.T.; Carter, S.K., Academic Press, 1980, p. 213-226.
28. Lomonossoff, N.G.P.; Butler, P.J.G.; Klug, A. J. Mol. Biol. 149 (1981), 745-760.
29. Royer-Pokora, B.; Gordon, L.K.; Haseltine, W.A. Nucleic Acids Res. 9 (1981), 4595-4609.
30. Mansy, S.; Chu, G.Y.H.; Duncan, R.E.; Tobias, R.S. J. Am. Chem. Soc. 100 (1978), 607-616.
31. Howe-Grant, M.E.; Lippard, S.J. Met. Ions. Biol. Syst. 11 (1980), 63 and references cited therein.
32. (a) Chottard, J.C.; Girault, J.P.; Chottard, G.; Lellemand, J.Y.; Mansuy, D. Nouv. J. Chim. 2 (1980), 551-553; (b) Chottard, J.C.; Girault, J.P.; Chottard, G.; Lellemand, J.Y.; Mansuy, D. J. Am. Chem. Soc. 102 (1980), 5565-5572; (c) Girault, J.P.; Chottard, G.; Lellemand, J.Y.; Chottard, J.C. Biochemistry 21 (1982), 1352-1356.

33. Marcelis, A.T.M.; Canters, G.W.; Reedijk, J. Recl. Trav. Chim. Pays-Bas. 100 (1981), 391-392.
34. Wang, J.C. J. Mol. Biol. 89 (1974), 783-801.
35. Mascharak, P.K.; Kuwahara, J.; Suzuki, T.; Sugiura, Y.; Lippard, S.J., submitted for publication.
36. Davis, Jr. H.L.; van Hoff, D.D.; Henney, J.E.; Rozencweig, M. Cancer Chemther. Pharmacol. 1 (1978), 83-90.
37. Umezawa, H. Bleomycin: Current Status and New Developments, Eds., Carter, S.K.; Crooke, S.T.; Umezawa, H.; Academic Press, 1978, p. 15ff.
38. Zwelling, L.A.; Kohn, K.W.; Ross, W.E.; Ewig, R.A.C.; Anderson, T. Cancer Res. 38 (1978), 1762-1786.

Is DNA The Real Target of Antitumor Platinum Compounds?

J.P. Macquet, J.L. Butour, N.P. Johnson, H. Razaka, B. Salles, C. Vieussens and M. Wright

Platinum compounds, particularly $\underline{cis}$-Pt$(NH_3)_2Cl_2$, represent a new class of effective antitumor drugs used clinically in cancer chemotherapy (1). The mechanism of action of these compounds is not yet elucidated. Antitumor activity and cytotoxicity have been correlated with the presence of a pair of $\underline{cis}$ labile ligands (2,3). In a $\underline{cis}$-Pt series, inert ligands modulate these activities whereas labile ligands influence toxicity in animals. Charged and neutral compounds as well as kinetically inert and very reactive ones were found antitumoral (2). At the cellular level, these electrophilic molecules bind to DNA, RNA and proteins (4). However, filamentation, mutagenicity, prophage and rec A protein induction, increased sensitivity in repair-deficient strains and inhibition of DNA synthesis observed with $\underline{cis}$-Pt$(NH_3)_2Cl_2$ indicate that DNA is a target (4). It is generally thought that inhibition of DNA synthesis is the perturbed DNA function responsible of the antitumor properties (for a review, see ref. 4).

In the first part of this study, two pieces of evidence argue against a correlation between a quantitative inhibition of DNA synthesis and antitumor activity. This does not mean that DNA is not directly or indirectly involved in the cell killing effect. The second part is concerned with Pt–DNA adducts isolated $\underline{in\ vitro}$ and $\underline{in\ vivo}$.

I. INHIBITION OF DNA SYNTHESIS BY CIS-DDP, TRANS-DDP AND [Pt(dien)Cl]Cl IN L1210 LEUKEMIA CELLS

The three above Pt(II) compounds were selected for two reasons. First, they exhibit different cytotoxicities (ID_{50} = 2.3 μM, 67 μM and 271 μM, respectively) and antitumor activities (T/C x 100 = 205 %, 116 % and 98 %, respectively) (2) in the L1210 leukemia cell line currently used for screening antitumoral drugs (5). Second, they are representative of the three different classes of DNA secondary structure perturbation observed for $\underline{in\ vitro}$ Pt–DNA interactions (6). The experimental procedure for measuring inhibition of DNA synthesis by these compounds has recently been reported (7).

Cells were treated with tritiated thimidine (1 hour) after two hours of contact with the Pt(II) compounds. Then, they were washed, sonicated and DNA extracted in order to determine the r_b values. The curves of Pt covalently bound at the cellular level were linear for cis- and trans-DDP until a concentration of 150 μg/ml and in the whole range studied. for [Pt(dien)Cl]Cl (2000 μg/ml). Trans-DDP was found to penetrate 8 times better than cis-DDP or [Pt(dien)Cl]Cl. This higher efficacy of penetration for the trans versus cis derivatives, which is also encountered in L1210 leukemia cells grafted in mice (6), is probably correlated with its higher partition coefficient (8). The inhibitory effect of each Pt(II) compound on DNA synthesis was plotted against r_b and a 50 % decrease of DNA synthesis corresponded to r_b values of 1.8×10^{-4}, 2.4×10^{-4} and 80×10^{-4} respectively for cis-DDP, trans-DDP and [Pt(dien)Cl]Cl. The cis-DDP lesions inhibit DNA replication in these experimental conditions only 1.3 times more efficiently than the trans-DDP lesions and 45 times more efficiently than the [Pt(dien)Cl]Cl lesions. It is interesting to mention that trans-DDP was also found to inhibit DNA synthesis in vitro (9), in E. coli (10,11) and in CHO cells (12). A recent study (13) with cis-DDP and $K_2[PtCl_4]$ (non-antitumoral) confirmed the fact that both compounds are able to reduce DNA synthesis to the same extent in two tumor cell lines. These results suggest that even if DNA is a target for antitumor and non-antitumor Pt(II) compounds, the biological parameter which can be correlated with the antitumor properties is not a quantitative inhibition of DNA synthesis.

II. INDUCTION OF GIANT POLYPLOID NUCLEI IN PHYSARUM POLYCEPHALUM BY PT ANTITUMOR COMPOUNDS AT CONCENTRATIONS WHICH PERMIT GROWTH AND DO NOT INHIBIT DNA SYNTHESIS

The plasmodium of the myxomycete Physarum polycephalum can be described as a flat giant cell (10 cm diameter) which contains 10^8 nuclei (14) showing a synchronous (15) semi-closed nuclear division (16,17) without cytokinesis. This myxomycete was used in order to check whether or not DNA could be the pharmacological target of Pt antitumor compounds. Chemicals which perturb nuclear division and the equipartition of chromosomes do not lead to imme- diate death of Physarum but to the formation of giant nuclei (18-20) which is in contrast to what happens in animal cells. The experimental procedure has been published elsewhere (21). Growth of synchronous plasmodia was estimated by the ratio of the surface covered by the plasmodia at various times to the surface of the plasmodia at the beginning of the experiment. Surfaces were determined using a Hewlett-Packard 9820A calculator equipped with a Hewlett-Packard 9864A digitizer. Nuclei were observed under phase contrast microscopy (15) and/or electron microscopy (22).

Abnormally large nuclei were observed when a single application of 100 nmoles of cis-DDP were spread on a plasmodium, with no growth inhibition. Under phase contrast microscopy one or several enlarged nucleoli were visualized. The main ultrastructural characteristic of these giant nuclei in electron microscopy was the frequent presence of masses of macrotubules not observed in control nuclei. The histogram of DNA content per nucleus of these polyploid nuclei was broader than the histogram which could be expected from control G2 nuclei. Such an effect could be due to a perturbation of the equipartition of chromosomes during mitosis occuring in the presence of the drug and/or to a loss of synchrony between nuclei during the polyploidisation process.

A delayed and lengthened mitosis was also observed when cis-DDP was applied before S phase which could be explained by a direct effect of cis-DDP on microtubules. We thus investigated the interaction of cis-DDP on the in vitro assembly of sheep brain tubulin at 37°C (23) and found an inhibition of microtubular assembly. However, trans-DDP was even a more potent inhibitor than cis-DDP. Since the observed perturbations of mitosis could be associated with some earlier perturbation of the cell cycle, we investigated the action of cis-DDP in the agar medium on the occurence of two significant cell cycle events : DNA synthesis (14) and the periodic increase of thymidine kinase synthesis (14,24). We failed to observe any significant differences in the incorporation of radioactive thymidine into an acid insoluble form during late G2 and S phase even after treatment for 8 hours in the presence of cis-DDP. The intensity of the peak of thymidine kinase synthesis was normal although its timing was delayed with mitosis in the presence of cis-DDP. The non-antitumor compound trans-DDP did not induce any large nuclei or growth inhibition even at concentrations as high as 5000 nmoles, larger amounts being limited by its water solubility (Fig. 1).

In order to check the possible correlation between the formation of polyploid nuclei in Physarum and antitumor activity in L1210 leukemia cells grafted in mice, at concentrations which had no inhibitory action on growth of plasmodium, we studied the effect of 26 Pt(II) and (IV) amine compounds on Physarum synchronous plasmodia (21). The minimum quantity of Pt compounds corresponding to polyploid nuclei (pn) and to growth arrest (ga) were deduced from figures similar to figure 1. All Pt compounds showing a T/C x 100 lower than 125 % gave a ratio ga/pn < 2.5. Alternatively, all antitumor Pt compounds gave a ratio ga/pn > 3. Some of these values are presented in Table I for Pt-chloroammine compounds.

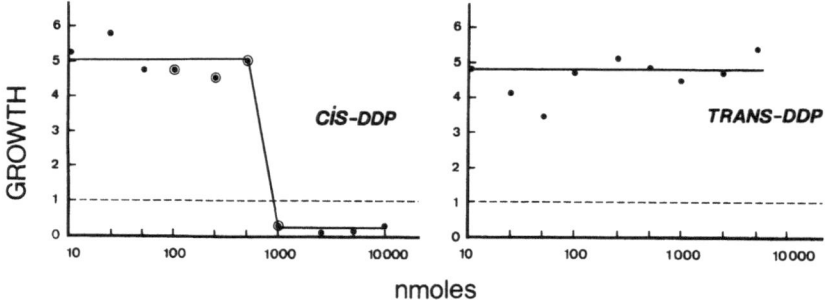

Figure 1. Induction of polyploid nuclei and effect on growth in <u>Physarum polycephalum</u> by <u>cis</u>-DDP and <u>trans</u>-DDP. abcissa : amount of Pt compound (nmoles) ; ordinate : relative increase in the surface area of the plasmodium after 48 h in the presence of drug. Points surrounded with a circle indicate the presence of polyploid nuclei. The horizontal dashed lines corresponded to the absence of growth.

TABLE I - RELATIONSHIP BETWEEN THE APPEARANCE OF POLYPLOID NUCLEI AND GROWTH ARREST IN <u>PHYSARUM POLYCEPHALUM</u> AND ANTITUMOR ACTIVITY IN L 1210 LEUKEMIA FOR A SERIES OF PLATINUM (II) CHLOROAMMINES COMPOUNDS

Platinum Compounds	nmoles of compound		Ratio ga/pn	$\frac{T}{C}$ x 100[c] (%)
	pn[a]	ga[b]		
$K_2[PtCl_4]$	-[d]	10,000	?[e]	110
$K[Pt(NH_3)Cl_3]$	1,000	5,000	5	146
cis-$Pt(NH_3)_2Cl_2$	50	750	15	205
$trans$-$Pt(NH_3)_2Cl_2$	-	> 5,000	?	116
$[Pt(NH_3)_3Cl]Cl$	5,000	10,000	2	108
$[Pt(NH_3)_4]Cl_2$	-	-	?	108

[a]pn = minimum amount of Pt compound leading to polyploid nuclei ; [b]ga = minimum amount of Pt compound leading to growth arrest ; [c]see ref. 2 ; [d]the hyphen indicates that no polyploid nuclei and/or no growth arrest were observed at the maximum amount of Pt compound used (10,000 nmoles for $K_2[PtCl_4]$ and $[Pt(NH_3)_4]Cl_2$ and 5,000 nmoles for $trans$-$Pt(NH_3)_2Cl_2$) ; [e]the question mark indicates that the ratio ga/pn cannot be calculated since no polyploid nuclei were observed.

It seems unlikely that the observed results could be due to a direct perturbation on microtubules since trans-DDP is even more effective than cis-DDP in inhibiting microtubule assembly. Our results indicate a correlation between antitumor activity and the appearance of giant nuclei at non-toxic doses which do not sensibly inhibit DNA synthesis. These polyploid nuclei have been previously observed in animal (25-29) and plant cells (30) after a cis-DDP treatment and seem to be due to the impairment of the separation of the two daughter nuclei in telophase. Sodhi (28) also observed in sarcoma 180 cells that the nuclei of a single giant cell communicated through thin nuclear strands and were enclosed in a common nuclear envelope. The hypothesis that the cytotoxic action of antitumor Pt-amine compounds on mitosis may be mediated by a qualitative effect on DNA replication cannot be rejected. This would explain mitotic delays when cis-DDP is applied before S phase. This study suggests that the initial toxicity of antitumor Pt-amine compounds is due to the perturbation of the mitotic machinery rather than to a gross inhibition of DNA synthesis (31,32).

III. CORRELATION BETWEEN GROWTH INHIBITION AND ANTITUMOR ACTIVITY IN L1210 LEUKEMIA CELLS

Recently (2) we have shown that in a series of 31 Pt compounds the presence of a pair of labile ligands in cis position was correlated with an $ID_{50} < 10$ μM in cultured L1210 leukemia cells independently of the charge and of the reactivity of the compound. Only two cis-Pt compounds were found inactive in L1210 leukemia cells grafted in mice and for these compounds antitumor activity was probably limited by their high toxicity toward mice. It was also found that in a series of cis-Pt(NH$_3$)$_2$ and cis-Pt(DAC) compounds ID_{50} depended essentially on the inert ligands rather than the labile ligands and the more cytotoxic compounds were the more antitumoral ones in the same tumor model. These correlations between cis-geometry, growth inhibition and antitumor activity are also confirmed by the relative in vivo activity of the cis-DDP-DNA, trans-DDP-DNA and [Pt(dien)Cl]Cl-DNA lesions which are reported in Table II.

At the highest tolerated dose in mice for the three above Pt compounds, 25 times more trans ($r_b = 8.3 \times 10^{-4}$) bind to DNA than cis ($r_b = 3.3 \times 10^{-5}$) and 8 times more trans than the dien compound ($r_b = 10^{-4}$) (6). In these conditions, cis-DDP is active (8 mg/kg, T/C x 100 = 205 %) but trans-DDP (40 mg/kg, T/C x 100 = 116 %) and [Pt(dien)Cl]Cl (70 mg/kg, T/C X 100 = 98 %) are inactive (2). At equivalent antitumor activity 200 times more trans-Pt-DNA than cis-Pt-DNA lesions are observed ([cis] = 1 mg/kg, T/C x 100 = 107 % ; [trans] = 40 mg/kg, T/C x 100 = 116 %) (for experimental see ref. 6).

TABLE II - BIOLOGICAL ACTIVITIES OF Pt COMPOUNDS IN LEUKEMIA CELLS

[PLATINUM]	CIS-DDP	TRANS-DDP	[Pt(dien)Cl]Cl
	INHIBITION (50 %) OF DNA SYNTHESIS		
Concentration (μM)	165	250	5 500
Penetration (Pt/cell x 10^{16}g)	250	3 600	9 000
Pt/nucleotide	1.8×10^{-4}*	2.4×10^{-4}	80×10^{-4}
	GROWTH INHIBITION		
ID_{50} (μM)	2.3	67	271
Penetration (Pt/cell x 10^{16}g)	0.86*	200	110
Pt/nucleotide	1.6×10^{-7}*	4×10^{-5}	5×10^{-4}
	ANTITUMOR ACTIVITY		
T/C x 100 (mg/kg)	205 (8)	116 (40)	98 (70)
Penetration (Pt/cell x 10^{16}g)	180	4 700	400
Pt/nucleotide (dose injected)	3.3×10^{-5} (8) 4.1×10^{-6} (1)*	8.3×10^{-4} (40)	10^{-4} (70)

* calculated

We have reported (7) that at a concentration corresponding to the ID_{50} value, no Pt could be detected in cultured L1210 cells for cis-DDP (ID_{50} = 2.3 μM). However, if a concentration of 67 μM cis-DDP (corresponding to the ID_{50} of trans-DDP) is used, 8 times less cis-DDP (25×10^{-16} g Pt/cell) is bound at the cellular level than trans-DDP (200×10^{-16} g Pt/cell). Since the Pt fixation in L1210 cells is linear until a concentration of 500 μM for cis- and trans-DDP, it is not unreasonable to extrapolate the Pt fixation for cis-DDP in L1210 cells at a concentration corresponding to its ID_{50} value. The calculation gives a value of 0.86×10^{-16} g Pt/cell (200×10^{-16} g Pt/cell obtained experimentally for trans-DDP at its ID_{50} value). If we admit that the ratios between the amount of Pt fixed at the cellular and at the DNA levels in cultured L1210 cells and in L1210 cells grafted in mice are similar, then an r_b of 1.6 x 10^{-7} is found for a concentration of cis-DDP corresponding to its ID_{50}. It must be noted that the above assumption is verified for the uncharged trans-DDP. Then a ratio of 260 (4.16 x 10^{-5}/1.6 x 10^{-7}) is obtained between the r_b value of trans-DDP and r_b value of cis-DDP at a concentration corresponding to ID_{50}. This value very close to the factor of 200 found in antitumor activity confirms the correlation between growth inhibition and antitumor activity for cis-DDP and trans-DDP in L1210 leukemia cells. Such a difference in biological activity between cis- and trans-DDP-DNA lesions led us to study the physical chemistry of Pt-DNA complexes (33) and the characterization of Pt-DNA adducts (34,35). The following sections report preliminary investigations on Pt-DNA-lesions in vitro and in vivo.

IV. THE STRUCTURE OF PLATINUM-DNA ADDUCTS FORMED IN VITRO

We have recently developed a method for the separation of adducts containing platinum and nucleic acid base(s) from Pt-DNA complexes by means of mild acid hydrolysis (34). These complexes can be purified by electrophoresis and chromatography and they can be identified by comparison with model compounds of known structure.

A recent study (35) of the monofunctional fixation of [Pt(dien)Cl]Cl on DNA shows that the preferred reactive sites are the most nucleophilic as in the case for fixation of platinum(II) compounds on nucleosides and nucleotides. This platinum compound binds exclusively at the N(7) position of guanine below r_b = 0.1. Above this r_b, fixation at N(7) of adenine was also observed. Above r_b = 0.3 denaturation of DNA exposes the N(1)position of adenine and the complex [[Pt(dien)]$_2$Ade]$^{+4}$, with fixation at N(1) and N(7), is formed. Physico-chemical studies of 7-[Pt(dien)Guo]$^{+2}$ revealed that platinum complexation at the N(7) position stabilizes the glycosyl linkage and lowers the pK N(1)-H from 9.2 to 8.0.

Electrophoresis of the hydrolyzed cis-DDP-DNA complex, r_b = 0.1, resolved four platinum-containing peaks, the major species accounting for about 50 % of the observed platinum (34) and migrating 1.29 ± 0.05 unit relative to Gua. Electrophoresis of the hydrolyzed model compound cis-[Pt(NH$_3$)$_2$(dGuo)$_2$]$^{+2}$ resolved two minor peaks and a major peak which contained 93 % of the observed platinum and comigrated (1.26 ± 0.02) with the major species from the platinum-DNA complex. The major product was subjected to paper chromatography (1M NH$_4$ acetate/EtOH, 35/65, v/v). A single product was observed which had the same R_f for the DNA adduct (R_f = 0.14 ± 0.02) and the model compound (R_f = 0.16 ± 0.01). Reaction of these two compounds with thiourea (35) liberated guanine. The extinction coefficients of the hydrolyzed model compound and the adduct were the same within experimental error. We conclude from this evidence that the major product observed after acid hydrolysis of cis-[Pt(NH$_3$)$_2$(dGuo)$_2$]$^{+2}$ corresponds to the major adduct formed between cis-DDP and DNA, r_b ≤ 0.1. The major adduct formed by cis-DDP and DNA appears to be fixation on the N(7) position of two guanine bases.

Trans-DDP-DNA complex (r_b = 0.1) was submitted to the same treatment as cis-DDP-DNA complex. Four platinum-containing peaks were separated by electrophoresis, the major one (50 % total Pt) being located at 0.80 ± 0.04 unit relative to Gua (34). Subsequent paper chromatography (5% HCOOH/EtOH, 75/25, v/v) on this peak revealed a major species (63 %) with R_f = 0.28 ± 0.03. The model compound trans-[Pt(NH$_3$)$_2$(dGuo)$_2$]Cl$_2$ was synthetized and characterized by its elemental analysis, NMR and IR spectra, electrophoresis, paper chromatography and mass spectrometry (FAB). Platinum binding sites were found to be the N(7) position of the two dGuo molecules. This compound was hydrolyzed as for the trans-DDP-DNA complex and submitted to electrophoresis and paper chromatography. Electrophoresis revealed one major peak (95 % of total Pt) located at 0.84 ± 0.04 unit relative to Gua, which migrated with a major species at R_f = 0.25 ± 0.03. We then conclude that the major species observed between trans-DDP and DNA corresponds to the fixation of platinum on N(7) position of two guanine molecules.

V. KINETICS OF FORMATION OF CIS-DDP-DNA ADDUCTS IN VITRO

We investigated the kinetics of cis-DDP-DNA adducts in vitro for r_b = 0.1 in order to possibly characterize intermediates species which could form and evolve with time. The experimental procedure is the same as above and the electrophoretic patterns observed after 30 mins., 6 hrs, 24 hrs, and 3 weeks are presented in figure 2. Only one of the two major peaks (≅ 1.30-1.35 unit) corresponding to cis-[Pt(NH$_3$)$_2$(Gua)$_2$]$^{+2}$, is always present between 30 mins. and 3 weeks, the second most important one (1.45 unit) being only observed after 24 hrs of reaction. It must be noted the presence of an important intermediate species after 24 hrs located at 0.78 unit whose intensity decreases with time. These intermediates are probably less charged species and could correspond to 1:1 Pt:base complexes.

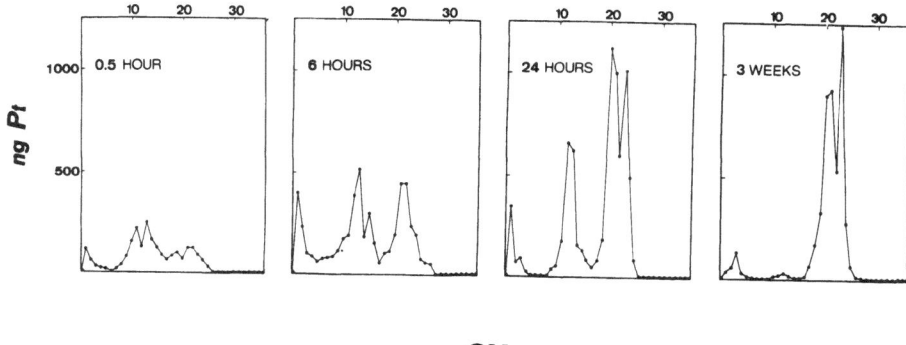

CM

Figure 2. Electrophoretic pattern of the kinetics of the in vitro cis-DDP-DNA interaction for r_b = 0.1 (experiment in duplicate).

The localization of the different Pt species is given below :

30 mins.	6 hrs	24 hrs	3 weeks
0.09* (11)**	0.06 (14)	0.06 (6)	0.14 (3)
0.68 (25)	—	—	—
0.81 (30)	0.78 (22)	0.78 (28)	0.75 (4)
1.15 (11)	0.93 (8)	—	—
1.35 (22)	1.34 (47)	1.28 (39)	1.31 (55)
—	—	1.44 (27)	1.46 (38)

* migration relative to Gua ; ** % Pt in the peak.

VI. CIS-DDP-DNA ADDUCTS IN VIVO

10^6 L1210 cells/ml (10^8 total) in exponentially growing phase were in contact with 20 μM cis-DDP for 5 hrs. Then, the cells were washed with 0.15 M NaCl solution (free platinum was followed by atomic absorption), counted with a Coulter counter (ZBI) and platinum covalently bound at the cellular level was measured by atomic absorption. A concentration of 200 x 10^{-16} g Pt/cell was found. After sonication DNA was extracted as already reported (7), dialyzed against 10mM NaClO$_4$, precipitated with 3 volumes of cold ethanol and 3 mg of DNA could be isolated. The corresponding r_b was 10^{-4}. The cis-DDP-DNA complex was then submitted to acid hydrolysis and electrophoresis. An amount of 100 ng Pt was deposited on the electrophoresis paper. The electrophoresis profile of Pt-containing species showed significant differences with that observed in vitro :

  - the two major peaks observed in vitro for an r_b of 10^{-4} (34) are absent. This means that cis-$[Pt(NH_3)_2(Gua)_2]^{+2}$ is not formed in vivo in our experimental conditions.

  - a significant amount of Pt is found toward the positive side of the electrophoresis, which correspond to minus charged species.

  - the platinum species migrating toward the negative part of the electrophoresis are located between the origin and the distance of Gua.

These results may indicate a different mode of fixation for platinum compounds on DNA in vitro and in vivo. This difference might be explained by reaction conditions which could allow ternary complexes between DNA, Pt and other nucleophiles in the cell nucleus. Indeed, we found that in vitro Pt-DNA complexes are able to bind ^{14}C-Guo (unpublished data). This interpretation is consistent with immunochemical studies which concluded that antibodies against cis-DDP-DNA complexes formed in vitro do not recognize Pt-DNA complexes isolated from the liver of rats which have been treated with cis-DDP (36).

VII. IS DNA THE REAL TARGET OF ANTITUMOR PLATINUM COMPOUNDS ?

Experiments which investigate the mechanism of action of antitumor compounds generally look for correlations between a biological activity and the antineoplastic response. Our results indicate that for platinum compounds such comparisons must be made at the r_b at which antitumor activity occurs in order to avoid complicating biological responses such as inhibition of DNA synthesis which occur at higher levels of DNA binding. We have presented two experiments which correlate antitumor activity with biological activity under these treatment conditions.

First, the growth inhibition of L1210 cells in culture (ID_{50}) is correlated with the antitumor activity ; in both cases the biological effect per DNA lesion is 200 times greater for cis-DDP than for the trans isomer. Both effects occur at $r_b \leqslant 10^{-5}$. The inhibition of DNA synthesis in these cells was a linear function of r_b until $r_b \cong 2 \times 10^{-4}$ and was not observed at $r_b = 5 \times 10^{-5}$(7). Hence, if DNA synthesis can be compared in cultured L1210 cells and in L1210 cells growing intraperitoneally in mice, the antineoplastic effects of cis-DDP occur in the absence of inhibition of DNA synthesis.

Second, platinum antitumor compounds, but not inactive compounds, form giant nuclei in Physarum. This effect occurs with cis-DDP at doses which do not inhibit DNA synthesis. This second experiment suggests that platinum antitumor compounds disrupt the partition of chromosomes during mitosis, an effect which would be lethal in most eucaryotic cells with an open mitosis but which causes giant nuclei in Physarum whose nuclear membrane remains intact during mitosis. A qualitative effect on DNA replication or a perturbation of the nuclear matrix (21,37) could be responsible for the antitumor activity of Pt compounds.

DNA is clearly a cellular target for Pt compounds, however we still do not know if it is one of the target(s) responsible for their antitumor properties. We believe that the investigation of giant nuclei formation and the nature of repaired and unrepaired DNA lesions in mammalian cells could give some insights into the molecular basis of the antineoplastic effect of platinum antitumor compounds.

ACKNOWLEDGEMENTS. We thank B. Attali (tubulin experiments), S. Cros (L1210 cells), J. Escalier (synthesis), A.M. Mazard (in vitro and in vivo Pt-DNA adducts) and A. Moisand (electron microscopy) for their expert technical assistance. The FAB study was kindly conducted by J.C. Promé and G. Puzo. The financial support of "L'Association pour le Développement de la Recherche sur le Cancer", "La Fédération Nationale des Centres de Lutte contre le Cancer" and "La Fédération Nationale des G.E.F.L.U.C." is gratefully acknowledged.

ABBREVIATIONS : dien = diethylenetriamine, $(H_2N-CH_2-CH_2)_2NH$; ID_{50} = median inhibitory dose, a drug concentration that decreases the growth rate of L1210 cells to 50 % of that of control ; r_b = number of Pt atoms bound per nucleotide ; DAC = trans(d,l)1,2-diaminocyclohexane ; T/C = mean survival time of treated leukemic mice/mean survival time of untreated leukemic mice (significant when T/C x 100 $\geqslant$ 125 %) ; FAB = Fast Atom Bombardment.

REFERENCES

1. Einhorn LH. 1981. Cancer Res 41, 3275-3280.
2. Macquet JP, Butour JL. 1983. J Natl Cancer Inst 70, 899-905.
3. Cleare MJ, Hoeschele JD. 1973. Bioinorg Chem 2, 187-210.
4. Roberts JJ, Thomson AJ. 1979. Progress in Nucleic Acid Research and Molecular Biology (Cohn WE, ed), 22, pp 71-133, Academic Press, New York.
5. Geran RI, Greenberg NH, MacDonald MM, Shumacher AM, Abbott BJ. 1972. Cancer Chemoth Rep 3, 1-103.
6. Macquet JP, Butour JL, Johnson NP. 1983. In "Platinum, Gold, and other Metal Chemotherapeutic Agents" (Lippard SJ, ed), ACS Symposium Series 209, pp. 75-100.
7. Salles B, Butour JL, Lesca C, Macquet JP. 1983. Biochem Biophys Res Commun 112, 555-563.
8. Hoeschele JD, Butler TA, Roberts JA. 1980. In "Inorganic Chemistry in Biology and Medicine" (Martell AE, ed), ACS Symposium Series 140, pp. 181-208.

9. Johnson NP, Hoeschele JD, Keummerle NB, Masker WE, Rahn RO. 1978. Chem-Biol Interactions 23, 267-271.
10. Alazard R, Germanier M, Johnson NP. 1982. Mutation Res 93, 327-337.
11. Kohl HH, Haghighi S, McAuliffe CA. 1980. Chem-Biol Interactions 29, 327-333.
12. Plooy AC, Lohman PHM. 1980. Toxicology 17, 169-176.
13. Hurwitz E, Kashi R. Wilchek M. 1982. J. Natl. Cancer Inst 69, 47-51.
14. Hütterman A. 1973. In "Physarum polycephalum : Object of Research in Cell Biology" Gustav Fischer Verlag, Stuttgart.
15. Guttes E, Guttes S. 1964. In "Methods in Cell Biology" (Prescott DM, ed), 1, pp 43-54, Academic Press, New York.
16. Guttes S, Guttes E, Ellis RA. 1968. J. Ultrastruct Res 22, 508-529.
17. Goodman EM, Ritter H. 1969. Arch Protistenk 111, 161-169.
18. McCormick JJ, Nardone RM. 1970. Exp Cell Res 60, 247-256.
19. Gull K, Trinci APJ. 1974. Protoplasma 81, 37-48.
20. Wright M, Moisand A, Tollon Y, Oustrin ML. 1976. C R Acad Sc (Paris) 283, 1361-1364.
21. Wright M, Lacorre-Arescaldino I, Macquet JP, Daffé M. Submitted for publication.
22. Del Castillo L, Oustrin ML, Wright M. 1978. Molec Gen Genet 164, 145-154.
23. Mir L, Oustrin ML, Lecointe P, Wright M. 1978. FEBS Lett 88, 259-263.
24. Wright M, Tollon Y. 1979. Eur J. Biochem 96, 177-181.
25. Aggarwal SK. 1974. Cytobiologie 8, 395-402.
26. Heinen E, Bassleer R. 1976. Chemotherapy 22, 253-261.
27. Heinen E, Bassleer R. 1976. Biochem Pharmacol 25, 1871-1875.
28. Sodhi A. 1977. J Clin Hematol Oncol 7, 569-579.
29. Sodhi A, Sarna S. 1979. Ind J Exp Biol 17, 1-8.
30. De Pauw-Gillet MC, Houssier C, Fredericq E. 1979. Chem-Biol Interactions 25, 87-102.
31. Harder HC, Rosenberg B. 1970. Int J. Cancer 6, 207-216.
32. Howle JA, Gale GR. 1970. Biochem Pharmacol 19, 2757-2762.
33. Macquet JP, Butour JL. 1978. Biochimie 60, 901-914.
34. Johnson NP. 1982. Biochem Biophys Res Commun 104, 1394-1400.
35. Johnson NP, Macquet JP, Wiebers JL, Monsarrat B. 1982. Nucleic Acids Res 10, 5255-5271.
36. Malfoy B, Hartmann B, Macquet JP, Leng M. 1981. Cancer Res 41, 4127-4131.
37. Roberts JJ, Pera MF. 1983. In "Platinum, Gold, and Other Metal Chemotherapeutic Agents" (Lippard SJ, ed), ACS Symposium Series 209, pp. 3-25.

Specific Binding of *cis*-Platinum Compounds to DNA and DNA Fragments

J. Reedijk, J.H.J. den Hartog,
A.M.J. Fichtinger-Schepman and A.T.M. Marcelis

1. INTRODUCTION

The reaction of cis-PtCl$_2$(NH$_3$)$_2$ (abbreviated cis-Pt) and related platinum compounds with DNA is believed to be the main cause
of the cytostatic activity of such compounds (1-4). After
administration the drug is transported through the body. The high
Cl$^-$ concentration in the blood (5) prevents the hydrolysis of
cis-Pt, which is a prerequisite for fast reaction. However,
hydrolysis does occur inside the cells after penetration through
the cell membrane. The following equilibria are accepted to occur.

$$\text{cis-PtCl}_2(\text{NH}_3)_2 \underset{}{\overset{\text{H}_2\text{O}}{\rightleftharpoons}} \text{cis-[PtCl}(\text{H}_2\text{O})(\text{NH}_3)_2]^+ \underset{}{\overset{\text{H}_2\text{O}}{\rightleftharpoons}} [\text{Pt}(\text{NH}_3)_2(\text{H}_2\text{O})_2]^{2+}$$

$$\updownarrow -\text{H}^+ \qquad\qquad \updownarrow -\text{H}^+ \quad \text{pK}_a = 5.6$$

$$\text{cis-[PtCl}(\text{OH})(\text{NH}_3)_2] \underset{}{\overset{\text{H}_2\text{O}}{\rightleftharpoons}} [\text{Pt}(\text{OH})(\text{H}_2\text{O})(\text{NH}_3)_2]^+$$

$$\updownarrow -\text{H}^+ \quad \text{pK}_a = 7.3$$

$$[\text{Pt}(\text{OH})_2(\text{NH}_3)_2]$$

SCHEME

The main species present under physiological conditions is calculated to be [cis-Pt(OH)(H$_2$O)(NH$_3$)$_2$]$^+$, but all species can react
with DNA. Although it is generally accepted that the N7 atom of
guanine is the primary binding site of Pt compounds, several
questions are still unanswered or subject of debate (6-13). Some
of these questions are:
1. Do all these Pt species react in the same manner with DNA?
2. Is a unique binding site present in DNA, determined by e.g.
   the tertiary structure and the neighbouring bases?
3. What is the effect of (local) pH, hydrogen bonding or charge
   effects on the kinetic and thermodynamic of the (initial)
   binding of Pt to guanine-N7 in DNA?

4. Can other atoms in guanine also bind to Pt (e.g. O6 or N1)?
5. After binding to N7, how large is the distortion of DNA when the Pt is present as a monofunctionally bound compound?
6. Knowing that cis-Pt amine compounds have two binding sites, is there a second binding to DNA, and if so, is this binding through chelation (to O6), intrastrand crosslinking, or interstrand crosslinking?
7. What is the effect of hydrogen bonding and/or neighbouring bases upon this second step? I.e. how easily can rotation about the Pt-N7 bond occur; which bases are in the right position to react (at the 3'-site, the 5'-site, purines, pyrimidines)?
8. What kinds of distortions occur in DNA after cis-Pt has reacted bifunctionally and what are the influences of neighbouring bases and phosphate groups on this distortion?

During the last couple of years our research has been directed mainly to the last 4 questions, although we have also studied some of the other questions (14-23). This paper will summarize our earlier results and combine these with the latest data. Special attention will be given to the formation of intrastrand crosslinks upon interaction of DNA and oligonucleotides, with cis-Pt compounds.

2. THE FIRST STEP

Early experiments, in which a mixture of nucleosides had reacted with cis-Pt$(NH_3)_2^{2+}$ (24), have already shown that under competitive conditions guanosine-N7 binding is highly favoured over binding to other nucleosides. Although a similar preference was found in competition experiments with nucleotides (8), this preference does not automatically occur in the case of DNA. In binding to DNA complication factors are:
- Watson-Crick base paring, making certain positions less accessible;
- effects of other species present around the DNA (proteins, cations);
- effects of neighbouring groups (phosphates, nucleobases) in

the DNA strand.

Molecular. models indicate that the N7-position of guanine in DNA is highly accessible for platinum. In fact the nearby located O6 atom may even assist the coordination of platinum by hydrogen bonding to the water (or amine) molecule, as shown in Figure 1.

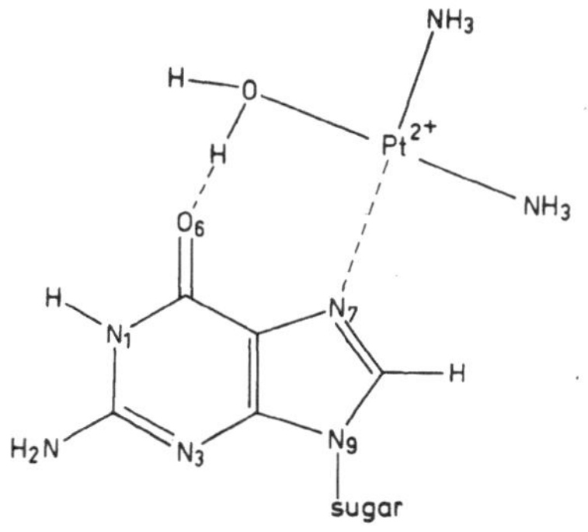

FIGURE 1. Schematic formation and possible structure of the adduct cis-Pt(NH₃)₂(H₂O)(G-N7), together with the used ring numbering system.

Up to now, all experimental data for mononucleotides, oligo-nucleotides and DNA point towards an initial binding to the N7 atoms of guanines (12,14,25). It is evident that not all guanine-containing fragments are equivalent and that some guanines react faster than other bases. This may depend upon the neighbouring bases and the influence and accessibility of phosphate groups. Several authors have shown that a 5'-phosphate group speeds up the reaction and even enhances the preference for N7 bonding. Further, we have shown very recently (26) that 5'-GMP reacts faster with cis-Pt(NH₃)₂²⁺ than 3'-GMP does. Apparently, a nearby negative 5'-phosphate group may enhance the interaction, or promote the approach of the [cis-Pt(NH₃)₂(OH)(OH₂)]⁺ ion. This may be attri-buted to a charge effect, or to a favourable hydrogen bonding.

Finally, it is known that cis-PtCl₂(NH₃)₂ reacts much slower with guanine residues than the aquated products. This is partly due to a slower ligand substitution process in case of Cl⁻ (a poor leaving group), but repulsion between O6 and Cl⁻ may also play a rôle.

In considering the first reaction step, one should also include the possible presence of dimeric and trimeric hydroxo-bridged species of the nature [(amine)₂Pt(OH)₂Pt(amine)₂]²⁺ (12). These species do occur after equilibration hydrolysis at concentrations above 0.1 mM Pt at neutral pH. The reactivity of these products with nucleotides has hardly been studied sofar, but they react much slower than the monomers (12). When Pt-compounds containing other amines than NH_3 are used (e.g. 1,2-diaminoethane, 2,2-dimethyl-1,3-diaminopropane) the reactions with nucleobases and derivatives are believed to be similar. It should be noted, however, that these reactions have been studied only in a few cases (21,22), but the results obtained sofar do not indicate that other products are formed in the first reaction step.

3. "PROLOGUE" OF THE SECOND STEP

When [cis-Pt$(NH_3)_2$]$^{2+}$ is reacted with an excess of 5'-GMP a product characterized as cis-Pt$(NH_3)_2$(5'-GMP)$_2$ is formed. At low temperatures and starting from the aquated Pt-product, a species cis-Pt$(NH_3)_2$(H$_2$O)(5'-GMP) has been detected by NMR spectroscopy (17). This species can react with another 5'-GMP, or with e.g. IMP or AMP (17,26). Before such a second reaction step can occur in DNA, quite some reorganization in the coordination sphere of platinum must take place. To understand how these processes occur, we have studied the process of rotation about the Pt-N7 bond as a function of the amine ligand. It appears that this rotation is fast in all cases (with reference to the NMR time scale), except when the amine nitrogen is tertiary (such as in tetramethylethylene diamine, tmed (11), or when a sterically bulky ligand like bis(2'-pyridyl)ethane, bpe, is used (11,17,26). In those cases the rotation is slow on the NMR time scale (for bpe only at low temperatures). So when a primary amine is used (this is the case in all Pt compounds with cytostatic activity), the Pt-N7 rotation is rather fast, so that - while rotating - a second nucleobase can be met (either interstrand or intrastrand) followed by binding through water substitution.

4. THE SECOND STEP

As discussed above cis-Pt$(NH_3)_2$$^{2+}$ has two reactive binding sites, so bifunctional binding has to be expected. Several species cis-Pt(NH$_3$)$_2$(L)$_2$ (L = mononucleoside or mononucleotide) have been studied, both in the solid state by X-ray crystallography and in solution by NMR spectroscopy (and other spectroscopic techniques). It has been found sofar that the mutual orientation of the bases is always "head to tail" (see Figure 2). Even when sterically bulky amines are used, the ligands keep their head-to-tail orientation, because that is the thermodynamically most favourable position. The rotation about the Pt-N7 bond, however, can be slowed down by steric effects of the amines (11,21,22,27).

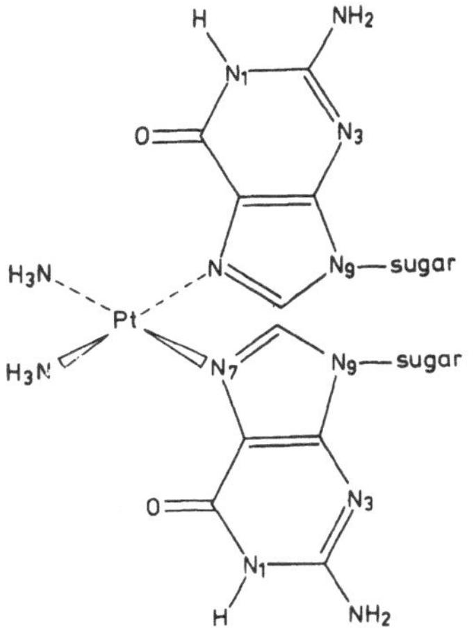

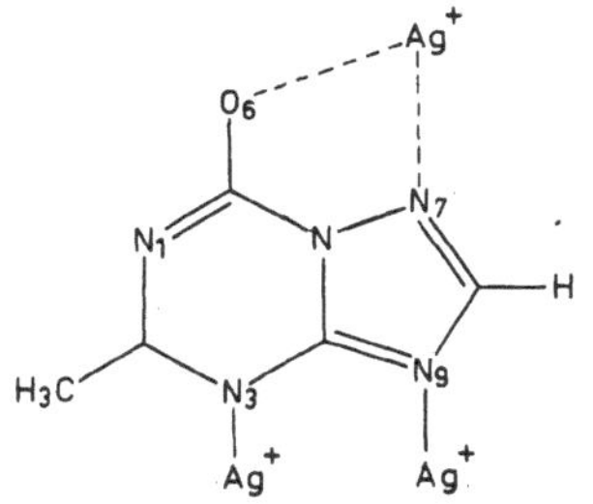

FIGURE 3. *Schematic structure of the Ag(I) salt of 2-methyl-5-azapurine (35). Dotted bonds are the long Ag-N and Ag-O bonds. The strongest bonds are to N3 and N9.*

FIGURE 2. *Schematic structure of cis-Pt(NH$_3$)$_2$(GMP)$_2$ with a head-to-tail arrangement of the nucleotides.*

When binding to DNA occurs via an intrastrand crosslink (i.e. two bases in the same strand), such head-to-tail orientations are impossible for neighbouring bases and only head-to-head (i.e. parallel orientation) is to be expected. Such a head-to-head orientation has not yet been observed in monomeric Pt-mononucleotide compounds (21).
Four possibilities have been proposed for the bifunctional binding:

1. Chelation through N7 and the O6 atom of the same guanine. This
   has been proposed by several investigators (28-30), and some
   experimental evidence from infrared spectra (a decrease in ν_{CO})
   (31) and photo-electron spectra (7) has been put forward.
   Geometric arguments, on the other hand, disfavour chelation
   (9,32). Although coordination of the C=O group is certainly
   possible, and has been found in a few compounds (33,34),
   chelation to one metal through both N7 and O6 in a related
   ligand has only been observed sofar for an Ag(I) compound of an
   anionic 2-methyl-5-azapurine (35)(see Figure 3). The experimental evidence that points to a weakening of the C=O bond and to
   the liberation of protons (from N1) upon platination of guanine
   at N7, might equally well be explained by changes in π-electron
   density distribution or by hydrogen bonding of H_2O or NH_3 to
   O6, (see also Figure 1).
2. Crosslinking between guanine-N7 and a protein surrounding the
   DNA. This possibility has been demonstrated to occur (36-38).
   It is agreed, however, that this type of bonding is only
   present for a few percent (38,39).
3. Interstrand crosslinking between the two strands of DNA (37).
   This binding type comprises less than 1% of the total amount
   of platinum bound to DNA in vivo (40).
4. Intrastrand crosslinking. This type of bifunctional binding to
   two bases in the same strand of DNA has been proposed by several authors, and is considered to be an important lesion for
   the anti-tumor activity of cis-Pt compounds.

The remaining part of this paper will deal with chemical and biochemical studies of the binding of Pt-compounds to oligonucleotides and DNA with special attention to intrastrand crosslinking
in oligonucleotides.

5. INTRASTRAND CROSSLINKING

The main questions to be answered in such studies are:
- Do Pt compounds, after initially binding to a guanine-N7,
  preferentially bind to a neighbouring base in the 5'-direction,
  in the 3'-direction or to a next-nearest neighbouring base?

- Does binding occur only, or specifically, to a (next) nearest
  neighbouring guanine, or also to the other nucleobases?
Biochemical studies (10,41,42) have shown that the action of a
restriction endonuclease is inhibited in DNA treated with cis-Pt,
when a $(dG)_4 . (dC)_4$ sequence is present near the cutting site.
It has been found that digestion of cis-Pt-treated DNA by
exonuclease III stops at sites with sequences $d(G)_n$ with $n = 2$ or
larger (43,44). These data suggest the presence of intrastrand
crosslinks at neighbouring guanines. Studies by Brouwer et al.
(15,16) have shown that base-pair substitutions in the lacI gen of
wild type E.coli bacteria, originate to a large extent from Pt-
adducts at GpCpG and GpApG base sequences.

   Fichtinger et al. (18) demonstrated in the enzymatic digest
of Pt-treated salmon sperm DNA, among other products, cis-Pt-
$(NH_3)_2 (pGpG)$. Recently, she also found the adducts cis-Pt$(NH_3)_2$-
(pApG) and cis-Pt$(NH_3)_2$(pTpGpG) (45), in which Pt is bound to N7
of the purines. Studies on oligonucleotide-Pt interactions in our
laboratories are focussing upon GpG- and GpCpG-containing nucleotides (X = C,A,G). Others have also been giving attention to e.g.
CpG, GpC, ApG and GpA oligonucleotides (25,46). In this paper we
only consider the studies on GpG-containing oligomers and on
GpCpG-containing trimers and tetramers.

   The smallest GpG-containing oligonucleotides are GpG, d(GpG)
and compounds containing an extra phosphate, i.e. pGpG and
d(pGpG). Studies by Chottard et al. (25,46,47) and us (19,23)
have shown that all these compounds yield chelates with cis-Pt-
$(NH_3)_2^{2+}$ through the N7 atoms.

   The structure of one of these adducts, i.e. cis-Pt(d(GpG)),
has been studied in detail by analysis of the high-resolution NMR
spectra under varying conditions. The results are summarized in
Figure 4 (19). It is clear that the stacking between the guanine
bases is decreased significantly upon chelation. Furthermore, the
conformation of the 5'-deoxyribose ring has been changed from an
"S"- to an "N"-type conformation, as a result of Pt binding. The
binding of d(CpGpG) to Pt is similar to that found for d(GpG) and
the GpG-unit seems to have the same conformation as described
above for the adduct with d(GpG) (Figure 4).

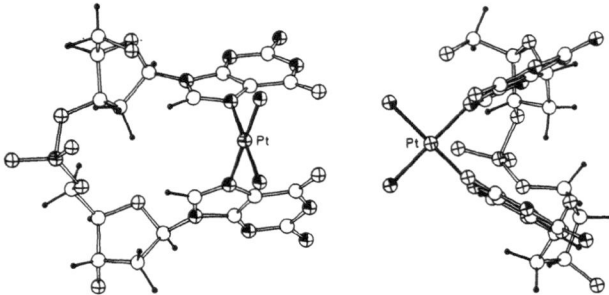

FIGURE 4.
Two projections of a possi-
ble conformer of cis-Pt-
(d(GpG)) as deduced from
NMR spectroscopy. (Taken
from ref. 19.)

Using d(CpCpGpG), a self-complementary oligonucleotide, which
shows significant duplex formation in dilute solution, some additional features are to be noted. First of all, the duplex formation has disappeared after binding of cis-Pt (23). Secondly, the
lack of high-molecular weight products after the reaction of
d(CpCpGpG) indicates that interstrand crosslinking is unlikely
under these conditions. Chottard and co-workers (48) have recently studied the reaction between cis-Pt and d(ApTpGpG). Also in
this case a chelate via the GpG-part has been observed as the
main product.

Three self-complementary hexanucleotides have been reacted with
cis-Pt so far, i.e. d(ApGpGpCpCpT), d(TpGpGpCpCpA) and d(CpCpAp-
TpGpG) (48-50). In all these cases no indication is found for a
double helix after reaction of the oligonucleotides with cis-Pt.
Detailed analysis of the NMR spectra of the products as a function
of pH, has shown that the main products in all cases are chelates
with cis-Pt through the N7 atoms of the two guanines in each hexa-
nucleotide (48-50).

Very recently, we have studied the reaction of the decanucleotide d(TpCpTpCpGpGpTpCpTpC) with cis-Pt. Analysis of the NMR
spectra of the base protons at pH values of 1-10, clearly shows
that also in this case a chelate via the N7 of both guanines is
formed.

Since the above-mentioned biochemical studies (15,16) have
shown that GpCpG sequences are prone to mutations, we have also
studied the reactions of GpCpG-containing tri- and tetranucleotides with Pt(II) compounds (20,51). Striking similarities between GpG- and GpCpG-Pt reaction products are:

- In both cases only chelation products through the N7 atoms of guanine are observed.
- In self-complementary oligonucleotides (such as CpCpGpG and CpGpCpG), the hydrogen bonding is broken upon chelation to cis-Pt.
- In all cases the major products are of low molecular weight, and therefore interstrand crosslinking is unimportant under these conditions.

On the other hand, both types of chelates (i.e. Pt(GpG) and Pt(GpCpG) are clearly different. First of all, only the latter adduct leads to base-pair substitutions in wild type E.coli cells (15,16). Secondly, the NMR results show that the (GpCpG)-Pt chelates have much more conformational freedom, than the (GpG)-Pt chelates have (52).

Whether one of these adducts is the most important lesion for the antineoplastic activity, is a still unanswered question.

6. CONCLUDING REMARKS

During the last couple of years both chemical and biochemical evidence has been put forward that two types of adducts, i.e. (GpG)-Pt and (GpXpG)-Pt are formed upon reaction of cis-Pt with DNA (see Figure 5). A competitive study of the binding of cis-Pt to a mixture of d(GpG) and d(CpCpG), or even to d(GpGpG) is therefore of great interest. This work is now in progress in our laboratories.

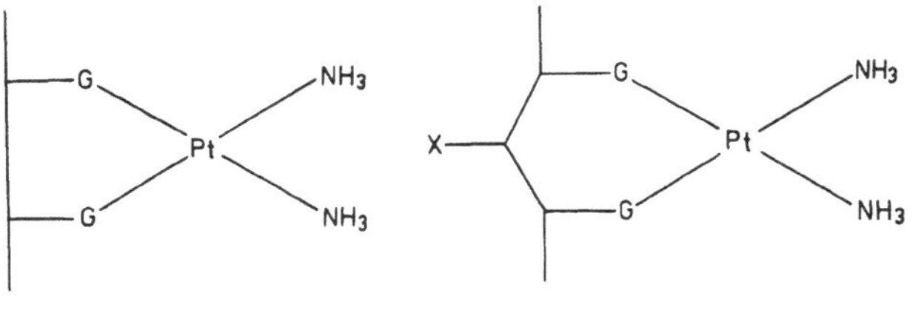

FIGURE 5.
Schematic representations of two possible intrastrand crosslinks in DNA, resulting from interaction with cis-Pt(NH₃)₂²⁺

What has become clear from studies of the interaction between oligonucleotides and platinum compounds is:
- Double strands are broken or disturbed up to at least two nucleobases separated from the Pt-binding site.
- Interstrand crosslinking seems to be a less frequent event.

- In case of chelation by a GpG-fragment, rather rigid chelates
  are formed with a fixed ribose conformation.
- Relatively flexible chelates are formed when chelation occurs
  through a GpCpG-fragment, although the distortion of the neighbouring bases may be significant (due to the bulge out of the
  C-group; see Figure 5).

For the future we expect that biochemical research in this area
will be focussed on the study of the formation and repair of
Pt-DNA lesions formed in vivo. However, classical analytical techniques, such as AAS, neutron activation analysis, etc. will not be
sensitive enough for the detection of these lesions. Therefore,
new methods for the detection of Pt in in vivo treated DNA have
to be developed. With immunochemical techniques it may be possible
to detect and even quantitate specific Pt-lesions formed in vivo
(see also ref.45). The fact that cis-Pt is administered in exactly known dosages to cancer patients offers the opportunity to
directly relate in vivo induction of Pt-DNA lesions in human
cells to the observed biological effects.

7. ACKNOWLEDGEMENTS

The authors are indebted to several colleagues and collabora-
tors, whose names appear as co-authors in the list of references,
for their valuable and stimulating contributions to the research
discussed in this paper. Prof.dr. J.H. van Boom and dr. G.J. van
der Marel are thanked for the synthesis of several oligonucleotides and for stimulating discussions.

The investigations were supported by grants from the Nether-
lands Foundation for the Fight against Cancer (KWF grant numbers
MBL-79-1 and 83-1) and the Netherlands Organization for the
Advancement of Pure Research (ZWO project number 11-28-17 of the
Foundation for Chemical Research).

The authors wish to thank the editor of Nucleic Acids Research
for the reproduction of a previously published drawing (Figure 4,
ref.19).

REFERENCES

1. Rosenberg B, Platinum Met.Rev. 1971, 15, 42.
2. Reslova S, Chem.-Biol. Interactions 1971/1972, 4, 66.
3. Johnson N.P, Hoeschele J.D, Kuemmerle N.B, Masker W.E, and Rahn R.O, Chem.-Biol. Interactions 1978, 23, 267.
4. Roberts J.J, in Marzilli G.L. and Eichhorn L.G. (Eds.), Metal Ions in Genetic Information Transfer, Elsevier/ North-Holland, New York 1981, 273.
5. Johnson, N.P, Hoeschele J.D. and Rahn R.O, Chem.-Biol. Interactions 1980, 30, 151.
6. Vestues P.I. and Martin R.B, J.Am.Chem.Soc. 1981, 103, 806.
7. Millard M.M, Macquet J.P. and Theophanides T, Biochim.Biophys. Acta 1975, 402, 166.
8. Mansy S, Chu G.Y.H, Duncan R.E. and Tobias R.S, J.Am.Chem.Soc. 1978, 100, 607.
9. Barton J.K. and Lippard S.J, Metal Ions in Biology 1980, 1 ,31.
10. Ushay H.M, Tullius T.D. and Lippard S.J, Biochemistry 1981, 20, 3744.
11. Cramer R.E. and Dahlstrom P.L, J.Am.Chem.Soc. 1979, 101, 3679.
12. Martin R.B. in: "Platinum, Gold, and other metal chemotherapeutic agents: Chemistry and Biochemistry", Lippard S.J. (ed), ACS, Symposium series no. 209, 1983, 231, Washington.
13. Clore G.M. and Gronenborn A.M, J.Am.Chem.Soc. 1982, 104, 1369.
14. Marcelis A.T.M. and Reedijk J, Recl.Trav.Chim.Pays-Bas, 1983, 102, 121 and references cited there.
15. Brouwer J, van de Putte P, Fichtinger-Schepman A.M.J. and Reedijk J, Proc.Natl.Acad.Sci.USA, 1981, 78, 7010.
16. Brouwer J, Fichtinger-Schepman A.M.J, van de Putte P. and Reedijk J, Cancer Research 1982, 42, 2416.
17. Marcelis A.T.M, van Kralingen C.C. and Reedijk J, J.Inorg. Biochem. 1980, 13, 213.
18. Fichtinger-Schepman A.M.J, Lohman P.H.M. and Reedijk J, Nucl.Acids Res. 1982, 10, 5345.
19. Den Hartog J.H.J, Altona C, Chottard J.C, Girault J.P, Lallemand J.Y, de Leeuw F.A.A.M, Marcelis A.T.M. and Reedijk J, Nucl.Acids Res. 1982, 10, 4715.
20. Marcelis A.T.M, den Hartog J.H.J. and Reedijk J, J.Am.Chem.Soc. 1982, 104, 2664
21. Marcelis A.T.M. Korte H.J, Krebs B. and Reedijk J, Inorg.Chem. 1982, 21, 4059.
22. Marcelis A.T.M, van der Veer J.L, Zwetsloot J.C.M. and Reedijk J, Inorg.Chim.Acta 1983, 78, 195.
23. Marcelis A.T.M, Canters G.W. and Reedijk J, Recl.Trav.Chim. Pays-Bas, 1981, 100, 391.
24. Robins A.B, Chem.-Biol. Interactions 1973, 6, 35.
25. Chottard J.C, Girault J.P, Lallemand J.Y, Chottard G. and Guittet E. in: "Platinum, gold, and other metal chemotherapeutic agents: Chemistry and Biochemistry", Lippard S.J. (ed), ACS, Symposium Series no. 209, 1983, 125; Washington.
26. Marcelis A.T.M, Erkelens C. and Reedijk J, Inorg.Chim.Acta, submitted.
27. Kleiböhmer W, Krebs B, Marcelis A.T.M, Reedijk J. and van der Veer J.L, Inorg.Chim.Acta., in press.
28. Rosenberg B, Biochimie, 1978, 60, 859.

29. Macquet J.P. and Butour J.L, Biochimie 1978, 60, 901.
30. Goodgame D.M.L, Jeeves I, Phillips F.L. and Skapski A.C, Biochim.Biophys.Acta 1975, 378, 153.
31. Hadjiliadis N. and Theophanides T, Inorg.Chim.Acta. 1976, 16, 77.
32. Sletten E, J.Chem.Soc.Chem.Commun. 1971, 558.
33. Swaminathon V. and Sundaralingam M. in :"CRC Critical Reviews in Biochemisty" (ed. Fasman G.D;), CRC Press, 1979, page 425.
34. Marzilli, L.G. in: "Metal ions in genetic information transfer" (eds. Eichhorn G.L. and Marzilli L.G.) Elsevier, North Holland, 1981, page 47.
35. Smith D.L. and Luss H.R, Photograph.Sc.and Eng. 1976, 20, 184.
36. Lippard S.J. and Hoeschele J.D, Proc.Natl.Acad.Sci.USA, 1979, 76, 6091.
37. Laurent G, Erickson L.C, Sharkey N.A. and Kohn K.W, Cancer Res. 1981, 41, 3347.
38. Erickson L.C, Zwelling L.A, Ducore J.M, Sharkey N.A. and Kohn K.W, Cancer Res. 1981, 41, 2791.
39. Pera M.F. Jr., Rawlings C.J. and Roberts J.J, Chem.-Biol. Interactions 1981, 37, 245.
40. Roberts J.J. and Friedlos F, Biochim.Biophys.Acta 1981, 655, 146.
41. Stone P.J, Kelman A.D, Sinex F.M, Bhargava M.M. and Halvorson H.O, J.Mol.Biol. 1976, 104, 793.
42. Cohen G.L, Ledner J.A, Bauer W.A, Ushay, H.M, Caravana A. and Lippard S.J, J.Am.Chem.Soc. 1980, 102, 3744.
43. Tullius T.D. and Lippard S.J, J.Am.Chem.Soc. 1981, 103, 4620.
44. Royer-Pokora B, Gordon L.K. and Haseltine W.A, Nucl.Acids Res. 1981, 9, 4595.
45. Fichtinger-Schepman A.M.J, poster at this conference.
46. Girault J.P, Chottard G, Lallemand J.Y. and Chottard J.C, Biochemistry 1982, 21, 1352.
47. Chottard J.C, Girault J.P, Chottard G, Lallemand J.Y. and Mansuy D, J.Am.Chem.Soc. 1980, 102, 5565.
48. Chottard J.C, Girault J.P, Guittet E, Huynh-Dinh T, Igolen J, Lallemand J.Y, Neumann J. and Tran-Dinh S, Inorg.Chim.Acta, in the press.
49. Girault J.P, Chottard J.C, Guittet E.R, Lallemand J.Y, Huynh-Dinh T. and Igolen J, Biochem.Biophys.Res.Commun. 1982, 109, 1157.
50. Caradonna J.P, Lippard S.J, Gait M.J. and Singh M, J.Am.Chem. Soc. 1982, 104, 5793.
51. Marcelis A.T.M, den Hartog J.H.J, van der Marel G.A, Wille G. and Reedijk J, Eur.J.Biochem. in press.
52. Den Hartog J.H.J, Altona C, van Boom J.H, Marcelis A.T.M, van der Marel G.A, Rinkel L.J, Wille-Hazeleger G. and Reedijk J, Eur.J.Biochem.; in press.

POSTER PRESENTATIONS

I-1   Pt(II) BINDING TO N-7 of ADENINE: EFFECTS ON LIGAND BASICITY AND STACKING PROPERTIES.
R. Beyerle-Pfnur and B. Lippert.

I-2   ALTERATION IN THE DNA, NUCLEOSOMES AND CHROMATIN STRUCTURES UPON INTERACTION WITH PLATINUM COORDINATION COMPLEXES.
C. Houssier.

I-3   N-15 AND Pt-195 NMR STUDY OF REACTIONS OF cis-Pt $(NH_3)_2$-$(H_2O)_2{}^{2+}$.
T.G. Appleton, C.A. Bowie, J.R. Hall and S.F. Ralph.

I-4   NUCLEOBASE DISPLACEMENT FROM Pt(II)-COMPLEXES BY CYANIDE: A SURPRISING RESULT.
G. Raudaschl and B. Lippert.

I-5   CHEMISTRY OF 1-METHYLURACIL AND MIXED 1-METHYLURACIL, 1-METHYLCYTOSINE-COMPLEXES OF cis-Pt(II).
B. Lippert.

I-6   ETHIDIUM BROMIDE AFFECTS THE BINDING MODE OF cis-DIAMMINE-DICHLOROPLATINUM (II) TO DNAS.
C.M. Merkel and S.J. Lippard.

I-7   EFFECTS OF cis-AND $trans$-DICHLORODIAMMINEPLATINUM (II), (DDP) ON NUCLEOTIDE LUMINESCENCE.
T.A. Taylor and H. Patterson.

I-8   CHARACTERIZATION OF THE INTERACTION OF cis-DIAMMINE DICHLOROPLATINUM (II) WITH DNA.
A. Eastman.

I-9   SEPARATION, IDENTIFICATION AND IMMUNOLOGICAL DETECTION OF ADDUCTS FORMED IN DNA AFTER EXPOSURE TO DIAMMINEDICHLOROPLATINUM (II).
A.M.J. Fichtinger-Schepman, P.H.M. Lohman and J. Reedijk.

I-10   THE STRUCTURE OF CHELATES, FORMED UPON REACTION OF cis-DIAMMINEDICHLOROPLATINUM AND OLIGONUCLEOTIDES CONTAINING d(GpCpG) AND d(GpG) UNITS, AS STUDIED BY HIGH FREQUENCY PROTON NMR.
J.H.J. den Hartog, C. Altona, J.H. van Boom, A.T.M. Marcelis and J. Reedijk.

I-11   COMPARATIVE ACTIVITY OF PLATINUM II COORDINATION COMPLEXES AND THEIR $trans$-HYDROXY PLATINUM IV ANALOGS AS INDUCERS OF BACTERIOPHAGE LAMBDA.
R.K. Elespuru and S.K. Daley.

I-12   THE MODE OF FIXATION OF cis- AND $trans$-DDP ON DNA *IN VITRO*.
N.P. Johnson, J.P. Macquet and C. Vieussens.

I-13   NUCLEOSIDE OXIDATION AND HYDROLYSIS INDUCED BY COORDINATED Ru(III).
M.J. Clarke and P. Morrissey.

I-14   [195]Pt NMR SPECTROSCOPIC STUDIES OF a-PYRIDONATE BRIDGED PLATINUM (II) COMPLEXES: DYNAMIC STEREO CHEMISTRY.
T.V. O'Halloran and S.J. Lippard.

I-15 A MODEL FOR THE INFLUENCE OF *cis*-DIAMMINEDICHLORO-PLATINUM (II) BINDING ON SV40 DNA AND MINICHROMOSOME.
W.M. Scovell.

I-16 *cis*-DIAMMINEDICHLOROPLATINUM (II) CROSSLINKS HIGH MOBILITY GROUP 1 AND 2 PROTEINS TO DNA IN MICROCOCCAL NUCLEASE ACCESSIBLE REGIONS OF CHROMATIN.
W.M. Scovell, N. Muirhead and L.R. Kroos.

I-17 DEGRADATION OF DNA-PLATINUM (II) COMPLEXES BY THE SINGLE STRAND SPECIFIC NUCLEASE S_1.
J.L. Butour and C.E. Vieussens.

I-18 INHIBITION OF DNA SYNTHESIS BY *cis*-$Pt(NH_3)_2Cl_2$, *trans*-$Pt(NH_3)_2Cl_2$ AND [Pt(dien)Cl]Cl IN CULTURED L1210 LEUKEMIA CELLS.
B. Salles, J.L. Butour, C. Lesca and J.P. Macquet.

I-19 EXAFS STUDIES OF PT-BASE MODEL COMPOUNDS AND $[(NH_3)_2 Pt(OH)_2P^+(NH_3)_2]_2^+$ BOUND TO DNA.
A.P. Hitchcock, M.L. Martins and C.J.L. Lock.

I-20 DNA REPAIR CHARACTERISTICS OF WALKER RAT CARCINOMA CELLS SENSITIVE AND RESISTANT TO *cis*-DIAMMINEDICHLOROPLATINUM II (CISPLATIN).
J.J. Roberts, C.J. Rawlings and F. Friedlos.

I-21 *cis*-PLATINUM MEDIATED CROSSLINKING TO DNA OF CHROMOSOMAL NONHISTONE PROTEINS IN HeLa CELLS.
Z.M. Banjar, R.C. Briggs, L.S. Hnilica, J.L. Stein and G.S. Stein.

I-22 NMR AND CYSTALLOGRAPHIC STUDIES ON A SECOND GENERATION CISPLATIN ANALOGUE.
J.C. Dabrowiak, M.S. Balakrishnan, J. Clardy, D. Van Duyne and L. Silviera.

I-1 Pt(II) BINDING TO N7 OF ADENINE: EFFECTS ON LIGAND BASICITY AND STACKING PROPERTIES.

Rut Beyerle-Pfnür[+] and Bernhard Lippert, Anorganisch-Chemisches Institut, Technische Universität München, 8046 Garching, F.R.G., present address: Stanford University, Department of Chemistry, Stanford, Ca.94305, U.S.A.

Apart from stereochemical aspects of nucleobase cross-linking through cis- and trans-Pt(II), alterations of the electronic structure of nucleobases as a consequence of platinum binding are of particular interest. This is so because both base pairing and base stacking, the two major forces for duplex stability, strongly depend on the electronic structure of the bases.

Using fully characterized model nucleobase complexes of cis- and trans-Pt(II) containing N7 bound 9-methyl-adenine we have detected two distinct changes in the behaviour of this purine base as a consequence of Pt binding:

1) The basicity of the N1 position for accepting a proton is decreased by 1.5-2 pK units. This means that the electronic complementarity for AT base pairing according to the Watson-Crick scheme is lost, and that the affinity of the adenine-N1 site to form a hydrogen bond with the proton of thymine-N3 is lowered.

2) Although there is base stacking between N7 platinated 9-methyladenine and free 9-methyladenine, the extent of this interaction is smaller than in the absence of Pt. No major differences between cis- and trans-Pt(II) binding have been observed in this respect.

Both findings suggest that binding to N7 of adenine (and most likely to guanine as well) provide a local destabilization of DNA, probably necessary for any subsequent reaction with a second nucleobase.

I-2 Alteration in the DNA, nucleosomes and chromatin structures upon interaction with platinum coordination complexes. C. Houssier, Laboratoire de Chimie-Physique, Université de Liège(B6), Sart-Tilman, B4000 Liège Belgium.

The interaction of various platinum coordination complexes with DNA, nucleosomes and chromatin has been investigated by circular and electric linear dichroism, thermal denaturation and Tb^{3+} fluorescence enhancement. Three cis-bidentate (cis-dichlorodiammine or cis-DDPt,diaminocyclohexane or dac-Pt, and ethylenediamine or en-Pt),one trans-bidentate (trans-DDPt) and monodentate (diethylenetriamine or dien-Pt) ligands were bound to the above biopolymers at low binding ratios (less than 0.1-0.2 Pt molecule per mononucleotide residue).

Cis-DDPt, en-Pt,dac-Pt and trans-Pt produced a drastic decrease of the negative electric dichroism in the 260 nm absorption band of the bases, for DNA as well as for its nucleoprotein complex. On the contrary, the electric dichroism of the complexes with dien-Pt revealed little changes for DNA but a profound alteration of the DNA arrangement in chromatin and nucleosomes. A condensation of the superhelical structure in the latter two molecules was evidenced by electron microscopy upon interaction with cis-DDPt.

The Tb^{3+} fluorescence enhancement used to reveal the occurrence of unpaired guanine residues in DNA,indicated the largest effect for cis-DDPt, the lowest one for dien-Pt and intermediate behaviors for en-Pt, trans-Pt and dac-Pt (in decreasing order).

The above results, together with the circular dichroism and thermal denaturation observations will be discussed in terms of the various possible modes of binding of Pt derivatives to DNA and chromatin, particularly in relation with the level of "denaturation" of the double helix, the formation of intrastrand and protein-DNA cross-links.

I-3 N-15 AND Pt-195 NMR STUDY OF REACTIONS OF CIS-Pt(NH$_3$)$_2$-(H$_2$O)$_2^{2+}$. Trevor G. Appleton*, Carol A. Bowie, John R. Hall and Stephen F. Ralph. * Department of Chemistry, University of Queensland, Brisbane, Australia 4067.

cis-Pt(NH$_3$)$_2$(H$_2$O)$_2^{2+}$ is a useful intermediate in the preparation of both (i) new compounds which might have anti-tumor activity and (ii) compounds which are "models" for the interaction of platinum complexes with complex biological molecules such as DNA.

Because ^{14}N (I=1) is a quadrupolar nucleus, which relaxes at an intermediate rate in most ammine-platinum complexes, ^{195}Pt and ^{14}N nmr have only limited usefulness when nitrogen has its natural isotropic composition. For ^{15}N-substituted compounds (I=½), ^{195}Pt and ^{15}N spectra are easily obtained. ^{195}Pt and ^{15}N chemical shifts, ^{195}Pt-^{15}N coupling constants, and splitting patterns in the spectra all provide useful information.

Initially, ^{195}Pt and ^{15}N nmr were used to study reactions between cis-Pt(^{15}NH$_3$)$_2$(H$_2$O)$_2^{2+}$ and common "weakly coordinating" oxygen-donor anions, A^{n-}, such as perchlorate (which does not coordinate), nitrate, sulfate, phosphate, and acetate. The simplest complex in each case is cis-Pt(^{15}NH$_3$)$_2$(A)(H$_2$O)$^{(2-n)+}$, with the ligand unidentate. With phosphate and acetate, further complex reactions occur, giving dimeric and oligomeric species, including highly colored mixed-oxidation state compounds.

Using NMR, the first platinum complexes with an O-bound unidentate amino acid have been characterized.

Compounds with O-donor ligands were prepared, for testing for biological activity, and characterized using nmr.

The usefulness and limitations of ^{15}N and ^{195}Pt nmr in investigating reactions with nucleosides and other complex ligands will be discussed.

I-4 NUCLEOBASE DISPLACEMENT FROM Pt(II)-COMPLEXES BY CYANIDE: A SURPRISING RESULT. Gabriele Raudaschl and Bernhard Lippert, Anorganisch-Chemisches Institut, Technische Universität München, 8046 Garching, F.R.G.

Treatment of platinated DNA with agents exercising a high kinetic trans effect or leading to very stable complexes (e.g. thiosulfate, thiourea, cyanide) has been applied to gain insight in the stability of cis-Pt(II)/DNA cross-links, and in an attempt to possibly reduce Cisplatin toxicity. Interestingly, a complete removal of cis-Pt(II) from DNA appears not to be possible.

Using ^{1}H NMR spectroscopy, we have examined the behaviour of a large series of fully characterized complexes of cis-Pt(II), trans-Pt(II) and (NH$_3$)$_2$Pt(II) containing the model nucleobases 9-ethylguanine,G, 9-methyladenine,A, 1-methylcytosine,C, 1-methyluracil,U, and 1-methylthymine,T, respectively, when treated with an excess of cyanide (c_{Pt}= 0.025 M, c_{CN} = 0.5 M, D$_2$O, pD 8, 30°C).

As a result, the kinetics of the nucleobase displacement by cyanide have been found to be extremely variable and in some cases completely unexpected. In general, N7 platined G and A, and N3 platinated C are replaced relatively quickly, while N3 platinated T and U are rather hard to replace. For example, while 50 % of N7 bound G is displaced within 15 min from trans-a$_2$PtG Cl$^+$, within 60 min from cis-a$_2$PtG Cl$^+$, within 4 h from cis- a$_2$PtG$_2^{2+}$ and from a$_2$PtG^{2+}, there is no replacement of U from cis-a$_2$PtU$_2$ even after 2 weeks (a= NH$_3$).

Factors responsible for these findings and the possible relevance for cis-Pt(II) interaction with DNA will be discussed.

I - 5 CHEMISTRY OF 1-METHYLURACIL- AND MIXED 1-METHYL-
URACIL,1-METHYLCYTOSINE-COMPLEXES OF cis-Pt(II).
Bernhard Lippert, Anorganisch-Chemisches Institut,
Technische Universität München, 8046 Garching, F.R.G.

Preparative, structural, and spectroscopic results
on a series of model pyrimidine base complexes of cis-
$Pt(NH_3)_2Cl_2$ will be presented.

They include 1:1-, 1:2-, and 2:2-complexes of
1-methyluracil, their distribution in solution after
reaction of cis- $[(NH_3)_2Pt\ OH]_2^{2+}$ with neutral 1-methyl-
uracil, and their reactions with heterometals. Special
attention will be paid to complexes of 1-methyluracil
containing metals coordinated to N3, O4, and O2
simultaneously, and to the different consequences of
head-head and head-tail arrangement of the uracil rings
in such complexes.

Reaction of the 1:1-complex of 1-methyluracil with
1-methylcytosine gives the mixed 1-methyluracil,
1-methylcytosine complex. Novel heteronuclear compounds
derived from this complex have been isolated and
studied.

ETHIDIUM BROMIDE AFFECTS THE BINDING MODE OF CIS-DIAMMINE-
I - 6 DICHLOROPLATINUM(II) TO DNAS. Carolyn M. Merkel and
Stephen J. Lippard. Columbia University, Department of Chemistry,
New York, New York, 10027, U.S.A. and Massachusetts Institute of
Technology, Department of Chemistry, Cambridge, Massachusetts, 02139,
U.S.A.

The binding of cis-diamminedichloroplatinum(II) (cis-DDP) to
DNAs is altered when the intercalator ethidium bromide (EtdBr) is
present during the platination reaction. The changes are manifest
in several ways. Plasmid DNAs show substantially less shortening
upon platination, as judged by electron microscopic and gel electrophoretic experiments. Moreover, the ability of cyanide ion to remove
bound platinum is greatly enhanced when platination is carried out in
the presence of EtdBr. The activities of certain nucleases are also
altered. For example, the single strand specific S1 nuclease has
greatly reduced activity against T7 DNA platinated with EtdBr present
as compared to DNA platinated in the absence of EtdBr. Exonuclease
III sensitive sites on the Hpa II/Hae III 165 base pair fragment from
pBR322are also altered when platination is carried out with EtdBr
present. The changes in cis-DDP binding are reversed when the Pt-DNA
complexes are reincubated following removal of EtdBr and free Pt.
These results are interpreted in terms of a model in which EtdBr
blocks a multifunctional binding mode of the cis platinum complex.
This mode can then be reactivated upon removal of the intercalator.

56

I-7 EFFECTS OF CIS- AND TRANS-DICHLORODIAMINEPLATINUM(II), (DDP), ON NUCLEOTIDE LUMINESCENCE. Todd A. Taylor and Howard Patterson. University of Maine, Orono, Maine. 04469, U.S.A.

The fluorescence and phosphorescence of simple nucleotides (2×10^{-4} M) can be observed at 77K in frozen saline solutions. We have found the luminescence to be a sensitive probe of metal binding to nucleic acids (metal = cis or trans-dichlorodiamineplatinum II (DDP), lanthanide ions or first row transition metals), base ionization, or the effects of base stacking. The intensity of the fluorescence and phosphorescence, as well as the phosphorescence lifetime has been measured as a function of the metal to base molar ratio. Our studies of dGMP with cis- and trans-DDP shows greater than a fifty percent reduction in the fluorescence and phosphorescence emission intensity from the base residue upon metal binding for both isomers. No observable effect is seen on the phosphorescence lifetime as is expected for a diamagnetic transition metal. The luminescence is unchanged by Mg(II), but for Mn(II) the metal paramagnetism and close association with the base changes the fluorescence and phosphorescence from that of the unbound residue. Binding of the 3'-5' dinucleotide of deoxyguanosine to cis- or trans-DDP also yields a reduction in the base emission intensity. In the case of cis-DDP binding a red shift in the fluorescence band maximum from the unbound base maximum is probably due to excimer fluorescence of base stacking. When Tb(III) or Gd(III) is added to 3'-5' dinucleotides of deoxyguanosine bound to cis or trans- DDP, differences in the luminescence spectra are observed. These results are consistent with intramolecular binding in the cis-DDP complex unlike in the trans-DDP complex. Further studies are underway for other dinucleotides.

I-8 CHARACTERIZATION OF THE INTERACTION OF cis-DIAMMINE-DICHLOROPLATINUM(II) WITH DNA. Alan Eastman, Dept. Biochemistry, Univ. of Vermont College of Medicine, Burlington, VT 05405

The effectiveness of cis-diamminedichloroplatinum(II) (cis-DDP) in treating a variety of human malignancies has led to extensive study of its mechanism of action. It is generally agreed that DNA is the critical cellular target with DNA-interstrand, DNA-intrastrand and DNA-protein crosslinks being variously implicated as the most significant lesion. Murine leukemia L1210 cells and a cis-DDP resistant subline were compared with respect to formation and removal of interstrand and DNA-protein crosslinks. The resistant cells tolerated much higher levels of these crosslinks suggesting that other lesions are more critical to toxicity. An equally active isomer of cis-DDP, [^{3}H]-cis-dichloroethylenediamineplatinum(II) (cis-DEP) has been synthesized and applied to sensitive and resistant cells. Both cell lines demonstrated identical time and dose dependent platination of DNA. To characterize the specific lesions in DNA a series of standards was first prepared. Both drugs were reacted with deoxyribonucleosides, the products separated by HPLC and characterized by $_3$H-NMR. Platination occured at N'-guanine, N^1, and N'-adenine and N^3-cytosine. The products resulting from reaction of [^{3}H]-cis-DEP with DNA, nucleic acid homopolymers and defined oligonucleotides were analyzed after enzyme digestion to deoxyribonucleosides. At low levels of modification of DNA, greater than 50% of the lesions were attributed to an intrastrand crosslink between two neighboring guanines; enzymatic removal of the phosphate between the two nucleosides being inhibited by the complex. At higher levels of modification, these sites became saturated and pronounced reaction occured at 4 other sites. These adducts were purified by HPLC, the platinum removed with 1 M thiourea and the nucleosides identified. They represented various crosslinks between adenosine and guanosine residues. Reaction was also demonstrated between two guanines separated by a third base but this was not a major lesion in DNA. An additional, more hydrophilic adduct was identified by denaturation studies as an interstrand crosslink but it represented about 1% of the total lesions at low levels of DNA modification. This frequency decreased at higher levels of modification. These platinum analogues were also reacted with M13 single stranded viral DNA and subjected to a DNA polymerase reaction using E. coli polymerase I (Klenow fragment). The products were separated by DNA sequencing gel electrophoresis. The major termination sites were observed to be one base before a guanine-guanine sequence. The polymerase also stopped at the same sequences after platination with a diaminocyclohexane derivative. Supp. by CA28599.

I-9 SEPARATION, IDENTIFICATION AND IMMUNOCHEMICAL DETECTION OF ADDUCTS FORMED IN DNA AFTER EXPOSURE TO DIAMMINE-DICHLOROPLATINUM(II) Anne Marie J. Fichtinger-Schepman*, Paul H.M. Lohman* and Jan Reedijk**. *Medical Biological Laboratory - TNO, P.O. Box 45, 2280 AA Rijswijk, The Netherlands and **Department of chemistry, Gorlaeus Laboratories, State University Leiden, P.O. Box 9502, 2300 RA Leiden, The Netherlands.

In our laboratories the working mechanism of platinum anti-tumor drugs is studied. These drugs are supposed to be active through their interaction with the DNA in the cell. Methods were developed to identify and quantitate the adducts formed in DNA treated with cis- or trans-diamminedichloroplatinum(II) (DDP). In order to prevent the spectrum of adducts to be altered by the continuation of reactions during purification and detection procedures, first (unreacted and) monofunctionally bound DDP was inactivated by reaction with NH_3, present in aqueous NH_4HCO_3. Secondly, DDP-treated DNA was degraded enzymatically to mononucleotides and Pt-containing (oligo)nucleotides. Then, these products were separated on a DEAE-Sephacel column at pH 7.5 into DNA adducts with monofunctionally- and bifunctionally-bound DDP. The latter category was shown to comprise Pt-containing oligonucleotides derived from interstrand crosslinks, together - when cis-DDP was involved - with products originating from intrastrand crosslinks on the base sequence pGpG and, presumably, on the sequence pGpXpG (X=G, C, A or T). This method offers the possibility to quantitate the various DDP-DNA adducts. Chromatography of the digested cis-DDP-DNA on a Mono Q column (FPLC) at pH 8.8 yielded adducts derived from intrastrand cross-links on the base sequence pGpG as well as on pApG, which were identified by ^{1}H-nmr.

To analyze the DDP-lesions in in vivo treated DNA, the current Pt analysis method (AAS) is too insensitive. To solve this problem, immunochemical techniques were set up. Antibodies, raised against the hapten cis-Pt$(NH_3)_2$GuoGMP by immunization of a rabbit, show almost absolute discrimination between Pt-labeled and free nucleotides and are specific for pG-Pt adducts. The immunochemical methods have an about 1000x lower detection limit for some cis-DDP-DNA adducts than AAS.

Acknowledgement: This investigation was supported by grants from the Koningin Wilhelmina Funds, Amsterdam, The Netherlands, Projects MBL 79-1 and 83-1.

I-10 THE STRUCTURE OF CHELATES, FORMED UPON REACTION OF cis-DI-AMMINEDICHLOROPLATINUM AND OLIGONUCLEOTIDES CONTAINING d(GpCpG) AND d(GpG) UNITS, AS STUDIED BY HIGH FREQUENCY PROTON NMR. Jeroen H.J. den Hartog, Cornelis Altona, Jacques H. van Boom, Antonius T.M. Marcelis and Jan Reedijk, Department of Chemistry, Gorlaeus Laboratories, State University Leiden, P.O.Box 9502, 2300 RA LEIDEN, The Netherlands.

Using high-frequency ^{1}H NMR spectroscopy at varying pH it was shown that in - for instance - d(CpCpGpG).cisPt and d(GpCpG).cisPt the N3 of cytidine can be protonated at low pH (pK_a = 4.5); the N7 of guanine (pK_a = 2.0) cannot be protonated, while the deprotonation of the N1 of guanine occurs among pH 8.5 (normal pK_a = 9.5). These observations clearly demonstrate the occurrence of N7-Pt-N7 chelates in several di-, tri- and tetranucleotides. Reaction products of d(GpG), d(CpGpG), d(CpGpCpG), d(GpCpG), d(CpGpCpG) and d(GpGpGpC) were analyzed in this way. These compounds are considered to be models for intrastrand crosslinks that are likely to occur in DNA.

Conformational analysis of d(GpG).cisPt reveals that the 5'-deoxyribose ring adopts a 100% C3'-endo conformation, while all other backbone bonds do not deviate significantly from normal B-DNA like values. The conformation of this chelate is significantly (but not completely) fixed by platinum binding. In d(GpCpG).cisPt, on the other hand, very much conformational freedom is apparent and no preferred conformation could be detected. However, from chemical shift considerations it is clear that the cytosine residue is largely destacked.

Details of the NMR results and conclusions about binding sites and possible conformations will be presented for several guanine-containing oligonucleotides.

Acknowledgements
The investigators were supported in part by the Netherlands Foundation for Chemical Research (SON) with financial aid from the Netherlands Organization for the Advancement of Pure Research (ZWO). Financial aid was also obtained through grants of the Koningin Wilhelmina Fonds (Dutch organization for fight against cancer), Amsterdam, The Netherlands (grants MBL 79-1; MBL 83-1; MG 79-68).

Reference
Jeroen H.J. den Hartog, Cornelis Altona, Jean-Claude Chottard, Jean Pierre Girault, Jean-Yves Lallemand, Frank A.A.M. de Leeuw, Antonius T.M. Marcelis and Jan Reedijk, Nucl.Acids.Res. 10 (1982), 4715.

I-11 COMPARATIVE ACTIVITY OF PLATINUM II COORDINATION COMPLEXES AND THEIR TRANS-HYDROXY PLATINUM IV ANALOGS AS INDUCERS OF BACTERIOPHAGE LAMBDA. Rosalie K. Elespuru and Sylvia K. Daley. NCI-Frederick Cancer Research Facility, PO Box B, Frederick, MD 21701

Results with Pt II and Pt IV complexes as inducers of bacteriophage lambda indicate that Pt IV compounds may not work as DNA damaging agents via generation of Pt II intermediates, a suggested pathway. Five dichloro, diammine Pt II compounds (diisopropyl, ethylenediamine and three ethylenediamine derivatives: hydroxymethyl, carboxy and N-hydroxyethyl) and their trans-hydroxy Pt IV analogs were tested as inducers of a lambda-lacZ fusion phage. Induction was measured quantitatively by the synthesis of B-galactosidase, product of the lacZ gene, five hrs after treatment with different doses of chemical. Although the inducing capacity of the Pt II compounds varied from strong to weak (based on the magnitude of induction observed), in each case the Pt IV analog induced greater quantities of enzyme than the Pt II compound. This is the reverse of expected results if induction were solely a consequence of Pt II-induced DNA interaction products. No concentration of Pt II compound could be found that would give levels of induction as great as that seen with the trans-hydroxy Pt IV analogs. Control experiments were run to rule out with reasonable certainty the possibility that the differences observed were a result of bacterial permeability or compound stability, solubility or toxicity. Experiments on a bacterial lysogen with a temperature sensitive repressor (λ cI$_{857}$) indicated little difference in enzyme expression during the induction process after treatment with Pt II or Pt IV complexes. Combination experiments with Pt II and Pt IV compounds present together did not provide evidence for additive effects. Rather, the Pt II compound inhibited the inducing capacity of the Pt IV analog.

Another type of experiment provides evidence for the presence of different DNA lesions after treatment with Pt IV as compared to Pt II complexes, that is, experiments on induction of a lysogen with a DNA repair deficiency (Δ uvrB). Dose response curves for induction with the repair-deficient strain shift to the left (toward lower doses), as compared with the wild-type, after treatment with Pt II compounds. This same response is observed after treatment with UV light, 4NQO and some other chemicals. However, in the case of the Pt IV compounds, the dose-response curves shift in the opposite direction, toward higher doses, in the repair deficient strain, as compared to wild-type. These data indicate that the DNA repair system plays an important role in the induction process after treatment with Pt IV but not Pt II complexes.

I-12 THE MODE OF FIXATION OF cis- and trans-DDP ON DNA in vitro. Neil P. Johnson*, Jean-Pierre Macquet and Claude Vieussens. Laboratoire de Pharmacologie et de Toxicologie Fondamentales, CNRS, 205 route de Narbonne, 31400 Toulouse Cedex, France.

The structure of the DNA lesion is often presumed to be responsible for the different biological activities of cis- and trans-Pt(NH$_3$)$_2$Cl$_2$ (DDP) and their different perturbations of DNA secondary structure and stability in vitro. In particular, it has been hypothesized that cis-DDP chelates two adjacent guanine bases whereas the trans isomer, by virtue of its geometry, can not.

In order to examine this hypothesis, platinum-DNA complexes (0.1 platinum per nucleotide) were hydrolysed under depurinating conditions and the resulting Pt-base adducts were characterized. Since hydrolysis cleaves the glycosyl linkage, these experiments provide no information about the positions of the bases on the DNA. The hydrolysis products were characterized by high voltage paper electrophoresis and paper chromatography. The ratio of nucleic acid base per platinum was determined using UV and atomic absorption spectroscopy and the base was identified after removal of platinum from the complex by thiourea.

Results indicate that after in vitro reaction of salmon sperm DNA with either cis- or trans-DDP, the major lesion is a 2:1 Gua:Pt adduct. The electrophoretic and chromatographic behavior of these adducts were compared with model compounds of known structures, (Pt(NH$_3$)$_2$(dGuo)$_2$)Cl$_2$. The principal lesion formed by both cis- and trans-DDP with DNA in vitro appears to be fixation of platinum at the N(7) position of two guanine bases.

I-13 NUCLEOSIDE OXIDATION AND HYDROLYSIS INDUCED BY COORDINATED Ru(III). M.J. Clarke and P. Morrissey Department of Chemistry, Boston College, Chestnut Hill, MA 02167

While it is often assumed that the oncological activity of Pt group transition metal ions is associated with their ability to chelate the heterocyclic bases on DNA, the presence of the metal ion may also enhance the reactivity of these bases. Chromatographic studies of the hydrolysis of Ru-dG (where Ru = $[(NH_3)_5Ru]^{3+}$ and dG = deoxyguanosine) indicated several unexpected products in addition to those derived from predicted reactions involving metal-ion catalyzed cleavage of the deoxyribose (dR) and dissociation of the G and dG ligands.
Two organic products have now been identified by their UV-Vis, IR and PMR spectra, HPLC and pK_a behavior to be 8-hydroxyguanine (GO) [2-amino-6,8-diketo(1H,7H)purine] and 8-hydroxydeoxyguanosine (dGO). These compounds are formed upon dissociation from the corresponding N-7 coordinated complexes of Ru(III), which have also been isolated in chromatographically pure solutions, characterized by their UV-Vis and PMR spectra and HPLC. Ru-dGO is unstable in neutral to mildly basic media but can be prepared in 55% yield in solution at pH 9.4 and isolated as the choride salt. The kinetics of the following reaction scheme have been monitored by HPLC and the various observed rate constants determined as a function of pH.

$$Ru\text{-}dG \underset{k_{14}}{\overset{k_{12}}{\rightleftharpoons}} \begin{array}{l} Ru\text{-}G + dR \xrightarrow{k_{28}} \begin{array}{l} Ru + G \\ Ru + dGO \end{array} \\ k_{13} \quad Ru\text{-}dGO \xrightarrow{k_{36}} \\ Ru + dG \qquad\qquad Ru\text{-}GO + dR \xrightarrow{k_{52}} Ru + GO \end{array}$$

In general, the various observed rate constants increase with increasing pH; however, k_{12} is independent of pH between pH 6-7 and then decreases in the range of the pK_a of Ru-dG (7.6). The metal ion serves as a general acid catalyst for sugar hydrolysis in the range pH 4-7; however, this effect is attenuated as the ligand becomes anionic. The autooxidation of coordinated dG probably involves the deprotonation of the C-8 site, facilitated by the proximity of the Ru^{3+}, followed by a 1e or 2e transfer to oxygen, possibly assisted by electron transfer through the metal ion. The oxidized species should be readily attacked by hydroxide followed by proton loss to yield Ru-dGO. Surprisingly, the loss of dR to yield the stable Ru-GO is base catalyzed. In conclusion: in addition to the mutation resulting from mere metal ion coordination to N-7 dG sites in nucleic acids, at least some metal ions can induce depurination and and autooxidation of dG sites, which may lead to other mutagenic effects.

I-14 ^{195}Pt NMR SPECTROSCOPIC STUDIES OF α-PYRIDONATE BRIDGED PLATINUM(II) COMPLEXES: DYNAMIC STEREOCHEMISTRY. Thomas V. O'Halloran and Stephen J. Lippard, Department of Chemistry, Room 18-207, Massachusetts Institute of Technology, Cambridge, MA 02139

Using ^{195}Pt NMR spectroscopy we have studied some ethylenediamineplatinum(II) dimers bridged by the pyrimidine analog, α-pyridone. These complexes serve as a model for the interaction of platinum antitumor drugs with nucleobases. A reversible isomerization of the bridging amidate ligand from a head-to-head to a head-to-tail linkage takes place. Kinetic studies revealed the stereochemical rearrangement to occur by an intramolecular, dissociative pathway. These results demonstrate that even the relatively inert linkage between platinum(II) and the nitrogen atom of a heterocyclic base can rearrange on a time scale close to that involved in the hydrolysis of cis-DDP ($t_{1/2}$ = 2 hr at 37°C), which is well within the half-life of the drug in the human body.

I-15 A MODEL FOR THE INFLUENCE OF CIS-DIAMMINEDICHLORO-
PLATINUM(II) BINDING ON SV40 DNA AND MINICHROMOSOME.
William M. Scovell, Department of Chemistry, Bowling Green State
University, Bowling Green, Ohio 43403, U.S.A.

The extent to which cis- and trans-$(NH_3)_2PtCl_2$ binding modifies
the structure of DNA is probed by high resolution gel electrophoresis and a battery of nucleases, including single- and multiple-cut
sequence specific restriction endonucleases, single-strand specific
S1 nuclease and less specific nucleases such as micrococcal nuclease
and DNAase I. These data reveal that although both isomers prefer
to bind to (G+C) rich regions in DNA, the modes of binding differ
for the two isomers with the cis-$(NH_3)_2PtCl_2$ modification on DNA
exhibiting a far more recognizable alteration in DNA structure than
that for the trans-$(NH_3)_2PtCl_2$ isomer. Cis-$(NH_3)_2PtCl_2$ binding
exerts a larger unwinding angle on supercoiled DNA than does the
trans-isomer, in addition to stimulating greater S1 nuclease sensitivity on a series of DNAs with different % (G+C) content. The
difference in the capability the two isomers have in producing S1
sensitive regions is most marked in DNAs with large tracts of adjacent guanines on the same strand. The binding of either isomer to
SV40 DNA inhibits site specific cleavage by six restriction endonucleases examined, with the relative inhibition for the series of
single-cut restriction endonucleases paralleling the number and the
relative positions of guanines in and adjacent to the recognition
sequence. These findings suggest that the Bgl 1 site, which is at
or near the origin of replication, and which is within the very
(G+C) rich regulatory region of the SV40 genome, is a hyper-reactive
site to $(NH_3)_2PtCl_2$ binding. A cis-$(NH_3)_2PtCl_2$ modification of the
genome in these regulatory sequences may be expected to directly
impair essential biological processes of Simian virus 40 (SV40) in
infected cells. The experimental findings and the proposal relating
the cis-$(NH_3)_2PtCl_2$ interaction with DNA to both structural and
functional alterations will be discussed in light of new findings on
the SV40 viral system and also chromatin structure.

I-16 CIS-DIAMMINEDICHLOROPLATINUM(II) CROSSLINKS HIGH MOBILITY
GROUP 1 AND 2 PROTEINS TO DNA IN MICROCOCCAL NUCLEASE
ACCESSIBLE REGIONS OF CHROMATIN. William M. Scovell, Nancy
Muirhead and Lee R. Kroos. Department of Chemistry, Bowling Green
State University, Bowling Green, Ohio 43403 U.S.A.

The anti-neoplastic agent, cis-$(NH_3)_2PtCl_2$ (cis-DDP), covalently modifies both DNA and proteins and is found to crosslink
these components in cellular chromatin, although the identity of the
proteins involved has not been determined. The proteins providing
the integrity to chromatin are of two types - the histone proteins
contained in the repeating nucleosome unit, in addition to the nonhistone chromosomal proteins (NHCP) which are non-randomly distri-
buted in the genome and are thought to contribute to both the
structural and functional heterogeneity of chromatin. To gain
further insight into chromatin structure, we reacted cis-DDP with
nuclei and observed a progressive crosslinking of (1) low mobility
group (LMG) proteins and also (2) the high mobility group (HMG) proteins 1,2 and E to DNA in micrococcal nuclease accessible regions of
chromatin. These findings imply that the HMG-1,2 and E proteins
directly interact with or are in very close proximity to DNA
segments which are sensitive to limited micrococcal nuclease
digestion.
These data are of interest on at least two counts. First, they
may reveal a novel mechanism by which cis-DDP inhibits DNA replication and other biological functions. Second, the data provide new
insights into chromatin structure and specifically the location of
the HMG 1 and 2 proteins in chromatin. A proposed model for the
protein-DNA interaction which we are currently evaluating will be
presented and discussed.

I-17 DEGRADATION OF DNA-PLATINUM(II) COMPLEXES BY THE SINGLE STRAND SPECIFIC NUCLEASE S₁. Jean-Luc Butour and Claude E. Vieussens. Laboratoire de Pharmacologie et de Toxicologie Fondamentales du CNRS, 205 route de Narbonne, 31400 TOULOUSE, FRANCE.

Physicochemical studies of the *in vitro* interaction of platinum (II) compounds with DNA indicate that they can be divided in three classes depending on the perturbations of the secondary structure of the macromolecule. The antitumoral compound *cis*-Pt(NH₃)₂Cl₂ and the non-antitumoral stereo isomer *trans*-Pt(NH₃)₂Cl₂ can form with the DNA bases bidentate complexes and also interstrand crosslinks. On the contrary, the monodentate non-antitumoral compound [Pt(dien)Cl]Cl, which cannot form crosslinks, has very little effect on the DNA secondary structure (1).
In order to determine if the covalent binding of platinum(II) compounds to DNA induces the formation of single stranded regions, we have examined the digestion of DNA-Pt complexes by the single strand specific nuclease S₁ of *Aspergillus oryzae*. The extent of digestion of the complexes was determined by the measurement of the acid soluble products liberated as described by Vogt (2).
For the three above Pt(II) compounds, we were not able to detect any acid soluble product for $r_b < 0.025$ (r_b = number of platinum atoms bound per nucleotide). When $r_b > 0.025$ for the *cis*, $r_b > 0.05$ for the *trans* and $r_b > 0.10$ for the dien, single stranded regions were recognized by the S₁ nuclease. The extent of digestion increases non-linearly as a function of r_b which indicates either that the formation of single stranded regions is a cooperative phenomenon requiring several platinum atoms or that different adducts are formed (3).
On the other hand the complete transformation of the DNA-platinum complexes in acido soluble products by the S₁ nuclease has been performed. The elution of these products through polyacrylamide gel indicates different profiles correlated with the nature of the platinum compound. Purification and characterization of these products are under investigation.

REFERENCES

1. MACQUET, J.P. and BUTOUR, J.L. Biochimie, 1978, 60, 901-914.

2. VOGT, V.M. in Methods in Enzymology (Grossman, L., ed.) 1980, Vol. 65, pp 248-255.

3. JOHNSON, N.P. Biochem. Biophys. Res. Commun. 1982, 104, 1394-1400.

I-18 INHIBITION OF DNA SYNTHESIS BY *CIS*-Pt(NH₃)₂Cl₂, *TRANS*-Pt(NH₃)₂Cl₂ AND [Pt(dien)Cl]Cl IN CULTURED L1210 LEUKEMIA CELLS. B. Salles, J.L. Butour, C. Lesca and J.P. Macquet. Laboratoire de Pharmacologie et de Toxicologie Fondamentales du CNRS, 205 route de Narbonne, 31400 Toulouse, France.

The inhibition of DNA synthesis by the antitumor compound *cis*-Pt(NH₃)₂Cl₂ in different experimental models is well established. However, no studies have clearly demonstrated the effect of the non-antitumor isomer *trans*-Pt(NH₃)₂Cl₂ on the inhibition of DNA synthesis in tumoral cells. This comparison is of great importance for a better understanding of the mechanism of action of the antitumor platinum compounds. We report in this study a comparison of the inhibition of DNA synthesis for the two geometrical bidentate isomers and for the monodentate [Pt(dien)Cl]Cl in a model used for screening potential antitumor compounds, the L1210 leukemia cells.
After a 2-hour exposure of the Pt drug with the cells, a linear relationship between the covalently bound platinum species (measured by atomic absorption spectrophotometry) in whole cells and the dose was obtained for the three compounds until a concentration of 0.5 mM. The efficacy of penetration is in the order $trans(8) > cis(1) \simeq dien(0.7)$, the corresponding r_b (number of Pt atoms bound per nucleotide) values being 20×10^{-4} for *trans*, 4.5×10^{-4} for *cis* and 4×10^{-4} for the dien derivative. Incorporation of ³H-methyl-thymidine was studied for 1.5 hours in exponentially growing L1210 cells which were previously treated for 2 hours with the Pt compounds at different concentrations and then centrifuged. In the case of *cis*-Pt(NH₃)₂Cl₂, the DNA replication is reduced to 50% of that of the control for $r_r = 1.8 \times 10^{-4}$, $r_r = 3.6 \times 10^{-4}$ for *trans*-Pt(NH₃)₂Cl₂ and $r_r = 95 \times 10^{-4}$ for [Pt(dien)Cl]Cl.
These results indicate that the *cis*- and *trans*-isomers inhibit DNA synthesis of L1210 cells with an efficacy two times better for the *cis*-isomer per Pt bound on DNA. If we admit that DNA is the pharmacological target of Pt antitumor compounds, these results suggest that inhibition of DNA synthesis is certainly not correlated with antitumor activity.

I-19 EXAFS STUDIES OF PT-BASE MODEL COMPOUNDS AND $[(NH_3)_2Pt(OH)_2$ $Pt(NH_3)_2]^{2+}$ BOUND TO DNA. Adam P. Hitchcock, M.L. Martins and C.J.L. Lock, Institute for Materials Research, McMaster University, Hamilton, Ontario, Canada, L8S 4M1.

$[(NH_3)_2Pt(OH)_2Pt(NH_3)_2]^{2+}$ (I) is produced from cis-Pt$(NH_3)_2Cl_2$ (II) (but not $trans$) in aqueous solution and is thus possibly involved in the anti-tumor activity of cis-platin. Our preliminary EXAFS studies [1] of the Pt environment of the complex of I with calf thymus DNA (1Pt:10bases) suggested that the dimer bound intact with a Pt-Pt distance slightly shorter than in I. Further, and definitive, EXAFS studies on both 1:10 and 1:20 complexes have failed to reproduce the initially observed Pt-Pt vector. We now conclude that the Pt hydroxy dimer (I) must dissociate during formation of the complex so that the distance between Pt atoms in the complex is not detectable by EXAFS. This indicates that although I may be present in cells and may react with DNA, the specific dimeric structure of I is not retained in the complex and is unlikely to be a critical factor in determining the bonding mode.

The average nearest neighbour distance in the complex of I and DNA will be compared to that of the complex of II with DNA, and to Pt-base compounds to suggest plausible bonding models. In addition the limits of detectability of Pt-Pt distances by EXAFS will be demonstrated by comparison of the Pt L_3 spectra of cis[(NH_3)_2Pt-(1-MeU)]_2(NO_3)_2 \cdot H_2O$, cis[(NH_3)_2(1-MeU)Pt(OH)Pt(1 MeU)Cl_2] \cdot ClO_4 \cdot H_2O$ and cis and $trans$ Pt$(NH_3)_2Cl_2$.

1. A.P. Hitchcock, C.J.L. Lock and W.M.C. Pratt, Inorg. Chim. Acta **66** (1982) L45.

This research is supported by NSERC (Canada) and the National Cancer Institute of Canada. The EXAFS spectra were obtained with the Cornell synchrotron light source, CHESS, a U.S. national facility supported by the N.S.F.

I-20 DNA REPAIR CHARACTERISTICS OF WALKER RAT CARCINOMA CELLS SENSITIVE AND RESISTANT TO CIS-DIAMMINEDICHLOROPLATINUM II (CISPLATIN). John J. Roberts, Christopher J. Rawlings and Frank Friedlos. Pollards Wood Research Station, Institute of Cancer Research, Nightingales Lane, Chalfont St. Giles, Buckinghamshire, England.

Studies on cultured cells have indicated the likely relevance of platinum DNA binding to cytotoxicity following their treatment with cisplatin. Moreover some, but not all observations suggest that the specific lesion associated with cytotoxicity could be the formation of an interstrand crosslink between opposing strands of DNA molecules. In order further to understand the possible importance of specific types of DNA damage in inducing toxic effects in cells, and also the basis of resistance to cisplatin, we have compared the formation and loss of total DNA bound adducts, DNA interstrand crosslinks and DNA protein crosslinks in two lines of Walker rat carcinoma cells sensitive and resistant to cisplatin and to other difunctional, but not monofunctional cytotoxic agents. Cisplatin binds to cellular macromolecules (DNA, RNA and protein) in a dose dependent manner and to the same extent in both cell lines. We noted from these binding studies that the Walker sensitive cells exhibit a unique sensitivity to DNA bound cisplatin while the so-called resistant cells have a sensitivity that approximates to that of many normal and other tumour cell lines. Total DNA bound adducts were lost from Walker sensitive and resistant cells at comparable rates. DNA interstrand crosslinks and DNA protein crosslinks were also formed in a dose dependent manner to an equal extent in both cell lines. Both types of crosslinks were also lost from the two lines of Walker cells at essentially similar rates. The small differences in manifestations of DNA excision repair as between sensitive and resistant Walker cells are therefore inadequate to account for the vast difference in their sensitivity to cisplatin. Other studies suggest that the two cell lines also do not differ in their ability to replicate DNA on a template containing damage induced by a difunctional alkylating agent, i.e. DNA daughter-strand gap (post replication) repair. Hence cytotoxicity induced towards sensitive and resistant Walker cells is not related to effects on DNA synthesis (i.e. sensitive cells can be killed by doses of agents that induce no, or only minimal effects on DNA replication). We can conclude that the unique response of sensitive cells to difunctional agents could be associated, either with the formation in sensitive but not resistant cells of certain types of crosslinks in those regions of chromatin that are associated with the regulation of cell division, or, if they are formed equally in both cell types, with their deficient repair in the sensitive cells.

63

I-21   CIS-PLATINUM MEDIATED CROSSLINKING TO DNA OF CHROMOSOMAL
NONHISTONE PROTEINS IN HeLa CELLS.   Zainy M. Banjar*,
Robert C. Briggs*, Lubomir S. Hnilica*, Janet L. Stein and Gary S.
Stein. *Department of Biochemistry, Vanderbilt University School of
Medicine, Nashville, TN 37232 U.S.A., and Department of Biochemistry
and Molecular Biology, University of Florida, Gainesville, FL 32610
U.S.A.

Immunization with dehistonized chromatin or isolated chromosomal
protein fractions elicits antisera which recognize not only the
individual antigens but also complexes of chromosomal proteins with
DNA. Based on complement fixation assays, we have found that various
crosslinking agents stabilized the antigenic nonhistone protein-DNA
complexes and rendered them non-dissociable in concentrated NaCl-urea
solutions. Using such antisera, we have investigated the crosslinking of chromosomal nonhistone proteins to DNA in isolated nuclei
or intact HeLa cells exposed to various concentrations of cis- or
trans-diaminedichloroplatinum (cis- or trans-PT). After incubation,
whole cells or isolated nuclei were dissolved in 2% buffered sodium
dodecyl sulfate (50 mM Tris-HCl, pH 8.0) and centrifuged at
110,000 x g for 24 hrs. The DNA pellets were rinsed with the SDS-Tris
buffer, dispersed in DNase I buffer, sonicated briefly and dialyzed
overnight against DNase I buffer. After digesting DNA with DNase I,
the released proteins were concentrated, electrophoresed and transferred to nitrocellulose sheets for immunochemical detection. Antisera to 0.35 M NaCl extracts and to the residual material of HeLa cell
nuclei were employed and the antigen-antibody complexes were
visualized by staining with peroxidase-antiperoxidase-diamino-
benzidine reagent. Both the cis- and trans-PT crosslinked significant numbers of chromosomal proteins to the DNA (as evidenced by
comparing similarly processed DNA pellets from untreated controls).
Cis-PT was found to be more efficient nonhistone protein-DNA
crosslinker than the trans-PT. There was little difference between
the protein patterns crosslinked by incubation in intact cells or
isolated nuclei, indicating that the isolation of nuclei did not
change significantly the relationships between chromosomal proteins
and DNA. Control experiments in which isolated nuclei were
crosslinked by gamma radiation or incubation with 1,3-bis(chloro-
ethyl)-1-nitrosourea (BCNU) showed similar but not identical crosslinking patterns. These crosslinking agents were less efficient,
however. We conclude that the cis-PT is a very efficient nonhistone
protein-DNA crosslinking agent and that some of its biological
effects on tumor cells may be the consequence of this phenomenon.

Supported by NIEHS Grant ES 00267.

I-22   NMR AND CRYSTALLOGRAPHIC STUDIES ON A SECOND GENERATION
CISPLATIN ANALOGUE.   James C. Dabrowiak, Department of
Chemistry, Syracuse University, Syracuse, New York 13210; M. S.
Balakrishnan, Bristol-Myers Laboratories, Syracuse, N.Y. 13201;
Jon Clardy, Gregory D. Van Duyne, and Linda Silviera, Department of
Chemistry, Cornell University, Ithaca, New York 14853.

The platinum complex, 1,1-diaminomethylcyclohexane (L) sulfato
platinum(II), $\underline{1}$, is a second generation Cisplatin analogue which is
currently in clinical trials in Europe. Dissolution of $\underline{1}$ in water
results in a lowering of the pH of the medium and the formation of
two platinum containing species. ^{1}H (360 MHz) and ^{195}Pt (77.252
MHz) NMR spectroscopic studies of $\underline{1}$ and of the related complex
Pt(II)(L)(NO₃)₂, $\underline{2}$, suggest that the species present in D₂O solution
at pD~3 are the complexes, Pt(II)(L)(H₂O)(SOₓ), $\underline{3}$, and
[Pt(II)(L)(H₂O)₂]$^{+2}$, $\underline{4}$. The ^{195}Pt NMR parameters (δ, relative to
K₂PtCℓ₆) for $\underline{3}$ and $\underline{4}$ are δ, 1835 ppm (Δν½, 820 Hz) and δ, 1860 ppm
(Δν½, 830 Hz) respectively. Raising the pD of the solution contain-
ing $\underline{3}$ and $\underline{4}$ to physiological values results in the formation of the
υ hydroxo-bridged dimer [Pt(II)(L)(OH)]₂$^{+2}$, $\underline{5}$, (δ, ppm,
Δν½ 400 Hz) and the cyclohydroxo-bridged trimer, [Pt(II)(L)(OH)]₃$^{+3}$,
$\underline{6}$, (δ, 1760 ppm, Δν½ 400 Hz). X-Ray crystallographic analysis of
$\underline{6}$ (NO₃)₃ confirmed the trimeric nature of the complex. Dissolution
of the isolated trimer in D₂O at pD~7 results in its slow partial
conversion to $\underline{5}$. At equilibrium the 5:6 ratio is 3:7. Allowing
guanosine to react with excess $\underline{5}$ and $\underline{6}$ in D₂O solution (pD~7)
for 2 days results in the formation of at least three species which
appear to contain platinum bound to the heterocyclic residue of
the nucleoside. The ^{1}H NMR chemical shift values for the H-8
proton of the new guanosine species are, 8:188, 8:290, and
8.343 ppm.

Section II

Pharmacology and Pharmacodynamics of Platinum Coordination Complexes in Cancer Chemotherapy

Chaired by C.L. Litterst

Overview
C.L. Litterst

Three areas of interest dominated the poster topics and discussion in the pharmacokinetics session. The first topic of interest was the pharmacokinetics of DDP analogs, particularly CBDCA and CHIP. CBDCA was studied in 4 animal species in addition to patients, and the correlation among the 5 species was quantitatively good and showed some major differences from DDP. For example, in dog, mouse and rabbit 90-100% of the administered dose was excreted in urine, whereas the urinary excretion of DDP is 50-70% for most species. CBDCA also differed from DDP in the kinetics of filterable platinum. There was no decrease in filterable platinum when CBDCA was incubated in vitro for 8 hours with plasma. During the first several hours after CBDCA administration to animals, filterable platinum and total platinum concentrations were equal and then filterable platinum declined at a greater rate than did total platinum. Filterable platinum was detectable for 4-6 hours after CBDCA administration, in contrast to 1-2 hours after DDP administration. In patients, urinary excretion of platinum after CBDCA was apparently 3 times greater than with DDP, and plasma filterable platinum levels were much more prolonged than with DDP. Protein binding of CBDCA in patients was quite variable, however, with a range of 0-60% bound 2 hours after treatment in 7 patients. In rats the amount of filterable platinum after CBDCA treatment was 80% of control values at the earliest time examined and remained at that level for several hours. This suggests the possibility of a saturable binding site in rat plasma proteins, which might become more obvious if lower doses were studied. Another alternative is that the treatment solution contained a contaminant that was avidly bound to plasma proteins. Plasma half times of total platinum after CBDCA were routinely greater for both elimination and distribution phases than were half times after DDP, but the prolonged final elimination phase appeared to be lacking. Plasma decay curves of total and filterable platinum in patients were complex, with unexplained secondary peaks occurring within the first hour after infusion.

Similar peaks have been observed following DDP, however (1). As might be expected, half times were variable from species to species and from one study to another, depending on the time that the determination was made. This reinforced the need for investigators to always identify the times over which distribution and elimination half times were determined when such calculations are presented. In general, platinum from CBDCA decayed in a bi- or tri-exponential manner in all species, including humans. Estimates of biliary excretion of CBDCA ranged from 0.5% to 14% of the dose in two different studies. Discrepant platinum uptake into RBC also was reported, ranging from essentially no uptake to relating mechanism of CBDCA-induced death to RBC binding by CBDCA. Of particular interest was the retention of platinum in kidneys of CBDCA-treated animals 4 and 6 days after treatment in two different studies. This result was in spite of the lack of CBDCA-induced renal toxicity, and thus forces us to wonder about the wisdom of our assumption that renal toxicity of DDP was related to platinum binding in the kidney.

CHIP, the platinum-IV analog, was studied in rats and dogs as well as in patients. Again, plasma half times were greater than those for DDP but without the very prolonged elimination phase observed with DDP. A striking finding was very high platinum levels in brain, which were exceeded by only two other of twelve tissues studied throughout the entire time course (0.25-13 days post-treatment). This might suggest the use of this analog in brain tumor therapy, where DDP has recently shown some promise. CHIP was the only of 4 analogs to bind to dog RBC's. The pharmacokinetics of other analogs (TNO-6 and JM-40) also were presented. TNO-6 had the lowest urinary excretion (32%) and highest tissue platinum retention of 4 analogs 6 weeks after dosing. One interesting poster suggested that although the final products of all platinum-nucleic acid interactions were the same, the different plasma half times and tissue distributions were the result of different reaction kinetics.

There were several excellent posters presented on how platinum pharmacokinetics were altered (or not altered) by various experimental variables, such as repeated dosing, whole body hyperthermia (WBH), renal failure, etc. Even though DDP is usually given on a daily x 5 schedule, the effect of multiple treatments on platinum excretion and toxicity has only recently been investigated in animals (2) and similar results were reported in an elegant study in patients that showed the excretion of platinum was decreased in multiple-treatment regimens. This correlated with higher plasma retention of platinum and a change in the plasma pharmacokinetic curve, perhaps due to accumulation of bound platinum species. Although platinum has been identified in brain and in brain tumors (3,4) after DDP administration, only now have pharmacokinetics of platinum in cerebral spinal fluid (CSF) been investigated. When an iv bolus of DDP was given to patients, platinum in CSF had a monoexponential decay with a half time of 43-51 minutes and maximum CSF concentrations were reached 15-30 minutes after dosing. When DDP was given ip to patients with ascites, elimination of platinum from ascites fluid was biexponential, with half times of 0.3 and 3 hours. Plasma concentrations were only 2.5% of the maximum ascites fluid concentration. These results encourage the use of DDP for intraabdominal cancers (5), with the expectation of relatively little systemic toxicity. DDP pharmacokinetics were found to be unaltered by WBH, but nephrotoxicity was potentiated, probably due to the stress of heating. CBDCA, however, when administered to patients with poor renal function produced a significantly higher area under the concentration-time curve than was observed in patients with normal renal function, thus demonstrating a slower rate of excretion in these patients. These results suggest the need for continued attention to the interaction between nephrotoxicity and compromised renal function, even in patients receiving CBDCA, which is not particularly nephrotoxic. In the same context, several speakers related poor success following the use of nephrotoxic aminoglycoside antibiotics as first-line therapy in cases of sepsis. Additional caution should be exercised in the use of these drugs in the presence of platinum-containing agents unless specifically indicated by the bacterial agents involved.

Finally, much interest was evidenced in the analytical determination of parent cisplatin as distinct from the determination of total or filterable platinum. Techniques discussed included neutron activation analysis (NAA), pulse polarography, various HPLC modifications, and fluorescence. Each method has specific advantages, but frequently the associated disadvantages outweigh the advantages. For example, the use of NAA is more sensitive than any technique except radioisotopes, but the long and complex sample handling might preclude this method for large numbers of routine samples or for work where rapid turn-around time was necessary. HPLC offers good separation but some means must be utilized to detect platinum quantitatively in isolated peaks. The post column reactor is rapid but presented no proof of chemical identity of the separated species, which is a common short-coming of much of the HPLC work, and work involving derivitization. For those laboratories with no access to sophisticated separation or identification equipment, Sternson concluded during his oral presentation that filterable platinum results closely enough paralleled cisplatinum results that the extra effort to separate cisplatinum was questionable, and thus filterable platinum analysis should suffice as a good approximation of cisplatinum levels. Related to the analytical determination of platinum-containing species is the need for additional care to be exercised in the choice of words when presenting kinetics or distributional data following the use of DDP. Investigators should take care to clearly distinguish between, for example, total platinum and cisplatinum distribution following DDP administration.

REFERENCES

1. Gullo JJ, Litterst CL, Maguire PJ, Sikic BI, Hoth D, Wooley PV. 1980. Cancer Chemother. Pharmacol. 5:21.
2. Litterst CL, Schweitzer VG. 1983. Cancer Chemother. Pharmacol. In Press.
3. Stewart DJ, Leavens M, Maor M, Feun L, Luna M, Bonura J, Caprioli R, Loo TL, Benjamin RS. 1982. Cancer Res. 42:2474.
4. Bonnem EM, Litterst CL, Smith FP. 1982. Cancer Treat. Reports. 66:1661.
5. Speyer JL, Myers CE. 1980. Recent Results in Cancer Research 74:264.

Plasma Pharmacokinetics, Urinary Excretion, and Tissue Distribution of Platinum Following IV Administration of Cyclobutanedicarboxylatoplatinum-II and *cis*-Platinum to Rabbits.
C.L. Litterst

1. INTRODUCTION

Cisdiamminedichloroplatinum (Cisplatin) is an effective agent in the treatment of several human cancers (3). Its clinical effectiveness is limited, however, by dose limiting toxicities such as renal failure, nausea and vomiting, and hearing loss (8,10). Ever since the clinical introduction of cisplatin in the early 1970's efforts have been underway to discover or develop additional platinum complexes that would have a greater therapeutic index, i.e. either greater antitumor activity with the same degree of toxicity, or less toxicity so that greater doses could be administered. It has been only recently that large scale clinical trials of several of the most promising analogs have been undertaken. Cyclobutanedicarboxylatoplatinum (II) (CBDCA; JM-8; NSC 241240) is one of the second generation analogs of cisplatin that is currently undergoing large scale clinical trials (1). In these early clinical studies, evaluation of the pharmacokinetics and renal excretion of this analog have been conducted but similar data have not yet appeared for animals. We have evaluted plasma decay, urinary and biliary excretion, and organ distribution of CBDCA at various times after a single IV administration of 2 different doses to rabbits and compared the behavior of CBDCA to cisplatin.

2. METHODS

CBDCA was adminstered iv to male New Zealand rabbits (2-3 kg) at either 2.5 or 12.5 mg/kg (3 mg/ml in 0.9% NaCl). Cisplatin was administered at 2.0 mg/kg (1 mg/ml in 0.9% NaCl). Arterial blood was drawn through a preimplanted polyethylene cannula at various times beginning 2 minutes after drug administration. Animals were placed into stainless steel metabolic cages to faciliate urine collection. At 1,4,24,96 hours after treatment, replicate animals (n=3) were killed by pentobarbital overdose and various organs and tissues removed for analysis. Filterable plasma platinum was determined using CF-50 filtration cones (Amicon Corp. Danvers, MA). Tissues were digested in nitric acid prior to analysis. Plasma, plasma ultrafiltrate, bile, urine, and tissue digests were analyzed for platinum content by flameless atomic absorption spectroscopy. BUN was determined at daily intervals after drug treatment. Plasma pharmacokinetics of total and filterable platinum were analyzed using an iteritive least squares computer program (5). Pharmacokinetic parameters were derived for each individual rabbit and mean values then calculated. Data are expressed as mean $\pm$ SD.

RESULTS

When a standard solution of CBDCA prepared in 0.9% NaCl was filtered through filtration cones, 98.5% $\pm$ 1.0% of the platinum was filtered, indicating that there was no binding or absorption of CBDCA by the filters. When CBDCA was incubated (37°) in vitro (6 ug/ml) with either dog or rabbit plasma, no change in plasma filterable platinum concentration was noted during an 8 hour incubation period (Figure 1). Cisplatin under similar incubation conditions (5 µg/ml) gave a continually decreasing amount of filterable platinum (Figure 1). This suggested that CBDCA does not undergo the same plasma protein binding observed with cisplatin. Representative plasma decay curves of total platinum and filterable platinum following adminstration of CBDCA at 2.5 and 12.5 mg/kg are shown in Figures 2 and 3, respectively. It can be observed that during the first 4 hours after treatment (Figure 2), total platinum followed a standard two compartment distribution and elimination. Disappearance of filterable platinum also appeared 2-compartmental. When plasma total and filterable platinum were examined from rabbits treated at 12.5 mg/kg, a third elimination phase became evident for total platinum, even though filterable platinum still disappeared in a biphasic manner. This high dose was necessary because by 24 hours after dosing with 2.5 mg/kg only trace concentrations of platinum were present in plasma, and filterable platinum was usually near the limits of detection of the assay by 4 hours after adminstration. No platinum was ever detected in plasma 4 days after dosing with CBDCA even at 12.5 mg/kg.

Figure 4 and 5 show comparable data for cisplatin. Plasma decay of total and filterable platinum was similar to that observed with other species (5), with half times that were less than those observed with CBDCA. Half-times for the distribution and elimination phases of total and filterable

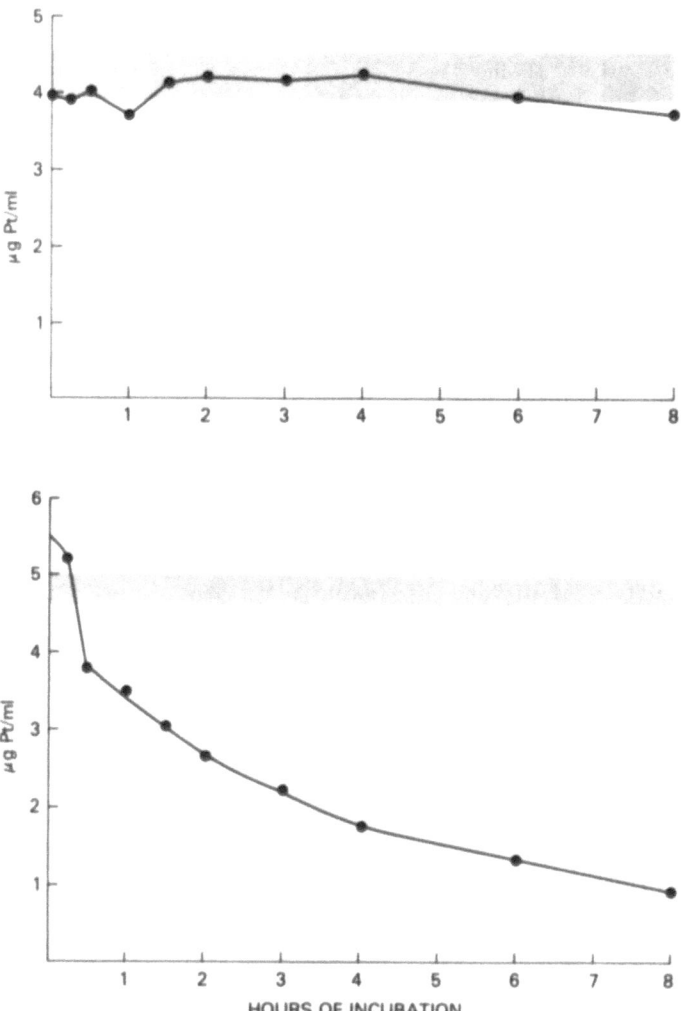

Figure 1. Filterable platinum from in vitro incubations of rabbit plasma with CBDCA (Top) or cisplatin (Bottom). Shaded area is the range of concentrations of total platinum in the incubates.

platinum following administration of CBDCA and cisplatin are shown in Table 1. The distribution half-times for the 2 doses of CBDCA were not significantly different (Student's t test, $P \leq 0.05$).

Table 1.   Half-time of total and filterable platinum after IV administration of CBDCA or cisplatin.

Drug	Dose	Platinum	Half-times (minutes)		
			A	B	C
CBDCA	2.5	Total	$13.3 \pm 4.1^*$	$69.3 \pm 15.7^*$	- - -
	12.5	Total	$18.3 \pm 2.9^+$	$62.5 \pm 2.5^+$	$888 \pm 118^{++}$
	2.5	Filterable	$5.1 \pm 0.5^*$	$28.2 \pm 7.7^*$	- - -
	12.5	Filterable	$8.9 \pm 2.6^+$	$29.9 \pm 2.8^+$	- - -
Cisplatin	2.0	Total	$4.5 \pm 2.2^{\ddagger}$	$46.7 \pm 24.2^+$	$2990 \pm 852^+$
	2.0	Filterable	10.6 ± 1.8	- - -	- - -

*, n=9; +, n=4; ‡, n=8; ++, n=2

Urinary excretion of platinum following administration of CBDCA was complete by 4 hours after treatment (Table 2) and 71% was excreted during the first hour after dosing. Total platinum excretion following cisplatin administration was much less complete and was similar to that observed in other species (2,6,9) with 57% excreted by 4 hours and 68% by 4 days (Table 3). Half of the total recovered platinum was excreted in the first hour. Table 2 shows distribution of total platinum in body tissues at various times after administration of CBDCA. Kidney had 3-5 times higher concentrations of platinum than any other tissues 1 hour after treatment. Concentrations of platinum in skin were next highest, followed closely by most other tissues. Concentrations in fat were quite variable and may have reflected incomplete or ineffective digestion.   By 4 hours after treatment, concentration of platinum in all tissues had declined and by 24 hours after dosing only liver and kidney had consistently detectable levels of platinum still remaining. Four days after treatment liver and kidney were the only tissues to contain any detectable platinum. It is of interest that liver platinum concentrations were unchanged between 4 hours and 4 days and kidney platinum concentrations were unchanged between 1 and 4 days.

CBDCA 2.5mg/kg RABBIT 11

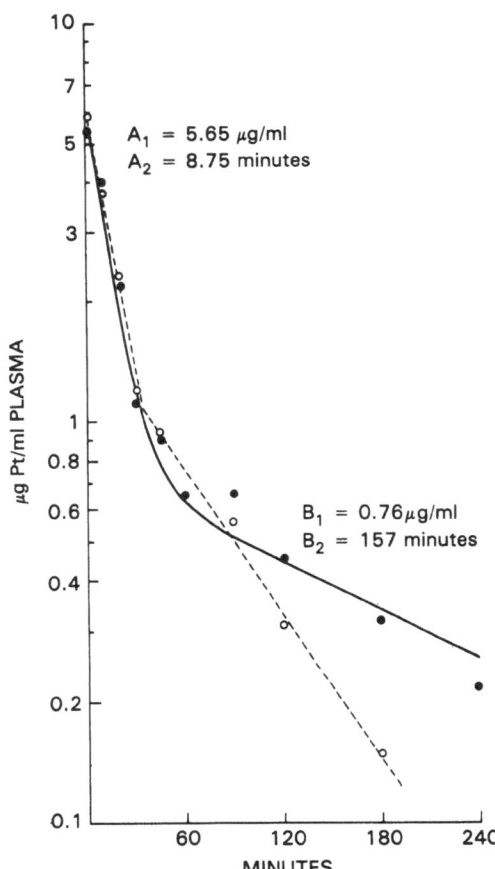

Figure 2. Plasma level of total (●——●) and filterable platinum
(O---O) after IV administration of CBDCA (2.5 mg/kg). Lines are computer-
generated fits to the experimental data points shown.

Table 2. Distribution of total platinum after IV administration of CBDCA (2.5 mg/kg). Data are µg Pt/g; X ± SD (n=3). Data in parentheses are from single animals dosed at 12.5 mg/kg.

	1 hr	4 hr	1 da	4 da
PLASMA	0.66 ± 0.19 (5.00)	0.17 ± 0.05 (0.79)	0.13 ± 0.02 (0.33)	(0) (0)
KIDNEY	2.24 ± 0.21 (22.8)	⌃ 1.32 ± 0.11 (6.65)	0.77 ± 0.14 (4.02)	0.61 ± 0.15 (1.49)
LIVER	0.60 ± 0.07 (5.34)	0.30 ± 0.10 (1.88)	0.29 ± 0.04 (0.91)	0.33 ± 0.06 (0.60)
LUNG	0.49 ± 0.07 (3.53)	0.27 ± 0.12 (1.13)	0.14 ± 0.20 (0.53)	0 (0)
COLON	0.49 ± 0.16 (1.95)	0.20 ± 0.04 (0.70)	0.11 ± 0.16 (0.51)	0 (0)
DUODENUM	0.55 ± 0.10 (2.07)	0.15 ± 0.05 (1.10)	0.10 ± 0.14 (0.53)	0 (0)
SPLEEN	0.47 ± 0.06 (2.32)	0.13 ± 0.03 (1.31)	0.14 ± 0.19 (0.56)	0 (0)
HEART	0.38 ± 0.14 (2.19)	0.21 ± 0.09 (0.53)	0.10 ± 0.14 (0.29)	0 (0)
TESTES	0.61 ± 0.02 (1.98)	0.22 ± 0.06 (0.39)	0.10 ± 0.12 (0.41)	0 (0)
SKIN	0.80 ± 0.04 (4.91)	0.30 ± 0.12 (1.97)	0.10 ± 0.14 (1.06)	0 (0)
MUSCLE	0.22 ± 0.12 (0.44)	0.15 ± 0.07 (0)	0 (0)	0 (0)
FAT	0.14 ± 0.12 (0.35)	0 (0)	0 (0)	0 (0)
BILE	0.64 ± 0.21 (2.74)	1.84 ± 0.51 (1.69)	1.53 ± 0.66 (9.09)	0.22 ± 0.05 (ND)
URINE (% dose)	71% ± 6% (67%)	105% ± 3% (99%)	101% ± 1% (89%)	102% ± 5% (102%)

Concentrations of platinum were detected in bile at all times after treatment, with highest concentrations 4 hours after treatment. This probably reflects the sustained levels of platinum in liver. Because of the high concentrations of platinum recovered very early in urine, fecal excretion probably is not of significance in the rabbit. The sustained biliary levels may reflect a small component of enterohepatic recirculation, as has been shown for cisplatin (2).

Concentration of total platinum in tissues following administration of cisplatin to rabbits is shown in Table 3. This distribution of platinum is similar to that observed in other species that have been studied (5), with highest and quite sustained platinum concentration in kidney and liver and sustained, but lower levels in liver, spleen, and skin.

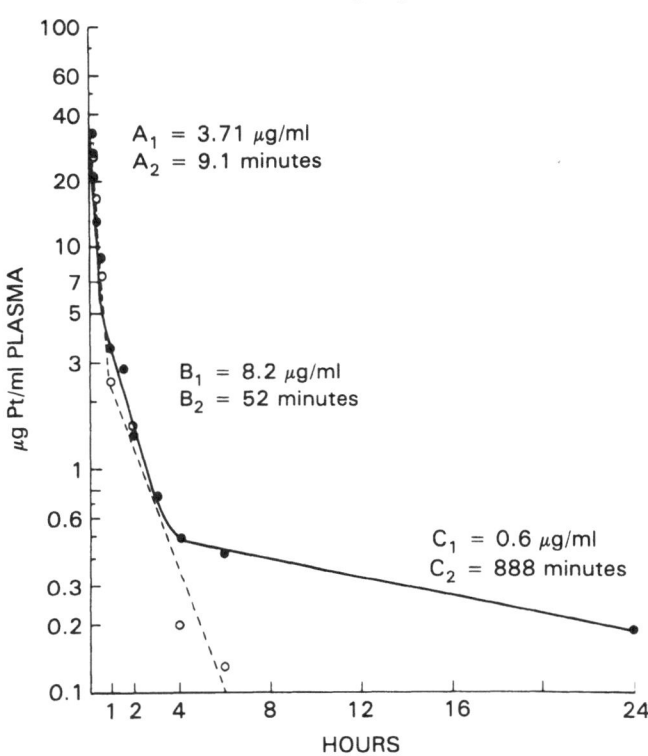

Figure 3. Plasma levels of total (●———●) and filterable (0---0) platinum after IV administration of CBDCA (12.5 mg/kg).

No elevations in BUN or signs of toxicity were detected at any time throughout the 4 days after treatment with either CBDCA or cisplatin.

Table 3. Distribution of total platinum after IV administration of cisplatin (2.0 mg/kg). Data are µg Pt/g; X ± SD (n=3).

	1 hr	4 hr	1 da	4 da
PLASMA	0.79 + 0.08	0.62 + 0.04	0.31 + 0.04	0.24 + 0.04
KIDNEY	3.30 + 0.53	2.66 + 0.17	3.27 + 0.13	2.49 + 0.28
LIVER	1.56 + 0.05	1.59 + 0.01	1.35 + 0.04	1.38 + 0.31
LUNG	1.01 + 0.02	0.60 + 0.04	0.61 + 0.03	0.45 + 0.03
COLON	0.88 + 0.01	0.70 + 0.03	0.65 + 0.12	0.52 + 0.06
DUODENUM	1.05 + 0.34	0.65 + 0.13	0.68 + 0.09	0.44 + 0.05
SPLEEN	0.83 + 0.12	0.90 + 0.13	0.90 + 0.29	0.62 + 0.09
HEART	0.55 + 0.11	0.45 + 0.04	0.60 + 0.01	0.34 + 0.02
TESTES	0.62 + 0.07	0.83 + 0.22	0.54 + 0.12	0.32 + 0.03
SKIN	1.22 + 0.12	1.19 + 0.10	1.15 + 0.08	0.77 + 0.14
MUSCLE	0.43 + 0.13	0.30 + 0.01	0.39 + 0.11	0
FAT	0.10 + 0.09	0.40 + 0.40	0	0
BILE	1.73 + 0.11	4.88 + 1.22	5.37 + 3.16	0.78 + 0.32
URINE (% dose)	32% + 6%	57% + 2%	64% + 4%	68% + 5%

3. DISCUSSION

The plasma pharmacokinetics and urinary excretion of total platinum following CBDCA administration are totally different than observed with cisplatin, with total urinary recovery by 4 hours after treatment, and nearly non-detectable plasma platinum levels by 24 hours. Urinary excretion data are consistent with data from patients, which show the kidney to be the major route of excretion (60% of the dose excreted in 24 hours) (1).

The in vitro incubation of CBDCA with plasma shows no spontaneous binding of CBDCA to plasma proteins, although the in vivo filterable platinum levels

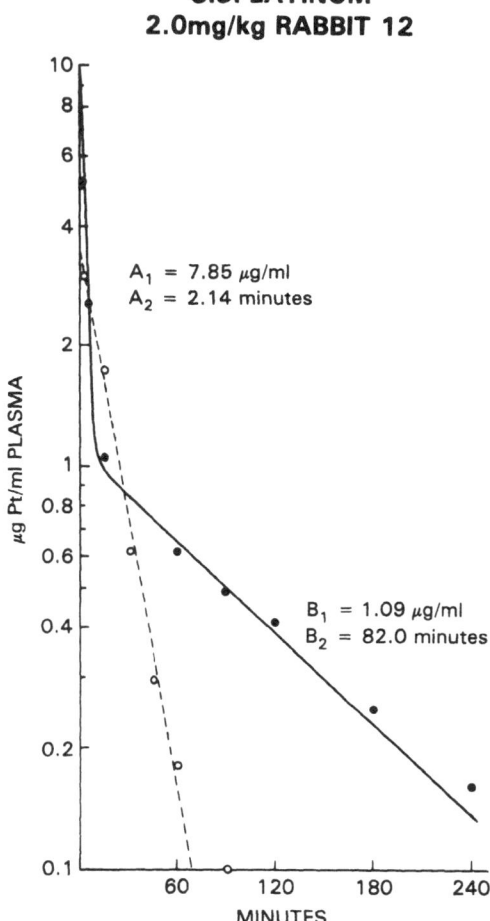

Figure 4. Plasma levels of total (●——●) and filterable (O---O) platinum after IV administration of cisplatin (2 mg/kg).

suggest that there may be some metabolic change during the first several hours after administration that results in appearance of a nonfilterable fraction. The nature of this metabolic alteration remains to be elucidated. Furthermore, although most tissues have no residual platinum by 24 hours after CBDCA administration, the sustained concentrations of platinum in kidney and liver suggest covalent binding of platinum in these tissues. The high standard deviation in Day 1 tissues and plasma reflects measurable concentrations in one animal but no measurable levels in the other two animals.

In summary CBDCA is much more completely cleared from the rabbit than is cisplatin, with a small percentage of possibly enzyme-mediated metabolism that results in binding of platinum to liver and kidney receptors resulting in sustained tissues levels throughout 4 days after administration. Filterable platinum following CBDCA administration closely paralleled total platinum levels during the first hour after treatment, but only small amounts of filterable platinum were present by 4 hours after treatment. It might be expected that CBDCA could be administered in multiple dose regimen with less cumulative toxicity than is observed with cisplatinum, but that typical treatment regimens utilized with cisplatinum such as hydration and diuresis would be unnecessary with CBDCA due to the very high urinary excretion, at least in the rabibit.

REFERENCES

1. Calvert, AH, SJ Harland, DR Newell, ZH Siddik, AC Jones, TJ McElwain, S Raju, E Wiltshaw, IE Smith, JM Baker, MJ Peckham & KR Harrap. Cancer Chemother. Pharmacol. 9: 140 (1982).
2. DeSimone, PA, RS Yancey, JJ Coupal, JD Butts, JD Hoeschele. Cancer Treat. Reports. 63: 951 (1979).
3. Durant, JR. In: Cisplatin, Current Status and New Developments (AW Prestayko , ST Crooke & SK Carter, Eds.) p.317 (1980).
4. Hoeschele JD & L Van Camp. Adv. Antimicrobial & Antineoplastic Chemother. II: 241 (1972).
5. Knott GD. MLAB - A Mathematical Modeling Tool. In: Computer Programs in Biomedical Research. Vol. 10 (3): 271 (1981).
6. Litterst, CL, TE Gram, RL Dedrick, AF Leroy & AM Guarino. Cancer Res. 36: 2340 (1976).
7. Litterst CL, IJ Torres & AM Guarino. Wadley Medical Bull. 7: 169 (1977).
8. Nakai, Y, K Knoishi, KC Chang, K Ohashi, N Morisaki, Y Minowa, A Morimoto. Acta Otolaryngol. 93: 227 (1982).
9. Pretorius RG, ES Petrilli, C Kean, LC Ford, JD Hoeschele, LD Lagasse, Cancer Treat. Rep. 65: 1055 (1981).
10. Schaeppi, U, IA Heyman, RW Fleischman, H Rosenkrantz, V Ilevaki, R Phelan, DA Cooney & RD Davis. Tox. Appl. Pharmacol. 25: 230 (1973).

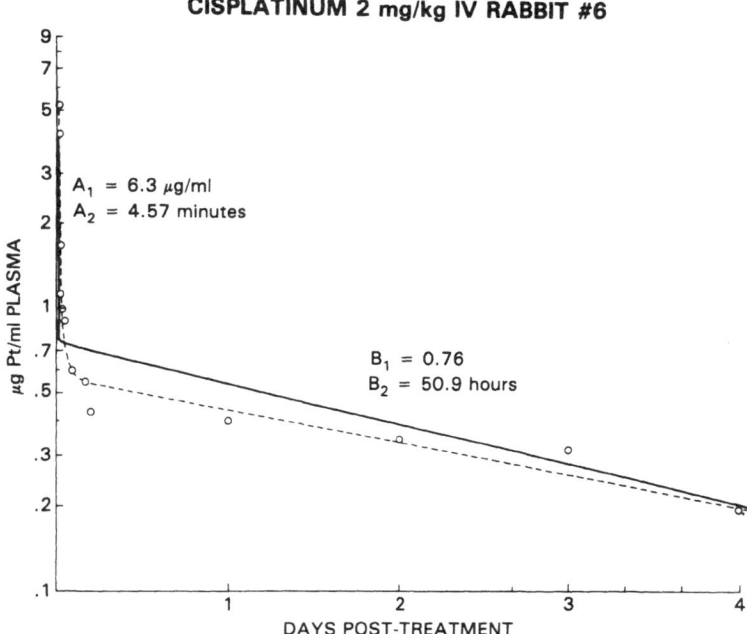

Figure 5. Plasma levels of total platinum after IV administration of cis-platin (2 mg/kg). Solid line is the computer-generated fit to the experimental data points shown.

Clinical Pharmacokinetics of Diammine [1,1-Cyclobutanedicarboxylato (2-)]-0,0'-Platinum (CBDCA)

P.V. Woolley, V.M. Priego, P.V.T. Luc,
A. Rahman and P.S. Schein

CBDCA is a second generation platinum coordination complex that
is presently in clinical trial. The principal advantage of this
agent over cis-diamminedichloroplatinum (II) (cisplatin) is a
reduction in its nephrotoxicity and acute gastrointestinal toxicity.
These features of the drug were initially described in preclinical
toxicologic studies and have now been confirmed in several Phase I
clinical trials (1-4). Clinical pharmacologic studies have been
performed as a part of several of these trials and this paper
summarizes the results obtained at Georgetown as well as two other
centers and draws comparison, where possible, to data for cisplatin.

Important pharmacologic features of platinum complexes have been
described for cisplatin in humans. After administration of cisplatin
as a bolus, platinum can be detected in plasma in two forms, free and
protein bound (5). The distinction between the two is usually based
upon the ultrafilterability of the free fraction. The clearance of free
platinum from plasma is very rapid, with a half life of 20-30 minutes
(5). By contrast total plasma platinum which includes the protein bound
species, is cleared in a biexponential process for which the $t_{1/2}$
of the first phase is 20-60 minutes and that of the second phase is
very long, usually 40-100 hours (5-7). Cisplatin forms stable
complexes with a spectrum of plasma proteins, including albumin and
transferrin, which is one of the reasons for the prolonged second phase
half-life of total plasma platinum (5). After a twenty four infusion
of cisplatin, all drug in the plasma is present in non-filterable
form and free drug cannot be detected (5). Occasionally more complex
pharmacokinetic profiles are seen. In particular a second peak of
total plasma platinum following the first phase elimination has been

described and attributed to either enterohepatic recirculation or "wash-back" from a tissue compartment (5). Cisplatin is partially eliminated from the body in the urine. Usually 20-30% of an administered dose appears in the urine in the first 24 hours.

These data provide a basis for comparison of cisplatin to CBDCA. At Georgetown we have studied the clinical pharmacokinetics of CBDCA during a Phase I trial in which patients received the drug once weekly for four conservation weeks. CBDCA was administered to these patients as a 30 minute infusion without prehydration or mannitol diuresis. Individual doses ranging from 20mg/m^2 to 150mg/m^2 were studied. Collection of plasma specimens and determination of platinum by flameless atomic absorption spectroscopy were performed as previously described (5). Table I below gives the peak levels of total plasma platinum and ultrafilterable platinum seen in these patients immediately after drug administration.

TABLE I

PEAK PLASMA LEVELS OF TOTAL AND ULTRAFILTERABLE
PLATINUM FOLLOWING A 30 MINUTE INFUSION OF CBDCA

PATIENT	DOSE (mg/m^2)	TOTAL PT (micromolar)	UF-PT (micromolar)
1	20	3.3	3.3
2	20	3.3	3.3
3	75	13.0	8.5
4	100	16.3	16.3
5	125	22.8	12.9
6	125	13.7	6.5
7	150	31.0	15.0

In general the disappearance of ultrafilterable drug from plasma consisted of one rapid phase with a half-life of a few minutes and at least one longer phase with a half-life of one to two hours. However several of the curves have been more complex and exhibited secondary peaks similar to those previously described for cisplatin. Figures 1a and 1b show the disappearance of total and ultrafilterable Pt for patient #1 who received 20mg/m^2 and patient #3 who received 75mg/m^2 of CBDCA. In each case the curves were well represented as the sum of three exponentials, the half-lives of which are given in Table II.

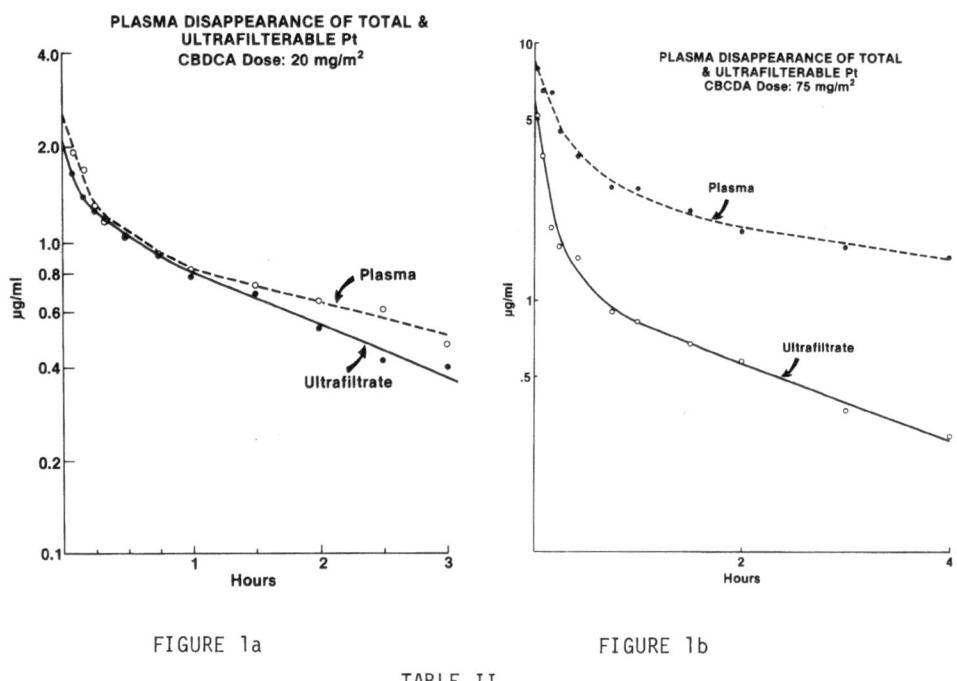

FIGURE 1a   FIGURE 1b

TABLE II

HALF TIME (MIN.) OF TOTAL AND UNLTRAFILTERABLE
PT IN PLASMA FROM CBDCA TREATED PATIENTS

Patient	Dose		$t_{1/2\ \alpha}$	$t_{1/2\ \beta}$	$t_{1/2\ \gamma}$
1	20 mg/m^2	Total	3.0	9.4	161
		UF	2.8	9.4	105
3	75 mg/m^2	Total	6.8	34	358
		UF	3.2	34.8	168

Patient #2, who also received 20 mg/m^2, showed first order disappearance of ultrafilterable Pt with a $t_{1/2}$ of 105 minutes. This may have been due to a delay in starting blood collection. This half-life agrees with the terminal phase of patient #1.

The patients treated at doses of 100-150 mg/m^2 were somewhat more complex because in some there was apparent second drug peak that occurred about 30 minutes after the end of the infusion. An example of this is shown in Figure 2 below.

PLASMA DISAPPEARANCE OF TOTAL AND
ULTRAFILTERABLE Pt [CBDCA DOSE: 125 mg/m^2]

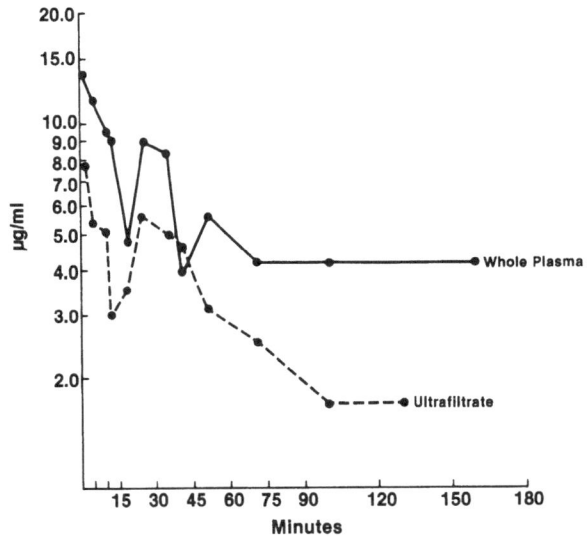

FIGURE 2

Whether or not a second peak appeared, the disappearance of Pt after CBDCA administration had a rapid initial phase, usually with $t_{1/2}$ less than 15 minutes and a terminal phase with a $t_{1/2}$ of 100-180 minutes, as shown in Table III.

TABLE III

HALF-TIMES (MIN.) OF TOTAL AND ULTRAFILTERABLE PT IN PATIENTS RECEIVING 100-180mg CBDCA /m^2

Patient		$t_{1/2\,\alpha}$	minutes $t_{1/2\,\beta}$	$t_{1/2\gamma}$	Comment
4	Total				No secondary peak
	UF	7	75	350	Ultrafiltrate and total Pt identical in disappearance
5	Total	8	45	--	Pronounced second peak.
	UF	7	45	--	About 1/3 of total plasma Pt ultrafilterable at·120 minutes.
6	Total	35	250	--	Probable second peak
	UF	35	250	--	About 1/3 of total plasma Pt ultrafilterable at 180 minutes.
7	Total	7	95	--	Probable second peak
	UF		95	--	Ultrafilterable and total Pt almost identical in disappearance.

A further feature of these pharmacokinetics was that the disappearance of ultrafilterable Pt was prolonged and generally paralleled that of total plasma Pt. In some cases, such as those of Patients 1,3,5 and 6, the ultrafilterable fraction fell more rapidly than whole plasma Pt, indicating that protein binding was occurring slowly over time. In other cases, such as patients 2,4 and 7 the disappearance of total and ultrafilterable Pt were virtually identical. In either situation the prolonged existence of ultra-filterable Pt in the plasma after CBDCA administration was in contrast to the rapid clearance of ultrafilterable drug and extensive protein binding after cisplatin administration. Table IV gives the approximate proportion of total Pt that was non-filterable, i.e. protein bound, after 2 hours for each of the patients studied.

TABLE IV

Patient	% protein-bound Pt after 2h
1	20
2	0
3	60
4	0
5	44
6	60
7	0

These results are in general agreement with those of other groups. Egorin, et al (3) from the University of Maryland Cancer Center have reported pharmacokinetics studies of CBDCA performed during a Phase I trial in which the drug was administered daily for 5 days. They observed that plasma concentrations of total platinum declined in a biexponential fashion with alpha and beta $t_{1/2}$'s of 26-49 minutes and 492 to 1188 minutes respectively. There were minimal amounts of platinum in plasma 24 hours after CBDCA administration. Plasma concentrations of ultrafilterable platinum declined in a biexponential fashion with alpha and beta $t_{1/2}$'s of 7.6-21.4 minutes and 102 to 236 minutes respectively. The majority of platinum in the plasma of patients receiving CBDCA was ultrafilterable. Ultrafilterable platinum accounted for over 70% of total plasma platinum for the first two hours after IV bolus administration of CBDCA, after which this percentage slowly declined to approximately 50%. Some secondary peaks were observed in this study. Another study of interest is that of Curt, et al (2) from the

National Cancer Institute, who have studied the pharmacokinetics of CBDCA during and after a 24 hour infusion of the drug. In patients treated with 320 mg/m^2 CBDCA over 24 hours, steady state concentrations of ultrafilterable drug of 10 micromolar were achieved. These disappeared from the plasma in a first order fashion after the infusion was stopped, the $t_{1/2}$ being 120-210 minutes. This is in marked contrast to reported results for cisplatin (5) showing no free drug after a 20 hour infusions.

The urinary excretion of CBDCA is more complete than is that of cisplatin. At least 40-70% of a dose is eliminated in the urine in 24 hours (1-3) as opposed to 15-25% of a cisplatin dose (5). It is further reported that the area under the concentration x time curve of CBDCA is a linear function of the dose (1,2).

CBDCA differs in its pharmacokinetics from cisplatin in that the ultrafilterable platinum species is present for prolonged periods of time in the plasma after either bolus or prolonged infusion. The elimination of the ultrafilterable species parallels that of total plasma platinum. While there is evidence that protein binding occurs over a period of time, much of the drug remains unbound and in some cases all plasma drug is filterable for 2-3 hours. While the studies in humans to date have not reported pharmacology in terms of parent compound, much of the ultrafilterable platinum probably represents intact CBDCA.

REFERENCES

1) Calvert, AH, Harland, SJ, Newell, DR, Siddik, H, Jones, AC, McElwain, TJ, Raju, S, Wiltshaw, E, Smith, IE, Baker, JM, Peckham, MJ, and Harrap, KR (1982): Early Clinical Studies with Cis-Diammine-1,1-cyclobutane Dicarboxylate Platinum II. Cancer Chemother. Pharmacol. 9:140-147.
2) Curt, GA, Grygiel, JJ, Weiss, R, Corden, B, Ozols, R, Tell, D, Collins, J and Myers, CE (1983): A Phase I and Pharmacokinetic Study of CBDCA (NSC 241240) Proc. Amer. Soc. Clin. Onc. 2:21.
3) Egorin, MJ, Van Echo, DA, Witacre, MY, Olman, EA and Aisner, J (1983): Phase I Study and Clinical Pharmacokinetics of Carboplatin (CBDCA). Proc. Amer. Soc. Clin. Onc. 2:28.

4) Priego, V, Luc, V, Bonnem, E, Rahman, A, Smith, F, Schein, P, and Woolley, P (1983): A Phase I Study and Pharmacology of Diammine-(1,1)-cyclobutane dicarboxylato (2-)-0,0'-platinum (CBDCA) Administered on a Weekly Schedule. Proc. Amer. Soc. Clin. Onc. 2:30.

5) Gullo, J, Litterst, C, Maguire, P, Sikic, BI, Hoth, DF, and Woolley, P (1980): Pharmacokinetics and Protein Binding of Cis-Dichlorodiamminoplatinum (II) Administered as a One Hour or as a Twenty Hour Infusion. Cancer Chemother. Pharmacol. 5:21-26.

6) Gormley, P, Bull, JM, LeRoy, AF and Cysyk, R (1979): Kinetics of cis-Dichlorodiamminoplatium. Clin. Pharmacol. Ther. 25:351-358.

7) Patton, TF, Himmelstein, KJ, Belt, R, Bannister, SJ, Sternson, LA and Repta, AJ (1978): Plasma Levels and Urinary Excretion of Filterable Platinum Species Following Bolus Injection and IV Infusion of cis-Dichlorodiamminoplatinum (II) in Man. Cancer Treat. Rep. 62:1359-1365.

Biliary Excretion, Renal Handling and Red Cell Uptake of Cisplatin and CBDCA in Animals

Z.H. Siddik, D.R. Newell, F.E. Boxall, M. Jones, K.G. McGhee and K.R. Harrap

1. INTRODUCTION

Since the discovery of its antitumour activity by Rosenberg et al (1), cisplatin has achieved global recognition in the clinical management of several neoplasms, particularly those of the ovary, testes and the head and neck (2). Its clinical application, however, can be severely curtailed by the onset of several dose-limiting toxicities, most important of which are nausea and vomiting, neurotoxicity, myelosuppression and, in particular, nephrotoxicity (2). In an effort to dispense with these toxic side effects, whilst retaining or even improving upon the antitumour activity of cisplatin, attention has focussed on the development of 'second generation analogues' (3). At The Institute of Cancer Research, this has resulted in identifying cis-diammine(1,1-cyclobutanedicarboxylato)platinum II (CBDCA, JM8) as a potential alternative to cisplatin in cancer chemo-therapy (3). The analogue has recently undergone phase I studies at The Royal Marsden Hospital (4), and phase II and III studies are currently in progress.

Cisplatin

CBDCA

An important preclinical feature of CBDCA, and an essential prerequisite selection criterion was its failure to elicit nephrotoxicity in animals (3,5). This significant deviation from the severe nephrotoxicity experienced with cisplatin has prompted us to identify pharmacokinetic features which may explain the difference in the nephrotoxicity of the two complexes. Since explanations for death in animals from lethal doses of CBDCA are as yet not evaluable, we have also investigated the potential of red blood cells as targets for CBDCA-induced toxicity.

2. PROCEDURE

Cisplatin and CBDCA, gifts from the Johnson Matthey Research Centre (Reading, England), were dissolved in normal saline immediately prior to use. Both compounds were administered iv to animals. ^{14}C-inulin was co-administered where necessary. Male and female Balb C$^-$ mice and female Wistar rats were used throughout. For short term experiments requiring serial sample collections, animals were anaesthetized with pentobarbital sodium and kept warm with heating lamps. Blood, bile and urine samples were obtained via cannulae placed in the carotid artery, the common bile duct, and the bladder, respectively. Freshly obtained anticoagulated rat whole blood was used for transport studies in erythrocytes. Plasma was isolated by centrifugation. Non-protein bound drug in the plasma or lysed red cells was determined following ultrafiltration using Amicon CF 50A membrane cones (6). All samples were kept at 0-4°C throughout.

The procedure for studying the uptake of cisplatin and CBDCA in kidney cortical (0.75 mm thick) and liver (1.0 mm thick) slices in Krebs-Ringer bicarbonate buffer, supplemented with sodium acetate (10 mM, for kidney) or glucose (5 mM, for liver), was described previously (7). ^{14}C-inulin was added to the media to enable the platinum content in the extracellular space to be subtracted from the total platinum content of the slice.

For haematocrit determinations, blood was obtained by venipuncture in the tail. For the transfusion studies, freshly prepared saline-washed (twice) red cells from donor rats were resuspended in saline (final haematocrit 0.45-0.55), warmed and transfused (16 ml/kg) via the tail vein.

Total platinum levels in the samples were determined directly as previously described (8). Kidney samples, however,

required digestion in 16 M nitric acid prior to analysis.
Unchanged CBDCA was determined on a Waters Associates HPLC at 255
nm using a spherisorb silica column and a 90% $CH_3CN/10\%$ H_2O (v/v)
mobile phase in the isocratic mode. ^{14}C was determined by
standard liquid scintillation spectrophotometric techniques. The
data, where applicable, were fitted to a two-compartment open
model using a non-linear least squares computer program. Further
pharmacokinetic analysis was performed using equations described
by Wagner (9).

3. RESULTS

3.1 Plasma binding and drug concentrations. Following
administration of cisplatin (2 mg/kg) to female rats , the drug
exists entirely in the free form for the first 5-10 min, (fig 1).
Thereafter, plasma binding increases rapidly so that by 60 min
free platinum is not detectable. CBDCA, on the other hand,
becomes reversibly bound to plasma to the extent of about 20%
immediately after its administration (20 mg/kg). This binding
remains constant during the first 60 min, but the free platinum

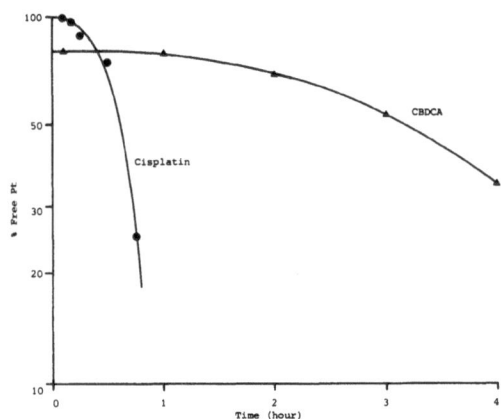

FIGURE 1. Decline in 'free' platinum in rat plasma in vivo

gradually decreases thereafter due to irreversible binding of CBDCA to plasma proteins. Conversion of CBDCA to other products is negligible during the first hour. The plasma decay curves of cisplatin (2 mg/kg) and CBDCA (20 mg/kg) are biphasic (fig 2), which give alpha and beta phase half lives for free platinum of 2 and 10 min respectively for cisplatin and 3 and 26 min respectively for CBDCA.

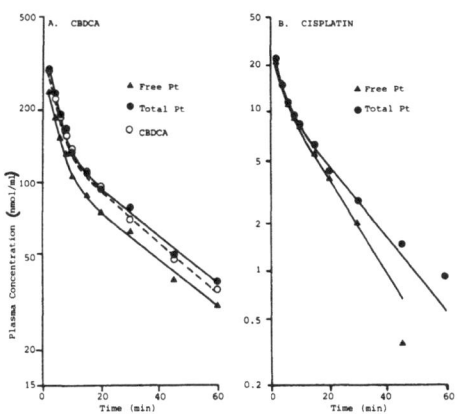

FIGURE 2. Plasma concentration-time curves for free and total drug.

3.2 <u>Renal platinum levels</u>. In female mice, the renal platinum concentration after administration of maximally tolerated doses of cisplatin (4 mg/kg) and CBDCA (80 mg/kg) can be described by biphasic decay curves with long terminal phases (fig 3a). The biphasic computer fit of the data over the first 10 days gave terminal-phase half-lives of 182 hours for cisplatin and 114 hours for CBDCA. The greater persistence of platinum in the kidney over that in the plasma results in kidney/plasma ratios of about 20-30 for both complexes by day 6 (fig 3b).

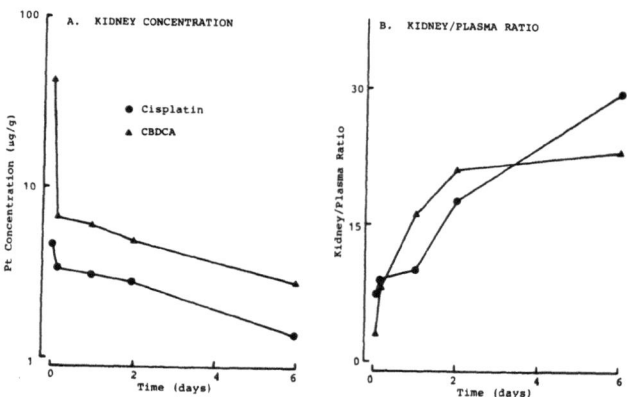

FIGURE 3.   Kidney concentration and kidney/plasma ratio of
platinum.

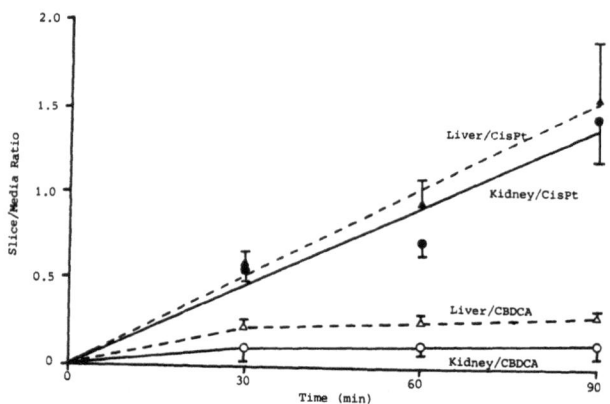

FIGURE 4. Uptake of cisplatin (100 μM) and CBDCA (100 μM) in
kidney and liver slices at 37°C.

3.3. Drug uptake in rat kidney and liver slices. Incubation of kidney and liver slices with cisplatin results in a time-dependent accumulation of platinum in both tissues as indicated by a linear increase in the slice/media ratios (fig 4). The ratios are similar for both tissues and exceed unity by 90 min post-incubation. The ratios for CBDCA in both tissues are much lower in comparison to cisplatin. Homogenisation of slices followed by protein precipitation with trichloroacetic acid indicate that the irreversibly bound platinum at 90 min in both tissues represents a major part (79-82%) of the total platinum content.

3.4 Urinary excretion. The kidney represents an important route for both cisplatin and CBDCA excretion in the mouse, with the major part of the total urinary platinum being excreted in the first 4 hours after drug administration (fig 5). Cisplatin excretion, however, is about half that of CBDCA. Excretion of the two complexes is not sex-dependent (data not shown). Furthermore, urinary excretion of the two platinum compounds in the rat is similar to that seen in the mouse (cf. table 1 and fig 5). In addition, the unchanged CBDCA in rat urine accounts for virtually all of the platinum excreted during the first 4 hours.

Table 1. Excretion of cisplatin and CBDCA in rat urine.

Compound	Dose (mg/kg)	% Dose in urine in 4 hours	
		Total platinum	Unchanged drug
Cisplatin	2	47	–
CBDCA	20	89	85

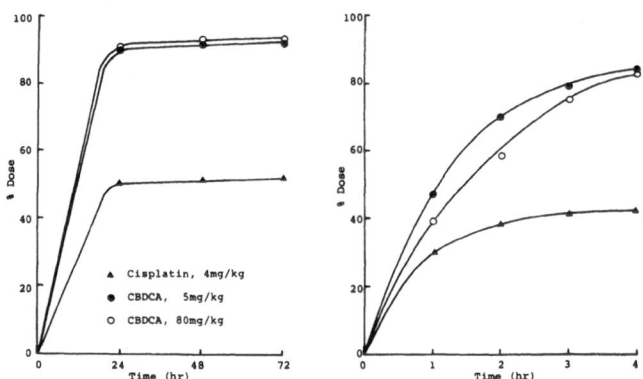

FIGURE 5. Excretion of cisplatin and CBDCA in mouse urine.

3.5. Biliary excretion. The rate of platinum excretion in rat bile is over two-fold greater for cisplatin than CBDCA (fig 6a). The cumulative % dose of platinum excreted in the first 6 hours is similarly greater for cisplatin than CBDCA (fig 6b).

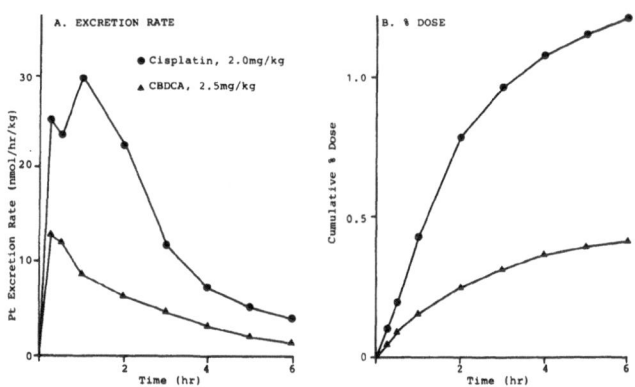

FIGURE 6. Biliary excretion of cisplatin and CEDCA in the rat.

Table 2. Concentration of platinum (µg/ml) in the mouse gall-bladder bile.

Compound	1hr	4hr	1d	2d	6d
Cisplatin	4.6	7.5	0.5	0.4	0.1
CBDCA	28	23	3.4	2.0	0.4

Biliary excretion, however, represents only 0.4-1.2% of the dose of the two complexes. In the mouse, examination of the gall bladder bile indicated that the platinum concentration reached a peak level at about 1-4 hours after cisplatin (4 mg/kg) and CBDCA (80 mg/kg) administrations, and, thereafter, declined progressively during the next 6 days (table 2).

3.6. Plasma, renal and biliary clearances. In the rat, plasma and renal clearances for both inulin, a marker for the glomerular filtration rate, and CBDCA are similar (table 3). Cisplatin renal clearance, on the other hand, is significantly greater than that of inulin (p<0.05). In addition, cisplatin plasma clearance is about two-fold greater than its renal clearance, and similarly greater than the plasma clearances of inulin and CBDCA. Biliary clearance of cisplatin, although much lower in comparison to plasma or renal clearance, is five-fold greater than that of CBDCA.

Table 3.   Clearances of CBDCA, cisplatin and inulin.

Compound	Clearance of free drug (ml/hr/kg)		
	Plasma	Renal	Biliary
CBDCA	618	558	3.2
Cisplatin	1566	738	16.2
Inulin	606	576	N.A.*

* Not assessed

3.7. <u>Changes in haematocrits</u>. Administration of cisplatin
(6.5 mg/kg) to rats causes a 15-20% drop in the haematocrit value
on days 7-14. This is followed by a recovery phase during the
next 14 days (fig 7). A lethal dose (8 mg/kg) of this complex,
however, causes haemoconcentration on day 4, and death a day
later possibly due to renal insufficiency. CBDCA (60 mg/kg),
on the other hand, causes a pronounced decrease (65-70%) in the
haematocrit by day 11. As with cisplatin, the haematocrit
values recover to normal levels between days 21 and 28. At
a lethal dose of CBDCA (80 mg/kg), the drop in the haematocrit
value by day 9 is even more severe, and death ensues a day later.

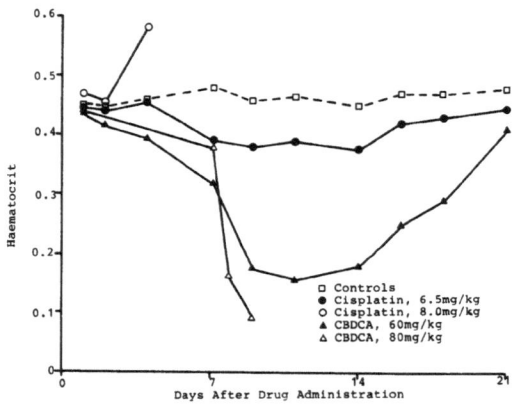

FIGURE 7. Changes in rat haematocrits.

3.8. <u>Platinum levels in rat erythrocytes</u>. The accumulation and
persistence of platinum in the red cells following <u>in vivo</u> (80
mg/kg) and <u>in vitro</u> (300 µM) exposure to CBDCA are indicated by
the high whole blood/plasma and red cell/plasma ratios,
respectively (table 4). The corresponding ratios for <u>in vivo</u> (10
mg/kg) and <u>in vitro</u> (30 µM) exposure to cisplatin are about
three-fold lower. The high blood/plasma ratios <u>in vivo</u> are
probably the result of a more rapid disappearance of platinum
from the plasma than from the red cells. <u>In vitro</u> studies with

whole blood indicated that the half-life for the irreversible binding of cisplatin in the plasma or the red cell is similar (table 4). Binding of CBDCA in the red cell, on the other hand, is three times faster than in the plasma.

Table 4. Uptake and binding in red cells and binding in plasma of cisplatin and CBDCA.

Parameter	Cisplatin	CBDCA
Blood/plasma Pt ratio in vivo at day 4	4	14
Red cell/plasma Pt ratio in vitro at 24 hr	1	3
$T_{1/2}$ (hr) for binding in plasma in vitro	1	13
$T_{1/2}$ (hr) for binding in red cells in vitro	1	4

3.9. Prevention of CBDCA-induced lethalities. Intravenous administration of 80 mg/kg CBDCA to rats results in deaths by days 9-10 (fig 8). A single transfusion of red cells on day 7 to rats given the lethal dose of CBDCA results in a delay in the time of death by 1-2 days. Transfusions on days 7,8,9 and 11, however, protects 85% of the animals from the drug-induced lethal event.

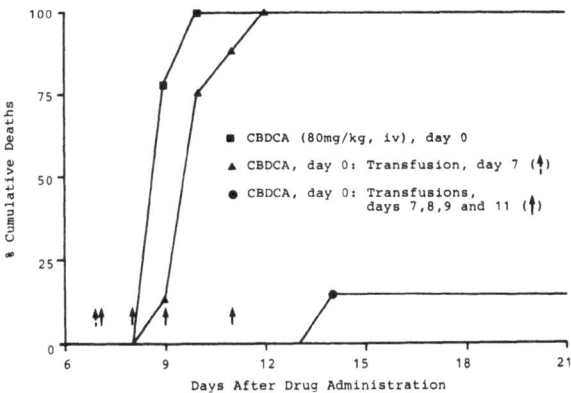

FIGURE 8. Prevention by red cell transfusions of CBDCA-induced lethalities.

4. DISCUSSION

The understanding of the underlying causes of cisplatin-induced nephrotoxicity would be of considerable importance, not only in the rational development of non-nephrotoxic platinum complexes, but also perhaps in the rational design of clinical protocols to limit the incidence of drug-related renal damage. The availability of CBDCA, a non-nephrotoxic cisplatin analogue (3,5), presents an ideal opportunity to examine whether the differences in the pharmacokinetics of the two compounds could provide us with a plausible explanation for the relative nephrotoxicities of these complexes. It is clear from the data that the lack of nephrotoxicity from CBDCA is not due to either a comparatively lower renal platinum concentration or to an appreciable biliary excretion of this compound. Indeed, the renal levels of cisplatin and CBDCA during the terminal phase are similar, and the biliary excretion of cisplatin itself is several-fold greater than that of the analogue. Furthermore, the low platinum concentration in the mouse gall-bladder bile indicates that platinum excretion via this route remains insignificant, even at the later times when the complex would probably exist as high molecular weight platinum species due to irreversible binding to macromolecules.

For both platinum complexes, the kidney plays a major role in their excretion, although excretion of cisplatin is about half that of CBDCA. In addition, the excretion of the latter compound is largely as the unchanged drug. What is clear is that, whilst urinary excretion of CBDCA is by glomerular filtration, excretion of cisplatin involves in addition an active renal secretory mechanism. The active urinary excretion of cisplatin is in agreement with the data previously reported (10, 11). Although active transport of cisplatin has been noted in rat kidney slices (10), the similarity in the uptake between the rat kidney and liver slices and the tissue binding studies indicate that transport of cisplatin at the concentration utilised is largely due to the drug binding intracellularly and not to an active transport mechanism. The data do, however, show that cisplatin uptake by kidney and liver slices is greater than that of CBDCA at an equimolar concentration. In vivo, the mouse renal levels of the two complexes are similar during the prolonged terminal phase, possibly because of the higher dose of CBDCA that was employed.

Another major difference between cisplatin and CBDCA is related to the plasma clearance of the compounds and the large discrepancy between plasma (total) clearance of cisplatin and its combined renal and biliary clearances. This suggests the existence of at least another major route of cisplatin clearance, thus distinguishing it from CBDCA. This additional clearance mechanism may well involve the rapid and extensive binding of the chemically unstable cisplatin to tissues, as has been seen here with the plasma proteins and kidney and liver slices. CBDCA, in comparison to cisplatin, has greater chemical stability and does not bind as rapidly to the plasma. Thus, the presence of tubular secretory mechanisms for cisplatin, probably resulting in high concentration of the compound specifically in the renal tubules (the target tissue (12)), in conjunction with its rapid binding to tissue could provide a basis for explaining the substantial nephrotoxicity of cisplatin compared with CBDCA.

The dose-limiting toxicity of cisplatin in animals is nephrotoxicity (12). Toxicity of this complex to red cells is not significant in the rat in spite of the high binding of the compound to the cells as has been demonstrated here and elsewhere (13). With CBDCA, however, erythropoenia is severe and can be correlated with the lethalities. This is confirmed by the observation that red cell transfusions can protect animals from CBDCA-induced lethalities. The major cause of erythropoenia with CBDCA is probably related to the high platinum content of the red cells in vitro and in vivo, resulting from the greater rate of irreversible binding of the drug in the erythrocytes than in the plasma. The gradient thus established promotes further entry of CBDCA into the cells by diffusion. The comparatively lower distribution of cisplatin in the red cells can be related to its similar rate of irreversible binding to both the cells and the plasma proteins. It therefore appears that the dose-limiting toxicity of CBDCA in rats is erythropoenia.

5. REFERENCES

1. Rosenberg B, VanCamp L, Trosko J Mansour VH.
    Nature 222: 385-386, 1969.
2. Prestayko AW, D'Aoust JC, Issell BF, Crooke ST.
    Cancer Treat Rev 6: 17-39, 1979.
3. Harrap KR, In: Cancer Chemotherapy, vol 1, pp 171-217
    Muggia FM (Ed). Martinus Nijhoff, Massachusetts, 1983.
4. Calvert AH, Harland SJ, Newell DR, Siddik ZH, Jones AC,
    McElwain TJ, Raju S, Wiltshaw E, Smith IE, Baker JW,
    Peckham MJ, Harrap KR.
    Cancer Chemother Pharmacol 9: 140-147, 1982.
5. Levine BS, Henry MC, Port CD, Richter WR, Urbanek MA.
    J Natl Cancer Inst 67: 201-206, 1981.
6. Litterst CL, Gram TE, Dedrick RL, LeRoy AF, Guarino AM.
    Cancer Res 36: 2340-2344, 1976.
7. Siddik ZH, Trush MA, Gram TE.
    Lung 157: 209-217, 1980.
8. LeRoy AF, Wehling ML, Sponseller HL, Friauf WS,
    Solomon RE, Dedrick RL, Litterst CL, Gram TE. Guarino AM,
    Becker DA.
    Biochem Med 18: 184-191, 1977.
9. Wagner JG. Fundamentals of Clinical Pharmacokinetics.
    Drug Intelligence Publications Inc. Hamilton,
    Illinois, 1975.
10. Jacobs C, McGarry K, Rich L, Weiner MW.
    Proc Am Assoc Cancer Res 23: 126, 1982.
11. Daley-Yates PT, McBrien DCH.
    Biochem Pharmacol 31: 2243-2246, 1982.
12. Madias NE, Harrington JT.
    Am J Med 65: 307-314, 1978.
13. Manaka RC, Wolf W.
    Chem Biol Interact 22: 353-358, 1978.

Biodistribution and Pharmacokinetics of 195mPt-Labeled *cis*-Dichloro-*trans*-Dihydroxo-*bis*(Isopropylamine) Platinum (IV), CHIP, In the Normal Female Fischer 344 Rat
J.D. Hoeschele, L.A. Ferren, J.A. Roberts ar 1 L.R. Whitfield

1. INTRODUCTION

The discovery and successful clinical application of the potent anti-tumor compound, cis-Dichlorodiammineplatinum(II), cis-DDP* has stimulated considerable interest in developing effective but less toxic second-generation platinum antitumor drugs. One such candidate drug is cis-Dichloro-trans-dihydroxo-bis-(isopropylamine)platinum(IV), cis-trans-[PtCl$_2$(OH)$_2$(i-PrNH$_2$)$_2$], (CHIP), the molecular structure of which is shown in Fig. 1. An important feature of this Pt(IV) agent is that in addition to exhibiting a generally milder clinical toxicity than cisplatin, the dose-limiting toxicity of CHIP is the more common myelosuppression rather than the less desirable nephrotoxicity. Also, CHIP has been reported recently to be more effective than cisplatin against both alkylating agent sensitive and resistant strains of the Yoshida sarcoma.[1] That CHIP is indeed a promising candidate drug is underscored by its selection by the National Cancer Institute as one of four new platinum analogs to enter clinical trials in the U.S.A.

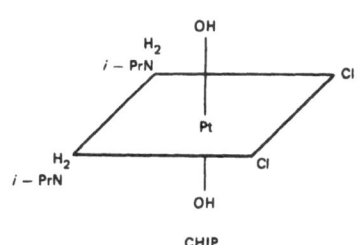

FIGURE 1. Molecular structure of CHIP

† ORNL is operated by Union Carbide Corporation under contract W-7405-eng-26 with the U.S. Department of Energy.
* Registered trademark is CISPLATIN.

As part of our continuing interest in platinum antitumor agents, we have developed a microscale synthesis for [195m]Pt-labeled CHIP and have studied the tissue distribution and pharmacokinetic properties of this radiolabeled agent in normal female Fischer 344 rats. The purpose of this paper is to report the details of the microscale synthesis, biodistribution, and pharmacokinetic studies of [195m]Pt-CHIP including a comparison with similar data for [195m]Pt-cis-DDP.[2]

2. MATERIAL AND METHODS
2.1. Microscale synthesis of [195m]Pt-labeled CHIP
2.1.1. [195m]Pt radiolabel. [195m]Pt ($t_{1/2}$ = 4.02d) was produced by neutron irradiation (n,γ) of highly enriched [194]Pt (97.41%) in the High Flux Isotope Reactor (HFIR) at Oak Ridge National Laboratory at a flux of 2.5 x 10[15] neutrons/cm[2]/sec. The high burn-up cross-section of [195m]Pt (13,000 barns) limits the specific activity to ~ 1.2 mCi of [195m]Pt/mg Pt metal. Details of the reactor production of [195m]Pt and hot-cell processing of irradiated targets are published elsewhere.[3] The [195m]Pt nuclide is an ideal radiolabel for studying the biodistribution and pharmacokinetic properties of Pt antitumor drugs because (1) [195m]Pt emits penetrating γ radiation (99 and 129 keV) which provides the capability of direct and sensitive detection (~ 2.7 x 10[2] disintegrations/min/ng Pt°) of Pt at low concentrations in biological specimens and (2) [195m]Pt decays directly to stable [195]Pt by isomeric transition, which simplifies quantitation by γ-ray spectrometry since no daughter activities are produced.

2.1.2. Reaction scheme. The eight-step reaction scheme for synthesizing [195m]Pt-CHIP is schematically outlined in Fig. 2.

Reaction conditions have been optimized at a 0.2 mmole reaction scale in order to obtain the highest yield and purity of CHIP. Steps 1, 2, 4, 5 (after substituting i-PrNH2 for NH4OH) and 6 are are carried out exactly as described in the refined microscale synthesis of cis-DDP.[3] Brief comments on the remaining steps are as follows:

(Step 3) A stoichiometric amount of KCl is added to the Na2PtCl4 solution from Step 2 and K2PtCl4 precipitated on adding 2 volumes of EtOH (absolute). The crude K2PtCl4(s) is dissolved in 0.1M HCl and then

1. Pt target + *aqua regia* + 2NaCl $\xrightarrow{\Delta, \text{ dryness}}$ $Na_2PtCl_6(s)$

2. Na_2PtCl_6 + 0.5 $N_2H_4 \cdot 2HCl$ $\xrightarrow{5°C \text{ 5 min; } 85°C}$ Na_2PtCl_4

3. Na_2PtCl_4 + KCl + EtOH $\xrightarrow{25°C}$ $K_2PtCl_4(s)$ → recrystallize

4. K_2PtCl_4 + 6KI $\xrightarrow{25°C}$ K_2PtI_4

5. K_2PtI_4 + 2A $\xrightarrow{25°C}$ *cis*-$PtA_2I_2(s)$

6. *cis*-$PtA_2I_2(s)$ + 2.2 $AgNO_3$ $\xrightarrow{60°C}$ *cis*-$[PtA_2(H_2O)_2]^{2+}$

7. *cis*-$[PtA_2(H_2O)_2]^{2+}$ + HCl $\xrightarrow{45°C}$ until Ag^+-free $\xrightarrow{60°C; \, 12M \text{ HCl}}$ *cis*-$PtA_2Cl_2(s)$

8. *cis*-$PtA_2Cl_2(s)$ + H_2O_2 (30%) $\xrightarrow{5 \text{ min; } 95°C}$ *cis-trans*-$[PtCl_2(OH)_2A_2]$(CHIP)

FIGURE 2. Scheme for the microscale synthesis of ^{195m}Pt-labeled-CHIP. Non-essential reaction products are omitted. Denotations: A for i-propylamine, Pt for ^{195m}Pt-labeled Pt.

reprecipitated with EtOH (absolute) as before. The use of pure K_2PtCl_4 instead of Na_2PtCl_4 generated in situ leads to a substantially purer CHIP product and usually eliminates the need to recrystallize the CHIP precursor, cis-Pt(i-PrNH_2)_2Cl_2.

(Step 8) The addition of 1 ml of 30% H_2O_2 to the yellow CIP residue from Step 7 followed by reaction at 95°C for 5 minutes converts the precursor to CHIP (crude). Reaction times longer than 5 minutes lead to reduction in the yield and quality of product. Under these reaction conditions at least five minute but detectable components are produced in this step.

2.1.3. Purification by preparative TLC. The crude ^{195m}Pt-CHIP was purified by preparative thin-layer chromatography (TLC) employing silica gel G (2000 μ thickness) as the support and a solvent mixture of Me_2CO: EtOAc:H_2O (45:45:10) as the developer. A saturated solution of ^{195m}Pt-CHIP in H_2O (1.5 ml at ~ 22 mg/ml) was loaded onto the TLC plate. After drying and development, the band containing CHIP was scraped off the plate and the CHIP eluted with MeOH. After evaporating the MeOH solution to dryness, the residue was dried in high vacuum at ambient temperature. TLC analysis of the purified CHIP (40% yield) using Whatman analytical LHP-K plates confirmed that the product was pure [single,

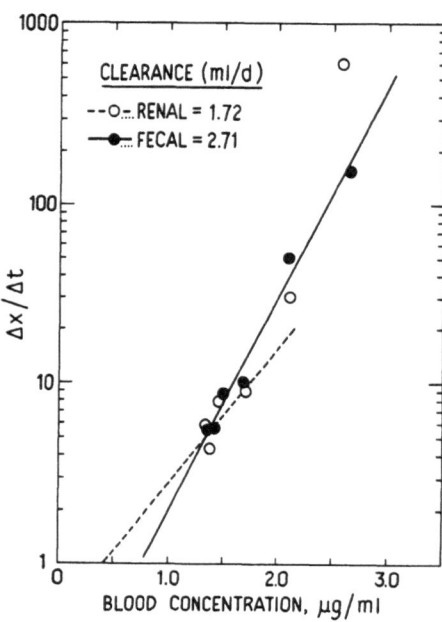

$1.0 \quad 2.0 \quad 3.0$
BLOOD CONCENTRATION, μg/ml

FIGURE 3. A graph of the $\Delta x/\Delta t$ vs [CHIP] in blood (μg/ml). x = amount of drug in urine or feces; t = time

homogeneous spot; R_f 0.43]. The uv-visible absorption spectra of the labeled and unlabeled reference samples were virtually the same. The molar absorptivities, ε, at the wavelengths of 206, 300, and ~ 384 nm are 2.8 x 10^4, 5.64 x 10^2, and 5.6 x 10^1 $\underline{M}^{-1}$ cm^{-1}, respectively.

Elemental, TLC, and spectroscopic analyses (^{13}C and ^1H-NMR) of a non-radioactive non-radioactive sample of CHIP which was prepared and purified as described above confirm that (1) the sample is pure (no extraneous peaks by NMR and TLC) and exists in the anhydrous form (i.e., no associated H_2O_2).

2.2. <u>Biodistribution studies</u>. The <u>in vivo</u> distribution studies were carried out in two separate experiments employing normal female Fischer 344 rats (137-175 g). Each rat received a single dose of ^{195m}Pt-labeled CHIP (7.5 mg drug/kg) <u>via</u> either the intraperitoneal (i.p.) or intravenous (lateral tail vein) route. Only four rats were treated i.v. ^{195m}Pt-CHIP was administered in saline (0.85% NaCl solution) and ~ 75-100 μCi of ^{195m}Pt was administered per rat. Rats were sacrificed at seven different times post-injection: 0.25, 1, and 6 h; 1, 3, 8, and 13 d. In general, a total of six to eight rats were used for each observation time. Fourteen tissues/organs were excised, rinsed with saline, and weighed. Urine and feces from four rats were collected in metabolism cages out to 8 d. ^{195m}Pt radioactivity was determined in the whole organ by means of an automatic gamma counter

(Packard, Model 522) set as follows: lower level at 390, window at 110, and a gain setting of 0.25 keV/channel.

2.3 Pharmacokinetic parameters. Clearance from the blood (Cl_b) and biological half-life ($t_{1/2}(b)$) were calculated according to model-independent methods described by Gibaldi and Perrier.[4] The apparent terminal-elimination phase rate constant (λ_z) was calculated by linear regression analysis using the 3 and 8 day post-injection data (Table 1).

TABLE 1. Pharmacokinetic parameters

Parameter	Value	Parameter	Value
$AUC_{0-\infty}$	31.9 µg d ml^{-1}kg^{-1}	Cl_b	236.1 ml min^{-1}kg^{-1}
λ_z	0.0676 d^{-1}	Cl_r	8.60 ml min^{-1}kg^{-1}
$t_{1/2}(b)$	10.4 d	Cl_f	13.5 ml min^{-1}kg^{-1}

Area under the blood concentration-time curve from time 0 to infinity ($AUC_{0-\infty}$) was calculated by the trapezoidal method with extrapolation to infinity. The apparent renal (Cl_r) and fecal (Cl_f) clearance values were determined from the slopes of graphs relating the natural logarithmic values of the incremental amount of drug in urine or feces/increment of time (i.e., $\Delta x/\Delta t$), respectively, plotted against the concentration of drug in the blood at the midpoint of the collection interval (cf. Fig. 3). Biological half-times $t_{1/2}(b)$ were also evaluated from a plot of the cumulative % dose of Pt excreted in the urine and feces as a function of time.

3. RESULTS AND DISCUSSION

3.1. Biodistribution data. The distribution and retention of ^{195m}Pt determined in 14 tissues as a function of time following administration of ^{195m}Pt-labeled CHIP to female Fischer rats is compiled in Tables 2 and 3. The data are expressed in terms of the % injected dose/organ and % injected dose/g tissue, respectively. The combined average uncertainity (mean % standard deviation) in these data is 13% for all tissues other than the stomach, small intestine, and colon. The combined average %

uncertainty for the latter three tissues is 31%. Unless stated otherwise, reference to the distribution data should be interpreted as the % injected dose/g tissue. Also, reference to the level or concentration of CHIP should be interpreted as the level or concentration of Pt, as measured by ^{195m}Pt, since the nature of the retained species is unknown. For purposes of data comparison, a retention of 1% of the injected dose/g tissue for a 0.15 kg rat corresponds to 0.27 µmoles or 5.2 µg Pt/g tissue.

Profiles of the tissue distribution of ^{195m}Pt-CHIP are shown in Figure 4. Examination of these data shows that there is initially a relatively rapid loss of ^{195m}Pt from all tissues followed by a slower loss out to 8 d for all tissues and blood with the exception of the spleen. Levels (% dose/g tissue) appear to rise anomalously between 8 to 13 d although the % dose/organ in general shows a uniform decline with time. The apparent increase results from the loss of organ weight without loss of the % Pt retained. Necropsy on Day 13 revealed nearly total fat depletion in the peritoneal cavity which may signal a potentially serious side effect. While the greatest ^{195m}Pt concentration is in the kidney and the lowest in the brain, the greatest amounts of

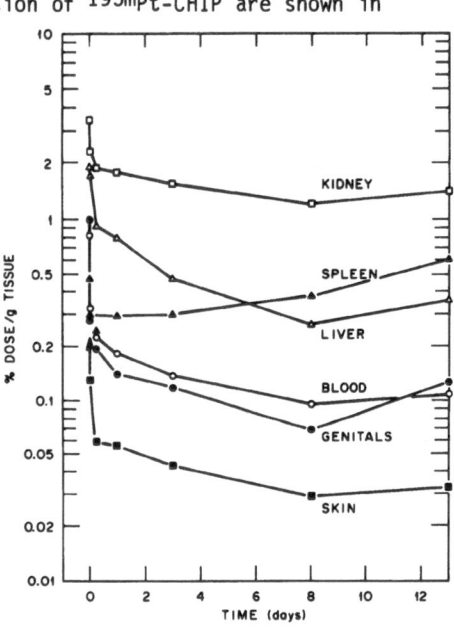

FIGURE 4 Distribution of ^{195m}Pt-labeled CHIP in selected tissues of the Fischer 344 (female) rat

^{195m}Pt CHIP are retained in the liver and kidney. Examination of the tissue distribution data at 24 h shows that the general order of decreasing tissue retention is:

Kidney > colon > liver > pancreas > spleen > stomach > blood > adrenals > small intestine > lungs > genitals > heart > skin > brain.

This order is to be compared with that for cis-DDP at 24 h[2] which is:

Kidney > genitals > liver > adrenals > spleen > bladder > lung >
pancreas > heart > brain (ten tissues).

TABLE 2. Distribution of [195mPt] in (female) Fischer 344 rat tissues[a,b]
as a function of time after administration (i.p.) of [195mPt]-labeled CHIP[c]

Time, Post-Injection	% Injected Dose/g Tissue							% Deviation (Mean)
	0.25 h	1.0 h	6.0 h	24.0 h	3.0 d	8.0 d	13.0 d	
Tissue								
Blood	0.778	0.378	0.232	0.194	0.139	0.109	0.110	9.95
Liver	1.67	1.87	0.899	0.739	0.476	0.257	0.367	12.0
Spleen	0.478	0.316	0.232	0.262	0.300	0.366	0.613	8.92
Pancreas	1.29	0.633	0.396	0.296	0.234	0.120	0.169	17.0
Stomach	0.299	0.199	0.0953	0.233	0.0500	0.0157	0.0240	51.6
S. Intestine	0.784	1.31	0.299	0.167	0.0535	0.0215	0.0275	31.0
Colon	0.225	0.0898	1.83	0.879	0.104	0.0411	0.0325	27.8
Adrenals	0.926	0.377	0.173	0.162	0.190	0.0845	0.180	18.9
Kidneys	3.46	2.73	2.03	1.74	1.56	1.32	1.43	11.4
Genitals	1.09	0.363	0.197	0.151	0.118	0.0679	0.125	22.3
Heart	0.328	0.190	0.129	0.107	0.0780	0.0518	0.0532	7.07
Lungs	0.663	0.306	0.192	0.151	0.101	0.0610	0.0655	10.7
Brain[d]	2.14	1.23	0.812	0.631	0.525	0.330	0.400	11.6
Skin	0.301	0.131	0.0588	0.0531	0.0438	0.0295	0.0330	14.5

a, b, c, d; see Table 3 for explanation.

A comparison of i.p. vs i.v. route for the 24 h data (Table 4) shows
that levels following i.p. injection are slightly but uniformly higher
than those following i.v. injection.

The persistence of [195mPt] activity in the tissues at longer times
(8 to 13 d) is consistent with the long $t_{1/2}$(b) of CHIP (and/or perhaps
a long-lived metabolite). Similar data were reported by Harrison, et
al,[5] who speculated that the higher tissue levels in their longer-term
studies could be artificially high due to the potential retention of
extraneous Ir daughter activity resulting from [191Pt] decay. While the
retention of Ir activity is possible, the two sets of data are in
qualitative accord, suggesting that the contribution of the Ir activity to
the total tissue activity may be less significant than was first thought.

TABLE 3. Distribution of [195m]Pt in (female) Fischer 344 rat tissues[a,b] as a function of time after administration (i.p.) of [195m]Pt-labeled CHIP[c]

Time, Post-Injection	% Injected Dose/Organ							% Deviation (Mean)
	0.25 h	1.0 h	6.0 h	24.0 h	3.0 d	8.0 d	13.0 d	
Tissue								
Blood	6.22	2.88	1.85	1.55	1.16	0.895	0.941	8.43
Liver	9.06	9.76	4.50	3.61	2.46	1.41	1.08	11.4
Spleen	0.185	0.121	0.0951	0.105	0.114	0.155	0.177	14.3
Pancreas	0.358	0.181	0.124	0.0992	0.0648	0.0507	0.0770	14.3
Stomach	0.670	0.443	0.173	0.418	0.082	0.0461	0.0390	29.8
S. Intestine	5.44	7.97	2.10	0.842	0.323	0.151	0.0990	21.0
Colon	1.53	0.659	11.2	5.65	0.820	0.279	0.145	27.5
Adrenals[d]	3.75	1.51	0.879	0.749	0.630	0.383	0.650	18.6
Kidneys	4.19	3.26	2.43	2.12	1.82	1.46	1.37	8.68
Genitals	0.468	0.144	0.0854	0.0687	0.0508	0.0303	0.0375	20.1
Heart	0.164	0.0932	0.0652	0.0533	0.0385	0.0271	0.0235	11.7
Lungs	0.499	0.254	0.167	0.126	0.0813	0.0553	0.0550	20.0
Brain[d]	3.40	2.00	1.31	1.04	0.850	0.550	0.600	18.0
Skin[e]	4.52	1.97	0.88	0.80	0.66	0.44	0.50	

[a] Rats ranged in weight from 137-175 g

[b] Eight rats/group except as follows: three and 13 d (four rats); 0.25, 1.0, and 6.0 h for stomach, intestine, colon, and skin (four rats)

[c] 7.5 mg/kg

[d] Divide data by 100 to obtain true values

[e] Based on 10% of body weight for a 150 g rat

A comparison of the tissue distribution of CHIP vs cis-DDP at 24 h postinjection (i.v.) shows that the tissue levels of CHIP are higher than those of cis-DDP in the colon, pancreas, liver (approximately twice as high) and to a lesser extent than that of the heart. Levels for all other tissues are either approximately the same or lower. If there is an association between tissue levels and chemotherapeutic effectiveness against cancers of the same tissue of origin, then CHIP might show a significantly better response than cis-DDP against colonic cancer since the levels of CHIP in the colon are approximately twice as high as those of cis-DDP.

Pt levels in the reproductive organs (uterus, fallopian tubes, ovaries) are substantially lower than for those of cis-DDP. On the same basis, then, one could speculate that CHIP may not be as potentially effective as cis-DDP against genito-urinary cancers. Although CHIP levels

TABLE 4. Distribution of ^{195m}Pt in (female) Fischer 344 rat tissues[a,b] 24 h after administration of ^{195m}Pt-labeled cis[dichlorotrans-dihydroxy-bis (isopropylamine)platinum(IV)], CHIP[c]

Route of Injection	I.P.	I.V.	Route of Injection	I.P.	I.V.
Tissue	% Dose g Tissue	% Dose g Tissue	Tissue	% Dose g Tissue	% Dose g Tissue
Blood	0.187	0.164	Adrenals	0.185	0.113
Liver	0.801	0.591	Kidneys	1.79	1.62
Spleen	0.297	0.202	Genitals	0.140	0.103
Pancreas	0.308	0.267	Heart	0.109	0.0985
Stomach	0.230	0.0908	Lungs	0.154	0.136
Intestine	0.166	0.102	Brain	0.0068	0.0070
Colon	0.967	0.669			

[a] 151-175 g

[b] Four rats/time period

[c] Dose = 7.5 mg/kg

in the kidney are higher than those of cis-DDP, CHIP is substantially less nephrotoxic suggesting that kidney toxicity is not solely a function of the amount of bound Pt in the kidney but rather is related to the intrinsic nature of the administered drug. Thus, one can continue to be optimistic about finding second-generation drugs which are less nephrotoxic.

The urine and fecal excretion data demonstrate that CHIP is excreted rapidly and exhibits at least biphasic excretion kinetics typical of most labeled Pt complexes studied to date. A semi-log plot of the cumulative % dose retained (urine plus feces) vs time is shown in Figure 5. Resolution of this curve into two components provides a graphical estimate of the fast (t1/2 = 8 h) and slow (t1/2 ≅ 15 d) phases. Loss of ^{195m}Pt-CHIP via the feces is considerably slower than via the urine and amounts to 23% of the injected activity on day 8. It is significant to note that the rate of fecal elimination is ten-fold higher for CHIP (23%) compared to cis-DDP (~2-3%).

3.2. Pharmacokinetics. Interpretation
of the radioactivity data obtained in
this study requires caution because
total rather than compound-specific
radioactivity in the blood, urine,
feces, and tissues was measured.
Interpretation of the pharmacokinetic parameters (Table 1) is
subject to the following assumptions/
limitations: (a) It was assumed that
absorption of CHIP from the peritoneal
cavity was complete. (b) The short
sampling period (8 days) relative to
the apparent $t_{1/2}(b)$ suggests that
the apparent $t_{1/2}(b)$ and the extrapolated area under the CHIP
concentration-time curve from 8 days
to infinity may be poorly determined.
Consequently, the value for Cl_b, which
is derived from the $AUC_{0-\infty}$ may also
be poorly estimated. A longer sampling

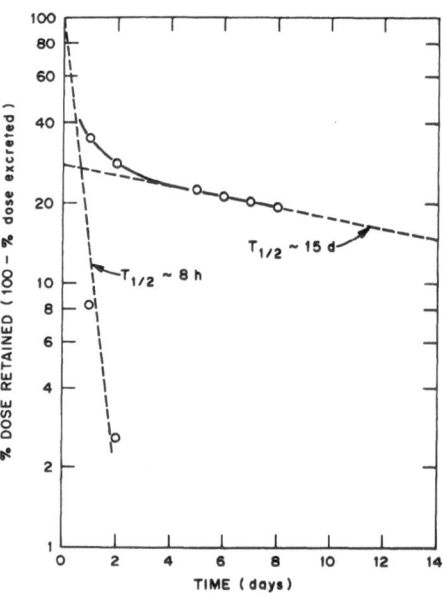

FIGURE 5   % Dose 195mpt-
CHIP retained in the rat;
graphical estimate of $t_{1/2}$ (b)

period was somewhat impractical in view of the short physical half-life of
195mpt (4.02 d); also, the need for such could not have been anticipated
a priori.

The concentration-time profile of CHIP in blood (figure not included)
shows an initially rapid decline in CHIP concentration followed by a
slower decline with an apparent $t_{1/2}(b)$ of 10.4 d. Comparison of the
renal and fecal clearance data (Fig. 3) shows that the fecal clearance of
CHIP is linear (i.e., first order) and that renal clearance is nonlinear.
The renal clearance data is, however, inconsistent with Michaelis-Menten
(capacity-limited) kinetics of renal elimination. The nonlinearity of
the renal clearance may be attributable to the relatively more rapid renal
elimination of CHIP during the early sampling periods (i.e., at high blood
concentrations) and less rapid renal elimination of a metabolite during
the later sampling periods (i.e., at low blood concentrations) and/or due

113

to a time-dependent decrease in renal function. The latter possibility
appears less likely since CHIP is much less nephrotoxic than cisplatin and
also because there was no apparent decrease in urine output with time.

REFERENCES

1. Shepard R, Kusnierczyk H, Jones M, and Harrap KR," Criteria for the
selection of second-generation platinum compounds," Br. J. Cancer (1980)
42, 668.
2. Hoeschele JD, Butler TA, and Roberts JA, "Correlations of physico-
chemical and biological properties with in vivo biodistribution data for
platinum-195m labeled chloroammineplatinum (II) complexes" Chapter 11
in A. E. Martell's Inorganic Chemistry in Biology and Medicine, ACS
Symposium Series No. 140, American Chemical Society, 1980.
3. Hoeschele JD, Butler TA, Roberts JA, and Guyer CE, "Analysis and
refinement of the microscale synthesis of the ^{195m}Pt labeled antitumor
drug cis-Dichlorodammineplatinum(II), cis-DDP, Radiochimica Acta (1982)
31, 27-36.
4. Gibaldi M, and Perrier D, "Pharmacokinetics," M. Dekker, Inc.,
NY (1982), 2nd.
5. Harrison R, McAuliffe CA, Zoki A, et al, "A comparative study of the
distribution in the male rat of platinum-labeled cis-dichlorodiammine-
platinum(II) cis-trans-dichlorodihydroxy-bis-(isopropylamine)platinum-
(IV), and cis-dichloro-bis (cyclopropylamine)platinum (II)," Cancer
Chemother Phamacol (1983) 10, 90-95.

Clinical Pharmacokinetics of *cis*-Dichloro-*trans*-Dihydroxy-*bis*(Isopropylamine)Platinum(IV)
L. Pendyala, J.W. Cowens, S. Madajewicz and P.J. Creaven

SUMMARY

The pharmacokinetics of total Pt, filterable Pt and unchanged drug were studied in patients receiving cis-dichloro-trans-dihydroxy-bis-isopropylamine Pt (IV) (CHIP) (20-350mg/m^2). Plasma decay of total Pt, and filterable Pt at doses $\geq$ 180mg/m^2 conform to a two compartment open model, with median half-lives of 69.3h and 33.0h, respectively. Plasma decay of unchanged CHIP and that of filterable Pt at doses 20-120 mg/m^2 conform to a one compartment model. The median half-life of unchanged CHIP is 1.17h. Urinary excretion of Pt ranges from 16-61% of the dose administered, at 24h. In addition to CHIP, two Pt containing species are seen in plasma and four in urine; one of these, less polar than CHIP, has been identified as cis-dichloro-bis-isopropylamine Pt II.

1. INTRODUCTION

Cis-dichloro-trans-dihydroxy-bis-isopropylamine platinum IV (CHIP) (Fig. 1), a quadrivalent, second generation platinum (Pt) complex, has been advanced to clinical trial because of its wide spectrum of activity and lack of renal toxicity in preclinical studies (1-5). In animals, the dose limiting toxicity was myelosuppression (4,6,7). In a phase I trial of widely spaced doses in which CHIP was administered as a 2h i.v. infusion, the maximum tolerated dose was found to be 350mg/M^2 with myelosuppression, particularly thrombocytopenia, being the dose limiting toxicity (8). No increase in serum creatinine or decrease in creatinine clearance was seen in this study. Initially, patients entered into this trial were hydrated with 2L of 0.5N saline over 12h before drug infusion at all the doses. This was omitted in some patients treated at the highest doses.

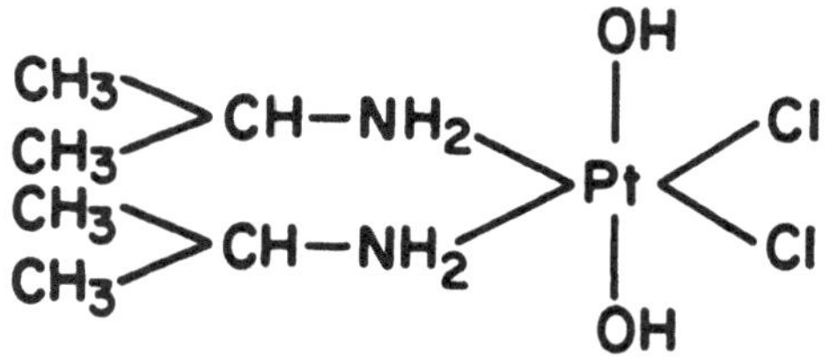

Figure 1. Structure of CHIP

The pharmacokinetics of CHIP during the phase I trial were studied both in patients who received pretreatment hydration and those who did not. The unchanged drug, filterable platinum and total platinum in the plasma were measured. In this paper we shall briefly review our experience to date with the pharmacokinetics of CHIP in man.

2. MATERIALS AND METHODS

2.1. <u>Sample Collection</u>. Blood (5-10ml) was collected at mid infusion, end infusion and at 0.08, 0.25, 0.5, 1.0, 1.5, 2, 4, 6, 12, 24h (and at 36 and 48h whenever possible) after the end of infusion. Blood was centrifuged immediately and plasma separated.

2.2. <u>Pt Estimations</u>. Duplicate 200μl aliquots of plasma were digested with 70% HNO_3. The residue was redissolved in an equal volume of 0.5% HCl; a 10-50μl aliquot of this digest was used for total Pt estimations by flameless atomic absorption spectrophotometry (FAAS) as previously described (9,10). The remaining plasma was ultrafiltered using Amicon CF25A ultrafiltration membranes. A 10-20μl aliquot was used directly for the measurement of filterable Pt species by FAAS. The remaining plasma ultrafiltrate was used for the measurement of unchanged CHIP. Urinary Pt was measured by FAAS directly.

2.3 <u>Measurement of Unchanged CHIP</u>. Unchanged CHIP was measured either by a previously reported high pressure liquid chromatography (HPLC) gradient elution procedure in conjunction with FAAS (9,10), or by a recently developed HPLC procedure with UV detection at 214nM. In the first procedure, fractions eluting from a C18 column during a 40min H_2O-MeOH gradient were collected and Pt in each fraction was measured by FAAS (10).

In the second procedure, separation of CHIP in plasma was carried
out on a Waters Associates μ Bondapak Phenyl Column with 10% methanol as
the mobile phase. At 1.5 ml/min flow rate the retention of CHIP was 5
min. Because of interference from the other plasma components at this
short wavelength, pretreatment of plasma ultrafiltrates was carried out
as follows: 0.5 ml of plasma ultrafiltrate was passed through 0.5-0.6ml
of a packed Dowex 2-X8 anion exchange resin (J.T. Baker), the column was
washed twice with 0.5 ml of distilled H_2O, and the washes were pooled
with the void volume. This procedure removed the majority of the
interfering plasma components with a 95.0 $\pm$ 5.1% recovery of CHIP as
evaluated in 24 separate analyses. An aliquot (25μL) of the eluate was
then injected into a Waters HPLC system. A chromatogram of the plasma
of a patient before and after receiving CHIP, using this procedure is
shown in Fig. 2. The detection limit of CHIP with this procedure is
0.5μg/ml of CHIP in plasma (0.24μg/ml of CHIP-Pt). Separation of CHIP
and other Pt species in urine was carried out by the HPLC gradient
elution procedure, in conjunction with FAAS, as described above.

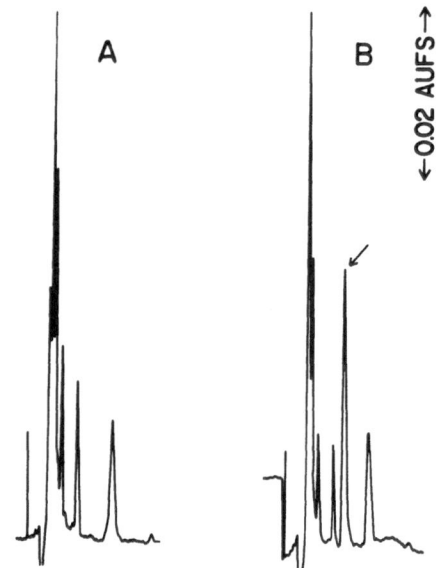

Figure 2.: HPLC separation of CHIP in plasma of a patient receiving the
drug (350mg/m^2) (Detection at 214nM). A. Plasma, before treatment. B. Plasma, 5 min after the end of infusion. The arrow indicates
CHIP. The peak shown here corresponds to 12μg/ml of CHIP in plasma.

2.4 <u>Data Analysis</u>. Plasma levels of unchanged CHIP, and filterable Pt at doses <180mg/m^2 were fitted to a one compartment open model using equation 1. Plasma levels of filterable Pt at doses >180mg/m^2 and that of total Pt at all doses were fitted to equation 2. Both these equations take into consideration the duration of drug infusion (11). By non-linear regression analysis using the computer program NONLIN or BMDP on a Univac 90/80, while fitting the plasma levels of the 3 species to the above equations, empirical parameters, A, α, B, β were generated and used to calculate all the other pharmacokinetic parameters[*] reported in this paper.

Equ. 1. $C_p = \dfrac{A(1-e^{\alpha T})e^{-\alpha t}}{\alpha T}$

Equ. 2. $C_p = \dfrac{A(1-e^{\alpha T})e^{-\alpha t}}{\alpha T} + \dfrac{B(1-e^{-\beta T})e^{-\beta t}}{\beta T}$

Differences between parameters were explored using Statistical Package for Social Sciences (SPSS) (12).

3. RESULTS

Plasma decay profiles of the 3 Pt species namely, total Pt, filterable Pt and unchanged CHIP in a patient receiving CHIP (350 mg/m^2) without pretreatment hydration is shown in Fig.3. The pharmacokinetic parameters derived for each of these species is given in Table 1. The pharmacokinetic characteristics of each of the species is described below.

3.1 <u>Total Pt</u>. Plasma decay of total Pt is biphasic, and fits a two compartment open model at all the doses studied (20-350mg/m^2). It has a short $t_{1/2}\alpha$ (median 1.01h) and a long $t_{1/2}\beta$ (median 69.3h) which appears to be a result of the extensive plasma protein binding of the Pt metabolites of CHIP. In all the patients studied 90-95% of the total Pt was protein bound by 12-15h after the end of CHIP infusion.

---

[*]Symbols used in this paper are defined as follows: C_p is the concentration of drug in plasma; t is the post infusion time; T is the duration of the infusion; $t_{1/2}\alpha$, $t_{1/2}\beta$ are half-lives for the α and β phase, respectively; CL is the plasma clearance; V_c is the volume of distribution of the central compartment, V_2 is the volume of the peripheral compartment; K_{12}, K_{21} are intercompartmental distribution rate constants, K_{10} is the elimination rate constant from the central compartment.

118

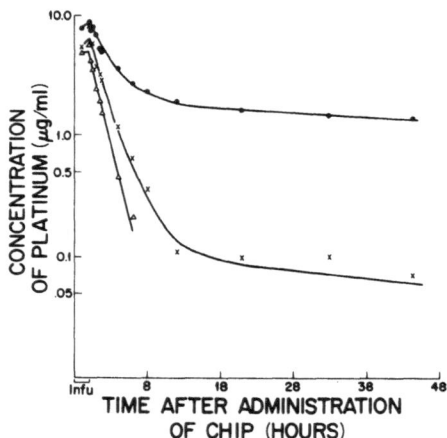

TIME AFTER ADMINISTRATION
OF CHIP (HOURS)

Figure 3.: Plasma decay of total Pt (-•-), filterable Pt (-X-) and CHIP-Pt (-△-) in a patient receiving CHIP (350mg/m^2). Data points shown are the experimental values, the curves are the computer generated least squares fits.

   The pharmacokinetic parameters shown in Table 1 are medians (with ranges in parentheses) derived from all the patients studied. Hydrating the patient before CHIP administration appears to affect some of the pharmacokinetic parameters but not others. The intercompartmental distribution rate constants, which are not affected by pretreatment hydration indicate larger k_{12} than k_{21}. The k_{10} of total Pt is smaller (median 0.06h^{-1}) than the other rate constants (k_{12} and k_{21}) and also smaller than that for filterable Pt.

   3.2 Unchanged CHIP. The plasma decay of unchanged CHIP is mono-phasic and fits a one compartment open model at all the doses (Fig. 3) (10). The median half-life of CHIP is short (median 1.17h) (Table 1). The decay curve shown in Fig. 3 is derived using the new HPLC method, which reduced the analysis time of CHIP decay in patients from 2 1/2 wks to 1 1/2 days and gave similar results to the previously used method. The median volume of distribution of unchanged CHIP is 24.7L (14.2-47.7L), similar to that seen with filterable Pt at doses <180mg/m^2; the plasma clearance is larger than that of the other 2 Pt species.

Table 1: A Summary of the Pharmacokinetic Parameters[a] in Patients Receiving CHIP

| Parameters | Total Pt (N=17) | Filterable Pt | | CHIP (N=13) |
		1-Compartment Model (N=5)	2-Compartment Model (N=9)	
$t_{1/2\alpha}(h)$	1.01 (0.34-2.23)	1.75 (1.45-2.05)	1.50 (0.84-1.93)	1.17 (0.64-1.38)
$t_{1/2\beta}(h)$	69.30 (32.1-124.0)	-	33.00 (12.8-54.6)	-
V_c (L)	12.80* (8.2-24.9)	28.10 (21.1-39.2)	26.50 (12.0-41.6)	24.70 (14.2-47.7)
V_2 (L)	57.30 (21.9-107.8)	-	318.50 (166.0-968.0)	-
CL $(L.h^{-1})$	0.85* (0.29-1.8)	11.60 (7.2-15.5)	11.00 (3.7-12.3)	17.80 (8.1-25.9)
$K_{12}(h^{-1})$	0.48 (0.23-1.61)	-	0.11 (0.07-0.44)	-
$K_{21}(h^{-1})$	0.12 (0.05-0.38)	-	0.03 (0.02-0.07)	-
$K_{10}(h^{-1})$	0.06 (0.03-0.13)	-	0.37 (0.22-0.58)	-

[a]Values reported are medians (range in the parenthesis)
*When the parameters were compared between patients who received prehydration and those who did not, significant differences were found (see text).
- Not applicable.

3.3 Filterable Pt. The pharmacokinetics of filterable Pt differed from those of unchanged CHIP and total Pt in that at lower doses (20-120 mg/m^2) it shows a monoexponential decay, conforming to a single compartment model, and at doses >180mg/m^2 the decay is clearly biexponential conforming to a 2 compartment open model. It is presumed that this dose dependent difference is due to limitations in detection of this species at later time points at lower doses. A summary of the pharmacokinetic parameters of filterable Pt fitted to one and two compartment models is presented in Table 1. The median $t_{1/2\alpha}$ of filterable Pt with 2 compartment fit is 1.5h (0.84 - 1.93h), and the $t_{1/2\beta}$ is 33.0h (12.8 - 54.6h), the latter being approximately half that for total Pt. A noteworthy feature of the pharmacokinetic parameters of filterable Pt compared to total Pt and unchanged CHIP is the large volume of the peripheral compartment , indicating a large tissue localization of this species. The intercompartmental distribution rate constants again indicate larger k_{12} than k_{21} as for total Pt. The elimination rate constant k_{10} however is much larger for filterable Pt (median 0.37h^{-1}), compared to that for total Pt (median 0.06h^{-1}) presumably because the plasma protein binding limits the excretion of the total Pt species. The plasma clearance of filterable Pt is greater than that of total Pt but lower than unchanged CHIP.

3.4 Effect of Omitting Hydration on Pharmacokinetics of CHIP. As indicated above, initially during the clinical trial, patients received 2L of pretreatment hydration. Because no renal toxicity was noted at myelosuppressive doses, it was decided to omit the hydration and was found not to alter the clinical toxicity of CHIP. The plasma decay profiles of the 3 Pt species are not different when hydration is omitted. However, a comparison of the pharmacokinetic parameters of the 3 platinum species between patients receiving hydration and those not receiving it, indicated a possible difference in V_c, V_2, and CL of total Pt. A statistical evaluation of these parameters using the Mann-Whitney test (12), indicated a significant difference in V_c and CL (P<0.05), and a suggestive difference in V_2 (P=0.07). With hydration the values for V_c, CL and V_2 were, 10.9L (8.2-18.8L), 0.76L.h^{-1}(0.29-1.10L.h^{-1}), and 44.1L(21.9-107.8L) respectively (N=11), while with no hydration the values were 21.3L(9.5-24.9L),

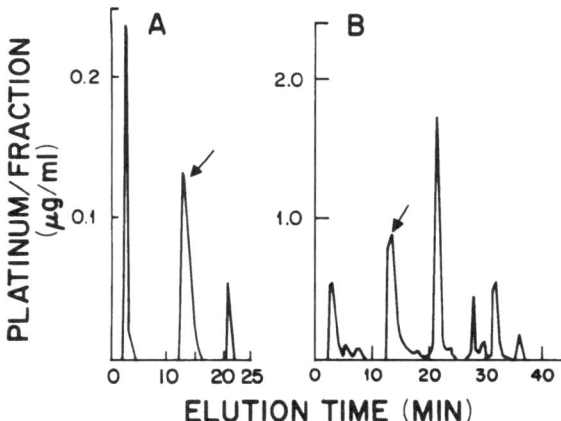

ELUTION TIME (MIN)

Figure 4.: CHIP and other Pt containing species in plasma (A) and urine (B) of a patient who received CHIP (40 mg/m^2). Arrows indicate CHIP. A. 15 Min after infusion; B. urine collected during infusion.

$1.08L.h^{-1}(0.75-1.8L.h^{-1})$, and $82.9L$ (56.4-104.0L),   (n=6).   The clinical significance of these differences in pharmacokinetic parameters of total Pt is unclear at this time.

3.5 Urinary Excretion of Pt. The urinary excretion of Pt is rapid initially but slows markedly by 10h. An overall excretion of 16-61% in the first 24h was found in a total of 25 patients studied. When renal clearance of total Pt was calculated for the patients for whom both plasma and urine data were available a pattern emerged similar to that suggested by Crom et al., for cisplatin (13). Although the renal clearance of Pt is initially high, it falls rapidly presumably because of the effect of protein binding and metabolism on renal excretion of Pt (10).

3.6 Separation and Identification of Other Pt Containing Species in Plasma and Urine. By H$_2$O-MeOH gradient elution on HPLC in conjunction with FAAS, CHIP was separated from other Pt containing species in plasma and urine. Two species, one more polar than CHIP and another less polar were detected in plasma (Fig. 4A). In urine, in addition to the two species detected in plasma (Fig. 4B), three more Pt containing species were detected. Although CHIP formed the bulk of non-protein bound Pt species initially, the polar Pt species increased with time and was the predominant species by 8-12h after CHIP administration in both plasma and urine. One Pt species eluting at 22min (present both in plasma and urine), has been identified by means of co-chromatography and mass spectrometry as the reduced form of CHIP namely cis-dichloro-bis-iso-propylamine Pt (II) (14).

4. DISCUSSION

Analysis of the pharmacokinetics of Pt containing species after infusion of CHIP revealed that the pharmacokinetics are linear (10) and that there is a marked difference between the pharmacokinetics of the three Pt species. Unchanged CHIP has a half-life of about an hour, while that for total Pt is about 3 days. Filterable Pt (at doses ≥ 180 mg/m^2) is intermediate between the total Pt and unchanged CHIP, having a half-life of about 33.0h. By 15h after the drug infusion, 90-95% of the Pt in plasma is bound to protein in plasma and as shown earlier, since CHIP itself does not bind to plasma proteins (9), the protein bound Pt must constitute CHIP metabolites.

Of the 3 Pt species measured the filterable Pt had a large volume of distribution of the peripheral compartment indicating tissue localiza-tion of some of the non-protein bound CHIP metabolites. In agreement with the observed half-lives of each of the Pt species, the plasma clearance of filterable Pt was greater than that of total Pt and that of unchanged CHIP was greater than that of filterable Pt. The inter-compartmental distribution rate constants (k_{12} and k_{21}) for both total Pt and filterable Pt indicate a rapid transfer of these species from central to the peripheral compartment, compared to that in the opposite direction. Pretreatment hydration has no effect on the pharmacokinetics of unchanged CHIP and filterable Pt, the two species presumably related to the activity.

It has been suggested by Tobe and Khokhar, that the quadrivalent Pt compounds may be reduced to the divalent form in a biological situation and that the divalent species may be the active species while the quadrivalent form is a novel way of administering an otherwise poorly

water soluble species (15). In our studies cis dichloro bis isopropylamine Pt (II) was identified as one of the Pt species found both in plasma
and urine. The significance of this finding with respect to the antitumor
activity or toxicity of CHIP is not known at this time.

The pharmacokinetics of total Pt and CHIP appear to be similar in the
different species studied. As in man, the total Pt conformed to a biexponential decay in rat and dog, with $t_{1/2}\alpha$ of less than 1h in both cases
and the $t_{1/2}\beta$ of 14h and 39.4h, respectively (6,7,9). The half-life of
UC-CHIP in dog was 0.3-0.5h as evaluated by urinary excretion rates (9).

The human pharmacokinetics of parent CHIP resemble those of parent
cisplatin, with a monoexponential decay and short half-life compared to
total Pt. The half-life of CHIP, however, appears to be 2-3 times longer than that of the reported values for cisplatin (16,17). The pharmacokinetics of total Pt after CHIP are similar to that reported after cisplatin, with a prolonged elimination phase (13,17-21). The pharmacokinetics of filterable Pt after CHIP up to doses of 120 mg/m^2 are similar
to those reported for cisplatin at similar doses, showing a monoexponential
decay. However, at higher doses of CHIP, the pharmacokinetcs of filterable Pt are markedly different, showing a biexponential plasma decay with
a prolonged elimination phase half life (median 33.0h). Whether or not
this represents a true difference between the two drugs or a dose effect
cannot be determined. The dose limiting toxicity after cisplatin is renal toxicity while that after CHIP is myelosuppression. Since plasma
decay of the two drugs show similar kinetics, it appears the difference
in toxicity may be a reflection of the differences of molecular interaction at the cellular level of non-protein bound metabolites, or the
unchanged drug itself.

5. ACKNOWLEDGEMENT

This work was supported by a USPHS Grant, CA-21071 from the National
Cancer Institute and by Bristol Laboratories, Syracuse, NY.

The expert technical assistance of Miss Mary Bajzik and the assistance of Mrs. Joan Solomon and Miss April Perry are gratefully acknowledged.

124

REFERENCES

1. Bradner WT, Rose WC, Huftalen JB. 1980. Antitumor activity of platinum analogs. In Cisplatin, Current Status and New Developments. Prestayko AW, Crooke ST, Carter SD, eds. Academic Press, Inc., New York, p. 171-182.
2. Cleare MJ, Hydes PC, Walerbi BW, Watkins DM. 1978. Antitumor platinum complexes: Relationship between chemical properties and activity. Biochimie 60: 835-850.
3. Connors TA, Cleare MJ, Harrap KR. 1979. Structure activity relationships of the antitumor platinum coordination complexes. Cancer Treat Rept 63: 1499-1502.
4. Mihich E, Bullard G, Pavelic Z, Creaven PJ. 1979. Preclinical studies of dihydroxy-cis-dichloro-bis-isopropylamine platinum IV (CHIP). Proc Am Assoc Cancer Res and Amer Soc Clin Oncol 20: 426.
5. Prestayko AW, Bradner WT, Huftalen JB, Rose WE, Schurig JE, Cleare MJ, Hydes PC, Crooke ST. 1979. Antileukemic (L1210) activity and toxicity of cis-dichloro-diammineplatinum (II) analogs. Cancer Treat Rept 63: 1503-1507.
6. Creaven PJ, Mihich E. 1981. Preclinical and clinical pharmacology in drug development. In New Leads in Cancer Therapeutics. Mihich E, Ed. GK Hall Medical Publishers, Boston, p. 1-26.
7. Pfister M, Pavelic ZP, Bullard GA, Mihich E, Creaven PJ. 1978. Dichlorodihydroxybisisopropylamine platinum IV, a new antitumor platinum complex. Pharmacokinetics in the rat; relation to renal toxicity. Biochimie 60: 1057.
8. Creaven PJ, Madajewicz S, Pendyala L, Mittelman A, Pontes E, Spaulding M, Arbuck S, Solomon J. 1983. Phase I clinical trial of cis-dichloro-trans-dihydroxy-bis-isopropylamine platinum IV (CHIP). Cancer Treat Rept (in press).
9. Pendyala L, Cowens JW, Creaven PJ. 1982. Studies on the pharmacokinetics and metabolism of cis-dichloro-trans-dihydroxy-bis-isopropylamine platinum IV in the dog. Cancer Treat Rept 66: 509-516.
10. Pendyala L, Greco W, Cowens JW, Madajewicz S, Creaven PJ. 1983. Pharmacokinetics of cis-dichloro-trans-dihydroxy-bis-isopropylamine platinum IV (CHIP) in patients with advanced cancer. Cancer Chemoth and Pharmacol. (in press).
11. Loo JK, Riegelman S. 1970. Assessment of pharmacokinetic constants from post infusion blood curves obtained after IV infusion. J Pharm Sci 59: 53-55.
12. Nie NH, Hull CH, Jenkins JG, Steinbrenner K, Bent OH. 1975. SPSS, Statistical Package for the Social Sciences, 2nd ed. McGraw-Hill Book Co., New York.
13. Crom WR, Evans WE, Pratt CB, Senzer N, Denison M, Green AA, Hayes FA, Yee GC. 1981. Cisplatin disposition in children and adolescents with cancer. Cancer Chemoth and Pharmcol 6: 95-99.
14. Pendyala L, Cowens JW, Creaven PJ. 1982. Metabolic studies in man of cis-dichloro-trans-dihydroxy-bis-isopropylamine Pt IV (CHIP): A new anticancer drug. Proc 13th Intern Cancer Congress, Seattle, 531.
15. Tobe M, Khokhar A. 1977. Structure, activity, reactivity and solubility relationships of platinum diamine complexes. J Clin Hematol and Oncol 7: 114-137.

16. Himmelstein KJ, Patton TF, Belt RJ, Taylor S, Repta AJ, Sternson LA. 1981. Clinical kinetics of intact cisplatin and some related species. Clin Pharmacol and Therap 29: 658-664.
17. Patton TF, Repta AJ, Sternson LA, Belt RJ. 1982. Pharmacokinetics of intact cisplatin in plasma. Infusion vs. bolus dosing. Int J Pharmaceutics 10: 77-85.
18. DeConti RC, Toftness BP, Lang RC, Creasey WA. 1973. Clinical and pharmacological studies with cis-diammine-dichloro-platinum (II). Cancer Res 33: 1310-1315.
19. Gormley PE, Bull JM, LeRoy AF, Cysyk R. 1979. Kinetics of cis-dichloro-diammineplatinum. Clin Pharmacol and Therap 25: 351-357.
20. Gullo JJ, Litterst CL, Maguire PJ, Sikic BI, Hoth DF, Wooley PV. 1980. Pharmacokinetics and protein binding of cis-dichlorodiammine platinum (II) administered as one hour or as a 20h infusion. Cancer Chemother and Pharmacol 5: 21-26.
21. Smith PHS, Taylor DM. 1974. Distribution and retention of the antitumor agent. [195m]Pt-cis-dichloro-diammine-platinum II in man. J Nucl Med 15: 349-351.

Disposition of Cisplatin *vs* Total Platinum in Animals and Man

L.A. Sternson, A.J. Repta, H. Shih, K.J. Himmelstein and T.F. Patton

Optimal clinical performance of antineoplastic agents is realized by maximizing cytotoxicity toward cancerous elements while limiting drug action on normal tissue. Effectiveness is controlled by the absorption, distribution and excretion characteristics of the drug as well as its biotransformation pattern. Biotransformation is a particularly important consideration in clinical utilization of chemically reactive molecules, such as cisplatin. Such compounds are known to rapidly degrade once in contact with blood components (1). This breakdown apparently results from nucleophilic displacement of chloride ligands by endogenous nucleophiles either directly or through aquated-platinum intermediates (2). Coordination of platinum with these nucleophiles yields complexes apparently exhibiting different spectra of biological activity and toxicity, and different distribution and excretion characteristics. Thus, a discussion of the clinical pharmacology and pharmacokinetics of cisplatin must be based on quantitative data describing the fate of the individual platinum species differing in ligand composition about the metal as well as an evaluation of the biological activity of these individual biodegradation products. Although the degradation reactions are apparently not enzyme-mediated, general "metabolic" pathways should be definable; the structure of specific reaction products, however, may vary among individuals, being determined by the nature and concentration of potential reactant molecules (those with available nucleophilic centers) which in turn are influenced by a variety of environmental, dietary and health factors. This chapter describes some of the sensitive analytical methodology developed in our laboratories to selectively monitor individual platinum-containing species and the application of that technology to begin to describe the disposition of cisplatin in man in clinically relevant situations and in animals.

ANALYTICAL METHODOLOGY

Methodology (for platinum-containing species) that responds to platinum irrespective of the ligands coordinated with it has been developed in our laboratory (3,4) as well as by others (5) and has been based primarily on atomic absorption spectroscopic determinations or radiochemical techniques (6,7) involving counting of ^{193m}Pt or ^{195m}Pt labels. Such measurements are useful in defining the distribution of total platinum species in various tissues as well as in establishing a mass balance of platinum when speciation based on ligand composition is to be carried out. Total platinum determination by atomic absorption has been plagued by imprecision, due to the dependency of the absorption signal on the sample matrix. This problem has now been overcome by digesting the sample directly in the atomic absorption furnace prior to atomization (4).

Still, the reactivity of cisplatin demands methodology allowing for discrimination among platinates. Following its administration, cisplatin rapidly (> 90% loss in 1-2 hr) and irreversible reacts with protein to form complexes devoid of cytotoxicity (as determined in cell culture experiments). Thus it is imperative to be able to discriminate between the free-circulating and protein bound fractions of platinum in plasma to make meaningful correlations between blood levels and activity and/or toxicity. This gross separation has been accomplished by centrifugal ultrafiltration (3,8). Subsequent fractionation of platinum species in the ultrafiltrate has required high efficiency liquid chromatography (HPLC).

Neutral and anionic divalent platinum complexes are retained on dynamic anion exchange columns prepared by adsorption of hexadecyltrimethylammonium bromide on the surface of octadecyl-silane bonded stationary phases (9,10). Retention is significant in pure water and can be decreased by increasing organic modifier concentration or ionic strength of the mobile phase or elevating temperature. Solute retention can also be controlled by the addition of electrolytes to the mobile phase (10), where salt-type and concentration determine whether retention increases or decreases relative to that observed in pure water.

However, even in the best situations, cisplatin coelutes with some biological components. The problem is exacerbated by the long retention of several other endogenous components. This problem could be overcome using a column-switching approach in which the dynamic anion exchanger was preceeded by a silica pre-column (11). These two columns exhibited different selectivities and could be exploited to achieve complete resolution of cisplatin and biological components. Chromatographic resolution of platinum-protein complexes, on the other hand, could only be achieved by reverse phase chromatography (12) using gradient elution with increasing amounts of organic modifier added to an initially aqueous mobile phase.

Although platinates in column effluent can be monitored by UV spectroscopy, the poor sensitivity of this technique toward these compounds (due to their low molar absorptivities) has led to the general use of off-line atomic absorption spectroscopy for platinum detection (9-12). Several highly specific, on-line HPLC detectors responsive to low levels of platinum-species have also recently been described. A polarographic detector incorporating a hanging mercury drop electrode, operated at 60° C at a potential of 0.00 V (vs Ag/AgCl), has been successfully utilized to monitor cisplatin in urine (13). By careful manipulation of cell parameters, the noise limited minimum quantities of cisplatin detected with this system was 70 pg injected. Unfortunately, detector response was highly dependent on the nature of the ligands coordinated to platinum.

A post-column reactor has also been designed in which platinates in column effluent are "activated" by mixing with dichromate solution and then allowed to react with sodium bi-sulfite (14). The resulting chromophoric products are detected spectrophotometrically at 290 nm. This detector offers sensi-tivity toward cisplatin (Fig. 1) similar to that observed using the electrochemical monitor, but also responds strongly to other

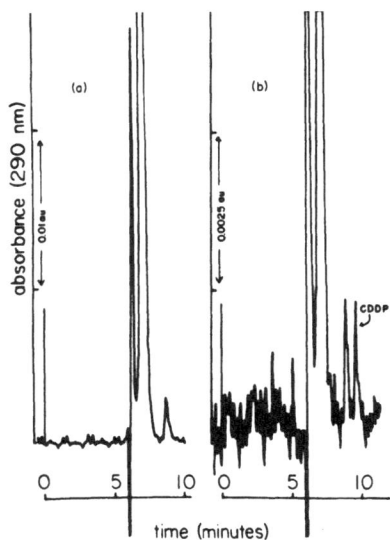

FIGURE 1. Post-column reactor response to plasma ultrafiltrate blank (a) and plasma ultrafiltrate containing cisplatin (equivalent to 5.1 ng of platinum). Chromatographic conditions: 100 X 4.6 mm, 5 μ Hypersil ODS column coated with HTAB; pH 5.0, 10 mM citrate with 10^{-4} M HTAB mobile phase; 1.0 ml/min, 290 nm.

platinates differing in ligand composition. These systems offer methodology capable of detecting low levels of various platinum complexes in biological fluids where emphasis is also placed on imparting high degrees of ligand specificity, thus permitting the execution of more detailed studies of the biodisposition of cisplatin and other platinum complexes.

Clinical Pharmacokinetics

The clinical pharmacokinetics of intact drug, total filterable platinum and total platinum were investigated in 24 patients after i.v. administration of cisplatin (10 min infusion) (15). Patients were studied at two commonly used dosage levels (50 mg/M^2) and 100 mg/M^2) and were further stratified with respect to the use of mannitol pretreatment to reduce nephrotoxicity.

The shape of the profiles for all three species was essentially identical for all patients in all four groups (Fig. 2).

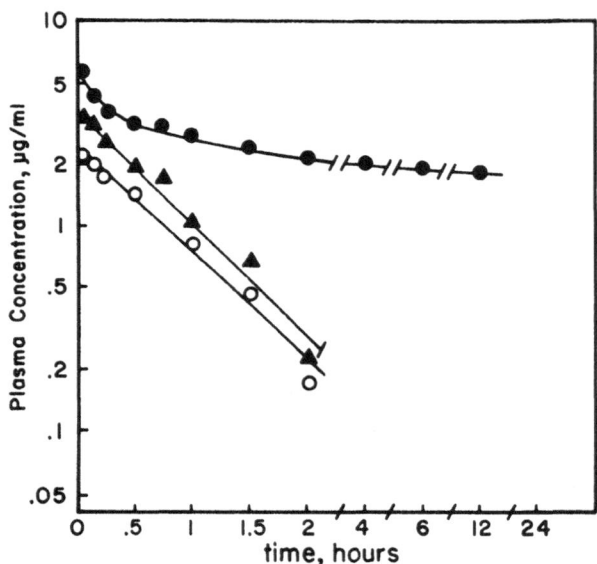

FIGURE 2. Plasma concentration-time profiles for total platinum (●), total filterable platinum (▲) and cisplatin (O) in a patient after administration of 100 mg/m² of cisplatin by rapid intra-venous injection (no mannitol pretreatment).

A tri-exponential curve best fit plasma levels of total platinum with distribution half-lives phases of 20 min and 1 hr (distribu-tion complete in ∿ 2 hr) and a terminal phase half-life of > 24 hr.   Cisplatin and total filterable platinum plasma levels declined monoexponentially with half-lives of ∿ 0.4-0.5 hr. Plasma concentration profiles of cisplatin paralleled but were somewhat lower than filterable species.   Levels were somewhat less than proportional to dose suggesting that sites to which platinum is bound or distributes are not saturated at observed levels.   For a given method of administration (with or without mannitol) there was no significant difference between the mean terminal slopes of total filterable platinum and cisplatin (P ≤ 0.05).   Thus, total filterable platinum levels may be a useful clinical indicator of cisplatin levels.   Total platinum values, however, bear little relationship to intact cisplatin levels and may be of questionable value in studies aimed at relating drug levels and cytotoxicity.   Ratios of cisplatin to total platinum decreased from ∿ 0.6 at the earliest sampling time (5 min post dose) to < 0.10, 2 hr after administration in all four groups of patients. This rapid and consistent decline suggests that either platinum species other than the parent drug, which predominate soon after administration, play a role in the manifested activity and toxicity (i.e., cisplatin is a "prodrug") or cytotoxic activity and toxicity potential is lost relatively rapidly following completion of cisplatin administration.

The ratios of cisplatin to total filterable platinum, however, remain relatively constant (∿ 0.6-0.8) for the entire time course over which both species could be monitored. It thus appears that a rapidly established equilibrium is maintained between cisplatin and filterable biotransformation products during the period over which they could be measured.

Urinary excretion of platinum was also monitored in the clinical setting (16). In the first 1-2 hr post infusion, ∿ 15% of the administered dose is excreted with > 90% of the urinary platinum present as cisplatin. Subsequent urinary excretion of platinum is slow and devoid of measurable quantities of parent drug. A number of other platinum-containing complexes were also found in the urine of patients following cisplatin administration. One of these has been tentatively identified as a 2:1 methionine: platinum(II) adduct, 1, by secondary ion negative ion mass spectrometry (Fig. 3) and comparison with synthesized material

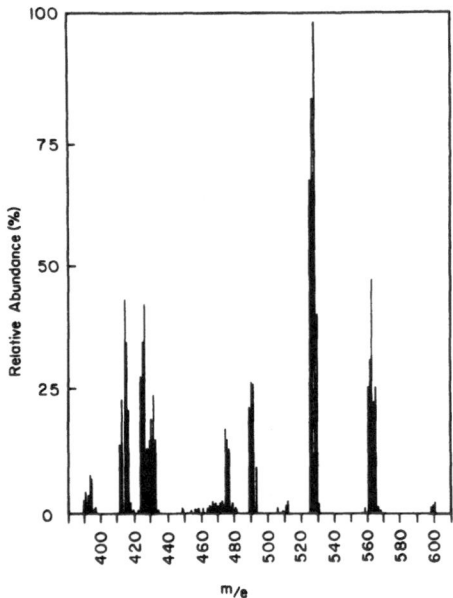

FIGURE 3. Negative-ion secondary-ion mass spectrum of the purified reaction product of cisplatin and methionine obtained in a glycerol matrix using Cs^+ ion bombardment.

(17). Electron impact, chemical ionization and field desorption techniques failed to yield discernible mass spectra of platinates; however, secondary ion or fast atom bombardment sources gave readily interpretable spectra (i.e., molecular ions and characteristic fragmentation patterns). These techniques appear to be of general utility in identification of metal-protein complexes (18,19). The methionine adduct, 1, has previously been shown to form directly from reaction of cisplatin with methionine (17), although its formation in vivo may involve other synthetic routes. It is presumed that additional biotransformation products are similarly formed by nucleophilic displacement of ligands coordinated with platinum and that that physical and chemical properties of the groups bonded to the metal determine its distribution characteristics, biological activity and toxicity.

In another series of five patients, receiving cisplatin (100 mg/M^2 i.v. over 10 min) for treatment of advanced or metastatic head and neck cancer, not only were blood levels measured, but accumulation of platinum in tumor tissue was also determined (by sequential biopsy from exophytic but not necrotic tumor) (20). Detectable amounts of platinum were found in tumor in all patients studied from 15 min to 24 hr post-infusion, with the highest concentration found 6 hr after dosing. As shown in Fig. 4, for a patient with a previously untreated posterior wall

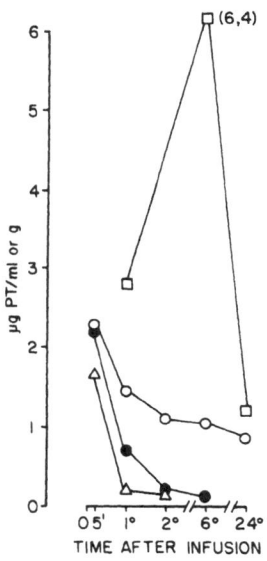

FIGURE 4. Concentrations of tumor platinum (□), total plasma Pt (O), filterable Pt (●) and cisplatin (Δ) in a patient with an esophogeal tumor, after receiving cisplatin (100 mg/m^2) by IV infusion. Plasma platinum is expressed as µg/ml and tumor platinum in µg Pt/g of tumor (wet weight).

squamous carcinoma, following cisplatin administration, tumor levels of 2.7, 6.4 and 1.4 µg/g of wet tissue were measured 1, 6 and 24 hr post-infusion, respectively. This patient had a partial clinical response to platinum therapy. The intratumor concentration was higher than could be explained on the basis of intravascular plasma platinum at the time of biopsy and suggests accumulation by the tumor. The cytotoxicity of the platinum (determined as total platinum) species concentrated in the tissue is not known, but is ostensibly covalently protein bound material.

Since the gross shape of the plasma concentration-time curves for the three species and the species ratios do not change as a function of method of administration, it was hypothesized that it may be possible to predict cisplatin levels regardless of the dosing schedule using a simple pharmacokinetic technique. The plasma drug level data from six patients who had received cis-platin (100 mg/M^2) without mannitol as a short i.v. infusion were used (15) to calculate the following mean pharmacokinetic parameters (21) for cisplatin: (mean dose = 180 mg) area under the plasma concentration time curve (0-120 min) = 104 µg min ml^{-1}, elimination rate constant = 2.48 X 10^{-2} min^{-1}, $t_{1/2}$ = 27.9 min, extrapolated plasma concentration at time zero = 31.3 µg/ml and volume of distribution = 57.5 liters.

Using these parameters, a hypothetical case was considered in which cisplatin was dosed (180 mg or 100 mg/M^2), 20% by bolus and 80% by 6-hour infusion (21). The bolus would serve as loading dose to achieve plasma levels of cisplatin which could then be maintained by the infusion. For a drug that declines from the plasma mono-exponentially such as cisplatin, plasma levels following combination bolus and infusion dosing can be described by Eq. 1:

$$C = C_o e^{-Kt} + \frac{k_o}{VK} (1 - e^{-Kt}) \qquad \text{Eq. 1}$$

where C is the plasma concentration at any time; C_o is the initial concentration following a single dose; K is the elimination rate constant; t is time; k_o is the infusion rate and V is the volume of distribution. At steady state, this expression simplifies to

$$C_{ss} = \frac{k_o}{VK} \qquad \text{Eq. 2}$$

which describes the plateau plasma levels, C_{ss}, for a drug given by i.v. infusion.

The hypothetical (calculated) values obtained using this treatment were compared to those obtained in 4 patients receiving 100 mg/M^2 of cisplatin by a combination of i.v. rapid infusion (20% of dose) and the remainder by a 6-hour infusion (15,21).

The calculated profile gave an AUC of 113 µg min ml^{-1} (5 min to end of infusion). The AUC's for the 4 patients studied here were 137, 132, 139 and 137. The agreement with prediction

is reasonable considering both patient variability and the variations in the infusion rates. Secondly, the hypothetical case
predicts plateau cisplatin levels of 0.28 µg/ml. The actual mean
plateau values for cisplatin in the 4 patients was 0.35 µg/ml.
Finally, the consistency of hypothetical and actual patient plasma
levels indicates that with a given dose, the pharmacokinetic
behavior of cisplatin is independent of the method of administration. Such predictability could be important ultimately in de-
signing dosage regimens of cisplatin based on therapeutic and
toxic drug levels.

Animal Pharmacokinetics

The disposition of cisplatin was also studied in male rats
administered the drug intravenously at doses of 1.5 or 2.5 mg/kg
of body weight. As shown in Fig. 5, cisplatin and filterable

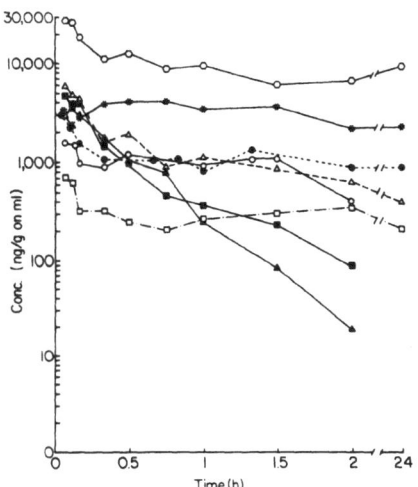

FIGURE 5. Platinum concentrations in rats administered cisplatin
(1.5 mg/kg) iv. Data points represent the average of at least 5
animals. (◯) kidney; (*) liver; (●) lung; (O) intestine; (△)
plasma (total Pt); (◻) muscle; (■) filterable platinum; (▲) cisplatin.

platinum plasma levels decline rapidly and in parallel to one
another, while total platinum plasma levels rapidly decrease
reaching a plateau after ∿ 1 hr. Levels were dose dependent but
not directly proportional to dose. Trends in plasma levels (22)
were identical to those observed in man (15). Platinum

determined as total platinum (irrespective of ligand coordinated with it) concentrated primarily in the kidney, with appreciable levels being found in liver, lung and intestines (Fig. 5) as seen by other investigators (23,24) as well. No significant accumulation of platinum was observed in brain tissue, in agreement with data reported by others (6,23). Speciation of the tissue bound platinum was not possible.

In summary, advances in analytical methodology and a greater understanding of the chemistry of platinum-containing antineoplastic agents is allowing for a more complete and rigorous description of the disposition of such drugs. This information will facilitate the design, evaluation and clinical utilization of cisplatin and its future generation analogs.

REFERENCES
1. Butour JL, Macquet JP. 1978. Europ J Biochem, 78, 455; 83, 375.
2. Repta AJ, Long DF. 1980, in "Cisplatin: Current Status and New Developments", Prestayko AW, Crooke ST, Carter SK, eds., Academic Press, New York, pp. 285-304.
3. Bannister SJ, Sternson LA, Repta AJ. 1978. Clin Chem, 24, 877.
4. Preisner D, Sternson LA, Repta AJ. 1981. Anal Letters, 14, 1255.
5. LeRoy AF, Wehling ML, Sponseller H, et al. 1977. Biochem Med, 18, 184 and references therein.
6. DeConti RC, Toftness BR, Lange RC, Creasy WA. 1973. Cancer Treat Rept, 33, 1310.
7. DeSimone PA, Yancey RS, Coupal JJ, Butts JD, Hoeschele JD. 1979. Cancer Treat Rept, 63, 951.
8. Bannister SJ, Sternson LA, Repta AJ, James GW. 1977. Clin Chem, 23, 2258.
9. Riley CM, Sternson LA, Repta AJ. 1981. J Chromatogr, 217, 405.
10. Riley CM, Sternson LA, Repta AJ. 1981. J Chromatogr, 219, 235.
11. Riley CM, Sternson LA, Repta AJ, Siegler RS. 1982. J Chromatogr, 229, 373.
12. Riley CM, Sternson LA, Repta AJ. 1982. Anal Biochem, 124, 167.
13. Bannister SJ, Sternson LA, Repta AJ. 1983. J Chromatogr, 273, 301.
14. Marsh KC, Sternson LA, Repta AJ. 1983. Anal Chem, submitted.
15. Himmelstein KJ, Patton TF, Belt RJ, Taylor S, Repta AJ, Sternson LA. 1981. Clin Pharmacol Ther, 29, 658.
16. Riley CM, Sternson LA, Repta AJ, Bannister SJ. 1982. J Pharm Pharmacol, 34, 826.
17. Riley CM, Sternson LA, Repta AJ. 1983. Anal Biochem, 130, 203.
18. Barber M, Bordoli RS, Sedgwick RD, Tyler AN, Bycroft BW. 1981. Biochem Biophys Res Commun, 101, 632.

19. Aberth W, Straub KM, Burlingame AL. 1982. Anal Chem, 54, 2029.
20. Mattox D, Sternson LA, vonHoff DD, Kuhn J. 1983, Arch Otolaryng, in press.
21. Patton TF, Repta AJ, Sternson LA, Belt RJ. 1982. Int J Pharm, 10, 77.
22. Himmelstein KJ, Patton TF, Repta AJ, Sternson LA. Unpublished data.
23. LeRoy AF, Lutz RJ, Dedrick RL, Litterst CL, Guarino AM. 1979. Cancer Treat Rept, 63, 59.
24. Robins AB, Leach MD. 1983. Cancer Treat Rept, 67, 245.

POSTER PRESENTATIONS

II-1   PHARMACOLOGICAL STUDIES OF *cis*-DIAMMINEDICHLOROPLATINUM AFTER
        REPEATED ADMINISTRATION.
        M. Sawada and T. Okinaga.

II-2   PHARMACOKINETICS OF FIVE PLATINUM COMPOUNDS IN DOGS.
        W.J.F. van der Vijgh, P. Lelieveld, I. Klein, L.M. van Putten and H.M. Pinedo.

II-3   PLATINUM DETERMINATION IN EXPERIMENT AND CLINICS.
        J. Drobnik, J. Kucera, V. Brabec, O. Vrana and V. Kleinwachter.

II-4   SLOW REACTING Pt DRUGS.
        J. Drobnik, D. Noskova, V. Saudek and M. Cervinka.

II-5   INTRA-ARTERIAL *cis*-PLATINUM (IACP), A RAT MODEL FOR PHARMACOKINETIC
        STUDIES.
        D. Lehane, M. Lane and H. Busch.

II-6   PHARMACOKINETICS OF CISPLATIN IN CSF OF MAN.
        J.P. Armand, J.P. Macquet and A.F. Le Roy.

II-7   PLATINUM BIOTRANSFORMATION PRODUCTS OF CISPLATIN IN URINE AND
        PLASMA.
        P.T. Daley-Yates and D.C.H. McBrien.

II-8   INTRAPERITONEAL CISPLATIN. A PHARMACOKINETIC STUDY IN PATIENTS
        WITH MALIGNANT ASCITES.
        J.A. Lopez, J.G. Krikorian, S.D. Reich, R.D. Smyth, B.F. Issell and F.H. Lee.

II-9   USE OF TERBIUM ION FLUORESCENCE ENHANCEMENT TO MONITOR THE EX-
        TENT OF INTRASTRAND CROSSLINKING IN A DEOXYDINUCLEOSIDE
        MONOPHOSPHATE BY *cis*-DICHLORODIAMMINE PLATINUM II.
        G.F. Leblond, P.M. Coussens and H.H. Patterson.

II-10   DETERMINATION OF FREE CISPLATIN IN THE PRESENCE OF DNA-CISPLATIN
        COMPLEX BY DIFFERENTIAL PULSE POLAROGRAPHY.
        V. Brabec, O. Vrana and V. Kleinwachter.

II-11   DEVELOPMENT OF A REACTION DETECTOR FOR PLATINUM ANTINEOPLASTIC
        COMPLEXES.
        K.C. Marsh, L.A. Sternson and A.J. Repta.

II-12   RENAL FAILURE WITH UNALTERED PHARMACOKINETICS IN THREE PATIENTS
        TREATED WITH *cis*-PLATINUM (DDP) AND WHOLE BODY HYPERTHERMIA (WBH).
        H. Gerad, M.J. Egorin, D.A. Van Echo, M. Whitacre, S. Ostrow and J. Aisner.

II-13   PHARMACOKINETICS OF *cis*-DIAMMINE-1, 1-CYCLOBUTANE DICARBOXYLATE
        PLATINUM II (CBDCA, JM8) IN PATIENTS WITH NORMAL AND ABNORMAL
        RENAL FUNCTION.
        S.J. Harland, D.R. Newell, Z.H. Siddik, R. Chadwick, A.H. Calvert and K.R. Harrap.

II-14   ALKALINE DENSITY GRADIENT ANALYSIS OF THE INTERACTIONS OF PLATINUM
        COMPOUNDS WITH POLYNUCLEOTIDES.
        M. Fesen, C.C. Lee and H.C. Harder.

II-15 COMPARATIVE EFFECT OF CISPLATIN, TNO-6, CARBOPLATIN, CHIP, AND JM40 IN A HUMAN TUMOR CLONOGENIC ASSAY.
W. Rombaut, M. Rozencweig, C. Sanders, Y. Kenis and J. Klastersky.

140

II-1 PHARMACOLOGICAL STUDIES OF CIS-DIAMMINEDICHLORO-
PLATINUM AFTER REPEATED ADMINISTRATION.

Masumi Sawada* and Tetsuji Okinaga. *Division of Gynecology, Department of Clinical Research, Research Institute for Microbial Diseases, Osaka University, Suita
City Osaka, Japan. and Development & Research Department Pharmaceuticals Division, Nippon Kayaku Bldg.Ichi-
bancho Tokyo, Japan.

Levels of cis-diamminedichloroplatinum(CDDP) were
determined in the serum and urine by the flameless
atomic absorption spectrophotometry. Samples were
obtained from 6 patients with ovarian cancer. The
patients were given CDDP in saline by infusion with
mannitol and furosemide every three weeks. The treatment schedules were as follows: A, 14-16 mg/body/day
x 5 days; B, 20 mg/body/day x 5 days; C, 50 mg/body
x 1 day.

The levels of CDDP in the serum of the patients
treated under schedules A and B became higher after the
repeated administration from day 1 through 5. In the
patients treated under schedules A and B, a more
complex serum elimination curve was seen, while a simple
biphasic clearance pattern was observed in the patient
treated under Schedule C. The concentration of CDDP in
the serum rose with the increase in doses. A measurable concentration of CDDP was still detected 14 days
after the end of administration.

The urinary recovery at 24 hours after administration of CDDP ranged from 17.0 to 21.0% under schedules
A and B. On the other hand, it was 55.3% under schedule C. The overall urinary recovery of CDDP ranged
from 25.3 to 35.3% which suggested the retention of
CDDP after repeated administration. The urinary excretion of CDDP and the concentration of CDDP in urine
showed close relation with urine volume per hour.

No significant elevation in the serum creatinine
or BUN were recognized in any patient.

The results suggested the significance of mannitol
or furosemide for preventing nephrotoxicity of CDDP.

II-2 PHARMACOKINETICS OF FIVE PLATINUM COMPOUNDS IN DOGS.

W.J.F. van der Vijgh, P.Lelieveld*, I.Klein, L.M.van Putten
and H.M.Pinedo. Research Laboratory of Internal Medicine and Department of Oncology, Free University Hospital, De Boelelaan 1117, 1007
MB Amsterdam and *REP-Institutes TNO, Lange Kleiweg 151, Rijswijk,
The Netherlands.

Five platinum drugs, CDDP, TNO-6, JM-40, CBDCA and CHIP were
each administered to individual dogs as an iv bolus injection in
dosages of 1.2, 1.0, 10, 12 and 10 mg/kg respectively. Three dosages
were given with an interval of three weeks. Platinum was analyzed in
plasma, plasma ultrafiltrate, RBC's and urine at regular times after
the first administration. Platinum concentrations also were measured
in tissues at necropsy six weeks after the third dosage. Platinum
concentrations were determined with flameless atomic absorption
spectrophotometry.The urine samples after the first administration
were analyzed for total protein concentration (Bradford's method).

Analysis of the platinum concentration-time curves by means of
curve-stripping revealed that half-lives of elimination were 3.5,
3.7, 3.5, 3.6 and 2.8 days when measured over day 1-5, half-lives of
distribution were 8.4, 8.4, 12.9, 11.2 and 27.2 min when measured
over 0-20 min after administration and the enterohepatic circulation
was 3.4, 3.5, 3.3, 14.3 and 7.2% of the dose for CDDP, TNO-6, JM-40,
CBDCA and CHIP respectively. There was no uptake of platinum in RBC's
except for CHIP. For this compound a maximum level of 4.4 ug Pt/ml
was obtained at 1 hour after administration.

The cumulative excretion of platinum in urine over the first 7
days was highest for CBDCA(95%) followed by JM-40(77%), CHIP(60%),
CDDP(51%) and TNO-6(32%). The reverse order was observed for the
amounts of platinum retained by the tissues as measured at necropsy.
Pronounced transient proteinuria was only observed for TNO-6 with
a maximum value at day 5.

It is concluded that the main difference between the platinum
compounds is presented by the cumulation of platinum in the tissues
which is inversely related to the cumulative excretion of platinum
in urine and not related to platinum concentrations in plasma.

CDDP = cis-diamminedichloroplatinum(II)
TNO-6= cis-1,1-di(aminomethyl)cyclohexaneplatinum(II)sulphate
JM-40= cis-ethylenediaminoplatinum(II)malonate
CBDCA= cis-diammine-1,1-cyclobutanedicarboxylateplatinum(II)
CHIP = cis-dichlorobis(isopropylamine)-trans-dihydroxyplatinum(IV)

II-3 PLATINUM DETERMINATION IN EXPERIMENT AND CLINICS

Jaroslav Drobník[1], Jan Kučera[2], Viktor Brabec[3], Oldřich Vrána[3], and Vladimír Kleinwächter[3]. [1]Institute of Macromolecular Chemistry ČSAV, 162 06 Prague 6, [2]Nuclear Research Institute 250 68 Řež near Prague, and [3]Institute of Biophysics ČSAV, 612 65 Brno, Czechoslovakia.

Platinum determination is a key problem in experimental and clinical pharmacology. It has still not been satisfactorily solved. We report a very accurate and absolute method based on radiochemical neutron activation analysis (RNAA), a versatile new method using differential pulse polarography (DPP), and modification of the reaction with diethyldithiocarbamate (DDTC).

RNAA: Dry samples sealed in quartz ampoules were irradiated 4 hours at 1×10^{13} thermal neutrons/cm^2/s. After 7 to 10 days the vials were crushed and extracted by perchloric and nitric acids. Au as carrier, Se as collector, V as catalyst and Cr(III) as indicator were added, and Se and Au were coprecipitated by ascorbic acid. Lines at 158.4 and 208.2 keV were measured in the precipitate. The detection limit was 3 ng and 10 ng could be easily measured in routine. Gold was the only element which seriously interfered since the background due to Na and Cl decayed before the analysis and bremsstrahlung of P and 158.8 keV line of Ca-Sc transmutation were eliminated by the separation of Au 199.

DPP: The biological samples were mineralized by dry combustion as recently described for atomic absorption, dissolved in aqua regia and Pt was derivatized to a bis-ethylenediamine complex which yields a catalytic current at a dropping mercury electrode measurable by DPP. The detection limit was 10 ng of Pt and 50 ng could be easily reached in routine. Certain simplification of the mineralization procedure is possible with urine.

Reaction with DDTC: DDTC-extraction can be used in limited applications only, since DDTC is not able to remove Pt from some very stable complexes. Direct spectrophotometry is possible, provided the DDTC-platinum complex is freshly extracted with chloroform.

II-4 SLOW REACTING Pt DRUGS

Jaroslav Drobník[1], Dagmar Nosková[1], Vladimír Saudek[1], and Miroslav Červinka[2]. [1]Institute of Macromolecular Chemistry ČSAV, 162 06 Prague 6, and [2]Dept of Biology, Faculty of Medicine, Charles University, 500 38 Hradec Králové, Czechoslovakia.

There are many second-generation platinum drugs which show an equal or better anti-tumor activity than cis-DDP; however, their in vitro hydrolysis and reactivity are incomparably slower. They include Pt(II) complexes with chelating leaving ligands and Pt(IV) complexes. Most of the administered drug is excreted unchanged by urine so that apparent LD and OD are quite high. However, considering the fraction retained in the body both values are very small. It can be shown that the final products of the reaction with important nucleophiles in the body are similar to those found with cis-DDP and Pt-ethylmalonato complex, but the kinetics of the reaction is different. The same is true for malpen. The effect on cells in culture is in good agreement with the in vitro chemical reactivity. The culture was followed by the time-lapse cinematography covering the one-week fate of cells after treatment with platinum drugs. It can be clearly seen that at concentrations comparable with those obtained in patients the cells stay alive, are not inhibited in mobility and grow in size. The only observable change is complete absence of nuclear and cellular division, which results in an enlargement of nuclei and cells. Possible implications for the mechanism of action will be discussed.

II-5 INTRA-ARTERIAL CIS-PLATINUM (IACP), A RAT MODEL FOR PHARMA-
COKINETIC STUDIES. Daniel Lehane, Montague Lane, and Harris
Busch, Dept. Pharmacology, Baylor College of Medicine, 1200 Moursund,
Houston, TX 77030, U.S.A.

Several clinical studies have suggested a marked increase in
therapeutic activity for IACP compared to intravenous cis-platinum
(IVCP) administration. However, there is little data to suggest the
optimum intra-arterial infusion conditions. We have developed an
animal model system to evaluate the therapeutic activity of IACP.
Male Holtzman rats weighing approximately 250 gm are innoculated with
5×10^7 Novikoff hepatoma ascites tumor cells as a 0.5 cc injection
administered intra-muscularly in the right thigh. Following tumor
inoculation, animals are examined daily until a readily identifiable
tumor nodule from 1 x 1 to 2.5 x 2.5 cm is identified. Measurable
tumors usually developed within 6 to 9 days. CP was administered IA
by catherization of the right common iliac artery through an abdominal
incision exposing the lower aorta. Hemodilution of arterially infused
drug was restricted by the use of a ligature placed around the right
common iliac artery which was drawn around the vessels allowing
partial occlusion proximal to the tip of the infusing needle. Therapeutic activity (TA) was defined by tumor growth rate. Tumor size was
measured in the 2 longest perpendicular diameters, and the product of
the the tumor diameters was plotted as a per cent of the original
tumor size. When IACP administration was compared to intra-peritoneal
(IP) CP administration at doses of 4, 5, and 6 mg/kg, a small therapeutic advantage was demonstrated for the IACP group measured by both
reduction in tumor size and survival. Lower doses of CP (3mg/kg)
were equally active by the IP, IV and IA routes of administration with
a minimal effect on tumor size and survival when compared to 0.9%NaCl
treated controls. When the rate of infusion of IACP was prolonged
from 1 to 15 min., the therapeutic activity was increased. When drug
hemodilution was reduced by temporary restriction of arterial blood
flow through the right common iliac artery, presumably limiting the
binding of active CP to plasma proteins and blood elements and reducing its inactivation, a marked increase was found in therapeutic
activity with a high cure rate observed even at 3 mg/kg of IACP.
These preliminary studies add support to the concept that the IA
administration of unbound, therapeutically active CP is associated
with an increased therapeutic response. Both the rate of IACP
infusion and the hemodilution of CP during infusion affect therapeutic activity of IACP infusions.

II-6 PHARMACOKINETICS OF CISPLATIN IN CSF OF MAN. J.P. Armand*,
J.P. Macquet** and A.F. Le Roy***. *Centre Claudius Regaud,
11 rue Piquemil, 31052 Toulouse Cédex, France ; **Laboratoire de
Pharmacologie et de Toxicologie Fondamentales du CNRS, 205 route de
Narbonne, 31400 TOulouse, France ; ***Biomedical Engineering and
Instrumentation Branch, Division of Research Services, Bdg 13, Rm
3W13, NIH, Bethesda, Md 20205, USA.

Preliminary clinical studies using cisplatin in the treatment of brain tumors are encouraging (1). It then became necessary
to quantify the amount of Pt which could cross the blood-brain barrier and also to determine the Pt species. In this study, we have
conducted the pharmacokinetic analysis of Pt in the cerebrospinal
fluid (CSF) and plasma in one patient after a systemic administration of cisplatin during two courses. The patient was a 41 year old
woman with an inoperable glioblastoma of the cerebellar peduncles.
She received an iv bolus (15 min) injection of cisplatin at a dose
of 80 mg/m2 (140 mg cisplatin) for two courses separated by four
weeks. Hydration was performed 4 hours before cisplatin administration with 2 liters of saline solution and continued after treatment
with 250 ml of mannitol. Pt was measured by atomic absorption spectrophotometry. Pt elimination from plasma followed two distinct phases with $t_{1/2\alpha}$ = 8.1 min and $t_{1/2\beta}$ = 95.8 hr for the first course
and $t_{1/2\alpha}$ = 25.1 min and $t_{1/2\beta}$ = 91.0 hr for the second course. CSF

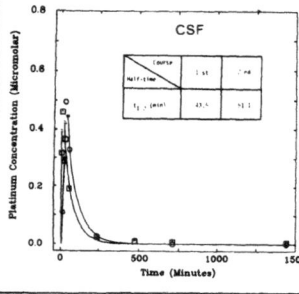

Pt depletion is represen-
ted by a single exponen-
tial (Fig.) with half-
times of 43.5 min and
51.1 min respectively
for the two courses. The
maximum concentration of
Pt (0.5 µM) in CSF was
obtained between 15 to 30
min after cisplatin admi-
nistration.

(1) A.B. Khan *et al.*
Cancer Treat. Rep. 66,
2013-2020, 1982.

143

II-7   PLATINUM BIOTRANSFORMATION PRODUCTS OF CISPLATIN IN URINE
AND PLASMA.   Peter T.Daley-Yates and David C.H.McBrien,
Biochemistry Department, Brunel University, Uxbridge, Middlesex
UB8 3PH, United Kingdom.

For rats treated with cisplatin the rate of appearance in
plasma and urine of platinum containing biotransformation products
has been investigated using our HPLC chromatographic procedure
(Biochem.Pharmacol. 32 181-184, 1983). At least seven platinum
containing peaks not attributable to cisplatin can be seen in both
plasma and urine only 1h after dosing at 15 mg/kg i.p. The predominant metabolites are those which elute in fractions 39-41 (species
C) and 60-62 (species F). Approximately 15 min after dosing species
C is the most abundant metabolite and accounts for between 15-20%
of the total free platinum in the plasma. At this time species F
accounts for only 4-5% of free plasma Pt the bulk of which is
unchanged cisplatin. By 2.5h post dosing cisplatin is no longer
detectable in the blood. At 3h post dosing species C and F are
50% and 30% of the free plasma Pt respectively. The change in
relative proportions of the two metabolites over this period can be
explained by the fact that C is actively secreted by the kidney
whilst F is reabsorbed. When cisplatin is incubated in vitro with
rat plasma the metabolites seen are the same as those seen in vivo.
However, in vitro F is the predominant metabolite. The importance
of soluble cisplatin metabolites in the development of cisplatin
nephrotoxicity is underlined by the results of the following
preliminary experiment. Metabolites were allowed to form by incubat-
ing rat plasma with 1 mg/ml cisplatin overnight under sterile conditions. Proteins of MW greater than 25,000 were removed by ultrafiltration and the filtrate injected into a rat to give a dose of
platinum equivalent to 2 mg/kg cisplatin. HPLC separation of the
filtrate showed that unchanged cisplatin was absent and F represented 54% of the total platinum. Nephrotoxicity was assessed by
BUN and urinary glucose. On day 5 post dose the treated animal
had a BUN value of 48 mg/dl whereas animals treated with 2 mg/kg
cisplatin had BUN values of 17 $\pm$ 4 mg/dl which is not significantly
different from controls. Urinary glucose showed a similar trend
and these preliminary results implicate cisplatin metabolites in
the development of the renal lesion.
(This work was supported by a grant from Bristol-Myers).

II-8   INTRAPERITONEAL CISPLATIN. A PHARMACOKINETIC STUDY IN
PATIENTS WITH MALIGNANT ASCITES.   Jose A. Lopez*, John G.
Krikorian, Steven D. Reich, Robert D. Smyth, Brian F. Issell, Francis
H. Lee. *Section of Medical Oncology, University Hospital, Boston
University Medical Center, Boston, MA. 02118; University
of Massachusetts Medical Center, Worcester, MA. 01605; Bristol
Myers Co., Syracuse, N.Y. 13201.

Pharmacokinetic modeling supports the intraperitoneal administration of cytotoxic agents as a potentially more effective strategy
of treating malignant diseases such as ovarian cancer, where the
peritoneal cavity is the major site of tumor spread. A Phase I study
of intraperitoneal cisplatin was therefore designed. Nine patients
with refractory malignant ascites from ovarian cancer and one patient
with peritoneal mesothelioma received a total of 16 treatment cycles
with 25 to 60 mg/m^2 of cisplatin administered in one liter of saline
over 15 to 30 minutes through an indwelling Tenkhoff peritoneal
dialysis catheter.   All patients with ovarian cancer had been
previously treated with systemic cisplatin. Total and free (ultrafilterable) platinum concentrations were measured in ascites, plasma
and urine by atomic absorption spectrometry. Peak total platinum
ascites concentrations ranged between 8 to 87 μg/ml and its elimination showed rapid (T_2/α 0.3 to 0.6 hrs) and slow (T_2/β 2 to 3 hrs)
phases. Maximum free platinum concentrations ranged between 3.9 to
24.2 μg/ml with half-lives ranging between 0.8 and 2.0 hours. A
direct correlation between ascitic fluid platinum concentrations and
dose was demonstrated. Peak plasma platinum concentrations at 1 to 6
hours after intraperitoneal infusion reached 2.4% of the maximum
values observed in ascites. The urinary excretion of platinum was
highly variable and consistent with the observed variability of
absorption from the peritoneum. There was minimal gastrointestinal,
bone marrow, and renal toxicity observed. Two episodes of sepsis
developed resulting from catheter manipulation. Two patients obtained a therapeutic benefit from this program. The intraperitoneal
route of administration is an effective method of obtaining sustained
free platinum concentration and deserves further clinical trials.

II-9   USE OF TERBIUM ION FLUORESCENCE ENHANCEMENT TO MONITOR THE
       EXTENT OF INTRASTRAND CROSSLINKING IN A DEOXYDINUCLEOSIDE
MONOPHOSPHATE BY CIS-DICHLORODIAMMINE PLATINUM II.

Gerard F. Leblond, Paul M. Coussens*, and Howard H. Patterson**.
Biochemistry Dept., University of Maine at Orono, Orono, Maine
04469, U.S.A., *Cell and Molecular Biology Dept., Penn State
University, State College, Pennsylvania 16802, U.S.A., **Chem-
istry Dept., University of Maine at Orono, Orono, Maine 04469,
U.S.A.

Qualitative comparisons of fluorescence emission, fluorescence
excitation, and ultraviolet light absorption profiles indicate that
terbium ions bound to stacked dimers of 2'-deoxycytidylyl-(3'-5')-
2'-deoxycytidine experience a greater fluorescence enhancement than
those bound to the unstacked species.
   By employing the van't Hoff method, to corrected fluorescence
versus temperature data, it is possible to quantitate the extent of
intrastrand crosslinking of a deoxydinucleoside monophosphate by the
bidentate platinum compound: cis-dichlorodiammine platinum II. The
errors and limitations of this method will be presented.

II-10   DETERMINATION OF FREE CISPLATIN IN THE PRESENCE
        OF DNA-CISPLATIN COMPLEX BY DIFFERENTIAL PULSE
POLAROGRAPHY. Viktor Brabec, Oldřich Vrána and
Vladimír Kleinwächter. Institute of Biophysics,
Czechoslovak Academy of Sciences, 612 65 Brno,
Czechoslovakia

Differential pulse polarography (DPP) was used to
investigate reactions of cis-dichlorodiammineplati-
num(II) (cis-DDP) with DNA. The use of this method is
based on the fact that most of Pt(II) complexes are
electroreduced at mercury electrodes at higher negative
potentials; on DPP curves cis-DDP yields a reduction
peak at -1.46 V (vs. Ag/AgCl). This peak appears only
when cis-DDP is not aquated in the solution and is not
bound to the polynucleotide. The height of this peak is
linearly dependent on the concentration of cis-DDP in
the range of 1×10^{-6} - 1×10^{-3} mol/l and is not influenced by the presence of DNA or the cis-DDP-DNA com-
plex. If, however, the reaction of DNA with cis-DDP is
followed in the medium, in which not all cisplatin
exists as the dichloro complex and thus is not polaro-
graphically reducible it is necessary first to stop the
reaction by adding sodium chloride to reach the concentration of chloride ions of 1 mol/l. The reaction mixture is then incubated for 2 hours at 25 - 30 °C and
only then DPP analysis is performed.
   The results of the investigation of reactions of
cis-DDP with DNA by means of DPP agreed very well with
those obtained by other methods currently used in quantitative analysis of cis-DDP binding to DNA. Moreover,
with the aid of DPP the reaction of cis-DDP with double-
-helical DNA was followed in the media containing
chloride ions at the concentrations higher than
0.08 mol/l. It was found that at 25 - 30 °C DNA reacted
with cis-DDP even in media containing sodium chloride
at the concentration of 0.3 mol/l. The kinetics of this
reaction was, however, markedly slower than that in the
medium in which cisplatin existed as an aquo complex.

145

II-11   DEVELOPMENT OF A REACTION DETECTOR FOR PLATINUM ANTINEO-
PLASTIC COMPLEXES. Kennan C. Marsh, Larry A. Sternson,
Arnold J. Repta, Department of Pharmaceutical Chemistry, Malott Hall
University of Kansas, Lawrence, KS, 66045, USA

In order to evaluate the clinical utility of platinum containing
antineoplastic agents, a suitable analytical methodology with selectivity and sensitivity at therapeutically significant levels was
desired. Preliminary distribution studies utilized atomic absorption
(AAS) to quantitate total platinum in biological fluids but subsequent studies demonstrated that these measurements did not provide
a valid description of CDDP pharmacokinetic behavior. Due to the
inherent reactivity of CDDP with water and other endogeneous nucleophiles (eg. methionine) and the poor detectability of the intact
drug($\sim$30-40μg/ml), a time-efficient, sensitive analytical method,
capable of separating platinum species prior to derivatization was
required to accurately characterize pharmacokinetic behavior.

A post-column reaction detector responsive to CDDP and other
platinum(II) antineoplastic agents has been developed. In this
reactor, CDDP was chromatographed on a solvent generated anion-
exchange HPLC system. A solution of potassium dichromate was added
to the column effluent immediately after exiting the column. After
$\sim$20 seconds reaction time, sodium bisulfite solution was added to
the flowing stream. The response at λ_{max}=290nm was quantitated
after a reaction delay of $\sim$4 minutes. Band broadening in the reactor
was minimized through the use of braided Teflon coils to provide
the reaction delay time. An online sensitivity of 40-60ng/ml for
the derivatized cis-dichloroplatinum(II) complexes (CDDP,Pt(en)Cl$_2$,
DACCl$_2$), of 250-300ng/ml for derivatized MAL and MALOH, and of 1200
ng/ml^2 for derivatized CBDCA and DACMAL was observed using reactor
conditions optimized for CDDP. In addition, the aquation reaction
of cisplatin and the loss of CDDP in plasma at 37°C could be monitored with this detector.

The sensitivity of the reaction detector to the cis-dichloro-
platinum(II) complexes is similar to that achieved using tedious
HPLC eluant fractionation followed by AAS. The post-column reactor
however, is a more time-efficient, matrix-independent system for the
direct, individual quantitation of platinum(II) antineoplastic
agents in plasma ultrafiltrate after HPLC separation. The response
of this simple, time-efficient reactor to a wide variety of platinum
(II) species suggests significant utility in the characterization of
the pharmacokinetic behavior of platinum(II) antineoplastic agents
in future clinical studies.

II-12   RENAL FAILURE WITH UNALTERED PHARMACOKINETICS IN
THREE PATIENTS TREATED WITH CIS-PLATINUM (DDP) AND
WHOLE BODY HYPERTHERMIA (WBH). H. Gerad, M.J. Egorin, D.A. Van
Echo, M. Whitacre, S. Ostrow, J. Aisner. University of Maryland Cancer
Center, Baltimore, MD.

Three previously treated patients (pts) with refractory melanoma,
mesothelioma and malignant fibrous histiocytoma were treated with DDP, 60
or 80 mg/m^2 and WBH (42.0-42.4°C.). WBH was induced with heated water
perfused nylon mesh body suits and warming blankets. A Tmax of 42.0-42.4°C
was maintained for 2 hours (hrs) during which time DDP was infused.
Mannitol, 37.5 gms as a 10% solution was given over 6 hrs, starting 4 hrs prior
to DDP. Hydration with 5% dextrose and half normal saline at a rate of 150
ml/hr began 8 hrs before warming. The hydration rate was 800-1200 ml/hr for
the duration of warming. After cooling to 37°C, hydration was tapered over
24 hrs to 150 ml/hr. A euthermic course of DDP was given to 2 pts 1 month
before administration with WBH to establish baseline pharmacokinetics. Pt 1
received 80 mg/m^2 and pt 3 received 60 mg/m^2 DDP. Prior to WBH,
creatinine clearances were 104 ml/min, 100 ml/min and 137 ml/min and serum
creatinines were 0.9 mg/dl, 1.1 mg/dl and 0.8 mg/dl in pts 1-3 respectively.
The serum creatinines peaked respectively on days 7, 12 and 12 at
concentrations of 2.7 mg/dl, 2.8 mg/dl and 13.6 mg/dl in the first 2 pts given
80 mg/m^2 DDP and the third given 60 mg/m^2. High frequency hearing loss
determined by audiogram, occurred in pt 2 and mild loss in pt 3. Serum
creatinines subsequently fell to 1.1 mg/dl (day 114) in pt 1, 1.9 mg/dl (day 82)
in pt 2 and 4.8 mg/dl (day 40) in pt 3. When the WBH-DDP pharmacokinetic
data are compared to the same or other pts given DDP euthermically, WBH
did not alter the peak plasma concentrations of total or ultrafilterable
platinum, the rapid t 1/2 of plasma nonprotein bound platinum, the percentage
of total plasma platinum that was unbound, the long t 1/2 for total plasma
platinum or the 24 hr renal excretion of platinum. Although WBH did not alter
the plasma and urinary pharmacokinetics of DDP, it potentiated the
nephrotoxic effects of DDP.

II-13 PHARMACOKINETICS OF CIS-DIAMMINE-1,1-CYCLOBUTANE
DICARBOXYLATE PLATINUM II (CBDCA JM8) IN PATIENTS WITH
NORMAL AND ABNORMAL RENAL FUNCTION Stephen J Harland,
David R Newell Z H Siddik, Ruth Chadwick, A Hilary Calvert and
Kenneth R Harrap. Institute of Cancer Research, and Royal Marsden
Hospital, Downs Road Sutton, Surrey, England

CBDCA is an analogue of cisplatin which is free of the latter's
nephrotoxicity (Calvert et al, Cancer Chemother. Pharmacol. 9:3,
1982) but which retains its efficacy. The limiting toxicity of
CBDCA is haematological and patients with poor renal function are
particularly susceptible to this. The pharmacokinetics following
a 1 hour infusion were studied in 25 patients receiving doses
between 20 and 520 mg/m'. Renal function was assessed in every
case by 51 Cr EDTA clearance. Total plasma platinum (Pt) and
free Pt (in plasma ultrafiltrates) were measured by atomic
absorption spectrophotometry. Intact CBDCA was measured by HPLC.
There was a linear relationship between dose and area under the
plasma concentration curve (AUC) for total Pt. Protein binding
during the first 4 hours was between 0 and 29%. It rose to 85-
9% by 24 hours. All the free Pt was in the form of CBDCA during
the first 4 hours. An early elimination phase for free Pt had a
half-life of 91 ± 6 (SE) mins, similar to that for CBDCA and
total Pt. Later half-lives of 279 ± 24 mins and >24 hours were
seen for free and total Pt respectively. $65 \pm 1\%$ of the
administered Pt appeared in the urine over the the first 24
hours. Patients with poor renal function have higher AUCs for
total Pt. Both renal and total clearance of free Pt correlated
significantly with glomerular filtration rate. These findings
justify the practice of reducing the dose of CBDCA in the
presence of renal impaiment. Renal clearance of free Pt
following CBDCA was 0.67 ± 0.05 51 Cr EDTA clearance, suggesting
that there was no tubular secretion of the drug as occurs with
cisplatin (Jacobs et al, Cancer Treat. Rep. 64: 1223, 1980).
This may account for the difference in nephrotoxicity.

II-14 ALKALINE DENSITY GRADIENT ANALYSIS OF THE INTERACTIONS OF
PLATINUM COMPOUNDS WITH POLYNUCLEOTIDES. Mark Fesen,
Christine C. Lee, and Harold C. Harder, Oral Roberts University,
School of Medicine, Tulsa, Oklahoma 74171, U.S.A.

When cisplatin (cis-Pt) reacts for 3 days with poly dG·poly dC
(dG·dC) in 2 mM NaCl, 2 mM MOPS, pH 7.2, a dose dependent hybrid
density band occurs upon alkaline (0.02 N NaOH) density gradient
centrifugation in Cs_2SO_4 midway between the low density dC and the
high density dG bands. This hybrid density band is physical chemical evidence of interstrand crosslink formation between dG and dC.
Plots of density (ρ) vs the Pt/base ratio (r_i) show that both the dG
and hybrid density bands increase in ρ while the dC band ρ remains
constant. This is consistant with an initial reaction by cis-Pt
with dG followed by a crosslinking reaction with the dC strand. Di-
ethylenetriaminechloroplatinum Cl (dien-Pt), a monofunctional platinum analogue, increases the ρ of dG without creating a hybrid density band. From a plot of the % dG·dC crosslinked vs r_i, the minimum
amount of cis-Pt required for corsslinking was $r_i = 0.017$. Calculations of the frequency of crosslinking range from a minimum of 1 in
15 but average 1 in 90 reactions. On the other hand, trans-Pt was
far more efficient in crosslining of dG·dC. Crosslinks were detect-
at r_i values as low as 0.001 and an extrapolation of a plot of %
crosslinks vs r_i goes through the origin. Thus potentially every
trans-Pt molecule creates a crosslink, but on the average 1 of every
7.4 reactions is a crosslink. CHIP creates crosslinks in dG·dC with
a frequency of only about 1/10 that of cis-Pt; the initial reaction
with dG is greatly reduced.
When cis-Pt is incubated with poly dA·poly dT (dA·dT) in 2mM
NaCl 50 mM $NaClO_4$, 2 mM MOPS, pH 7.2 3 days, and spun in alkaline
Cs_2SO_4 significant Pt binding to the dA strand occurred at $r_i \geq 0.05$
which increased in ρ as r_i increased. No hybrid density band occurred in dA·dT. However at $r_i \geq 0.2$ the initially lower density dA
band began to cosediment with the initially higher density dT band,
thereby indicating some type of interstrand interaction. There was
no increase in the density of dT following incubation of single
stranded dT with cis-Pt. Dien-Pt treated dA·dT caused a progressive
increase in the ρ of the dA band without co-sedimentation with the
dT band as the ρ of the dA band surpasses that of the dT band.
Postincubation of cis-Pt treated dG·dC in 5 mM KCN for three
days did not reverse either the crosslinks or platinum binding to
dG; but postincubation in 0.5 N NaOH did reverse the crosslinks
without affecting binding to dG. In contrast, 5 mM KCN removed all
cis-Pt bound to dA·dT. These results will aid our future studies.
(Supported in part by USPHS grant CA-25736.)

II-15 COMPARATIVE EFFECT OF CISPLATIN, TNO-6, CARBOPLATIN, CHIP, AND JM40 IN A HUMAN TUMOR CLONOGENIC ASSAY. W. Rombaut, M. Rozencweig, C. Sanders, Y. Kenis, J. Klastersky. Institut Jules Bordet, Brussels, Belgium.

A modified double-layer Hamburger and Salmon cloning assay was utilized to compare cisplatin, TNO-6, carboplatin, CHIP and JM40. These analogs were tested in a total of 34 tumor samples freshly obtained from patients with a variety of nonhematologic malignancies, mainly ovarian cancer (9), breast cancer (9) and unknown primaries (5). One-half of the patients had received prior chemotherapy which consisted of cisplatin regimens in 7. Solid specimens were mechanically disaggregated to obtain single cell suspensions and no conditioned media were used.Cell viability was determined by trypan blue dye exclusion; 500,000 viable nucleated cells were seeded per plate. Colonies were defined as aggregates of 40 cells or more and counted manually after 3 weeks of incubation. The median number of control colonies per plate per tumor type was 116 (70 - 2575). All drugs were dissolved in water. Tumor cells were exposed for 1-hr at concentrations of 0.1 and 1.0 µg/ml of cisplatin and TNO-6 as well as at concentrations of 1.0 and 10.0 µg/ml of carboplatin and CHIP. JM40 was always tested at a concentration of 1.0 µg/ml. Sensitivity to at least one of these compounds was found in 11 samples including 5 ovarian cancers, 1 breast cancer and 1 unknown primary. In the table, cell kill is expressed as ++ (> 70%), + (> 50%, < 70%) or 0 (< 50%). No antitumor activity could be detected with JM40. Sample # 2 had been obtained in a patient previously treated with cisplatin.

	Sample #										
	1	2	3	4	5	6	7	8	9	10	11
cisplatin	+	0	+	++	0	+	+	0	+	0	0
TNO-6	++	0	+	+	0	+	+	+	0	0	0
carboplatin	++	++	+	+	0	+	0	0	0	+	0
CHIP	0	++	++	0	++	0	0	+	0	0	+

The data indicate that a similar overall response rate in vitro may be expected with all these derivatives. In individual samples, antitumor effect was comparable for cisplatin and TNO-6 whereas it was strikingly different for cisplatin and CHIP. Combinations of these latter drugs should be investigated. Larger numbers of comparative tests are needed to confirm our preliminary findings. These experimental data remain to be validated by comparative clinical trials.

SECTION III

TOXICOLOGY OF PLATINUM COORDINATION COMPLEXES IN CANCER CHEMOTHERAPY

Chaired by M.P. Hacker

Overview
M.P. Hacker

The most common toxicities observed with cisplatin administration are nausea, vomiting, renal tubular damage, ototoxicity, peripheral neuropathy, myelosuppression, tetany and allergic reactions. The objective of this session was to bring together investigators actively involved in research cn platinum toxicity in order to present data generated in their laboratories and to discuss the possible mechanisms of these toxicities.

Dr. Richard Borch discussed some of the novel and exciting work that his group has been doing with the effect of the chelating agent diethyldithio carbamate (DDTC) on platinum toxicity and efficacy. Since their initial observation that DDTC could diminish or even prevent the nephrotoxicity of cisplatin, they have extended their studies into other toxicological aspects of cisplatin and have found some rather encouraging results with this combination of drugs.

An area of research receiving an increasing amount of interest is the role of circadian rhythm on the toxicity and efficacy of anticancer drugs. In his presentation, Dr. Hrushesky presented data that his group has generated in experimental animals and in the clinic on the importance of circadian variation in platinum toxicity. He reported that the time during the day that cisplatin is administered may play a role in the severity of toxicity one could expect to see.

Cisplatin has been referred to as the most nauseating drug ever used clinically and has actually resulted in patients refusing subsequent courses of cisplatin because of the nausea and vomiting. Dr. Schurig discussed a new animal model, i.e. the ferret, that his group is currently using to screen compounds for emetic potential. Data generated to date indicate that the ferret is an excellent qualitative predictor of platinum induced emesis and may play an important role in delineating the mechanism of this serious toxicity.

A major emphasis of the research reported was directed towards the nephrotoxicity of cisplatin. Data were presented that cisplatin infusion produced effective renal plasma flow in spite of the fact that all patients received pre- and post-hydration 0.9% NaCl. This immediate effect on renal perfusion may help explain the delayed decrease in GFR noted in patients 21 days after cisplatin infusion.

An interesting observation implicating iron in cisplatin-induced nephrotoxicity was also presented. Using electrol probe analysis and FAAS on kidneys taken from rats receiving weekly doses of cisplatin, only slight increases in Pt concentration were noted with time, whereas there was a surprisingly large increase in Fe. It was proposed that the nephrotoxicity may be in part due to an accumulation of insoluble Fe salts. Platinum concentrations as well as metabolites of cisplatin, CBDCA, and CHIP in plasma and urine taken from conscious rats suggest that the renal handling of these complexes differed depending upon the complex studied and the metabolites of each complex. While certain platinum complexes were actively secreted by the renal tubules, others were merely filtered at the glomerulus and still others are filtered and later resorbed.

Cisplatin-induced changes in BUN and creatinine clearance values were correlated with changes in K^+ and Ca^{++}. Hypocalcemia was noted just prior to the development of tetany. Hypokalemia was transient and occurred following each course of Pt.

The results of Phase I studies were reported for CHIP, PHIC, and CBDCA. When administered as a single IV injection per week for 4 weeks, the dose-limiting toxicity for CHIP was thrombocytopenia. Other toxicities were nausea, vomiting, and diarrhea and the MTD was calculated to be 95 mg/m^2. Similar toxicities were noted using a dosing regimen of 5 daily doses repeated every 3 weeks, but the MTD was 45 mg/m^2/day. Partial responses were reported in 2 patients and stable disease in another. PHIC was administered daily for 5 consecutive days repeated every 4 weeks and, as with CHIP, thrombocytopenia was the dose-limiting toxicity. While nausea, vomiting, fever, and phlebitis were noted but not considered to be dose-limiting, the MTD was reported to be 1200 mg/m^2. In a related study, PHIC was shown to be nephrotoxic to baboons at a dose of 100 mg/kg. It would appear that although much less nephrotoxic (on a mg/kg basis) than cisplatin, PHIC does cause damage to the kidneys. Patients received CBDCA either for 5 consecutive days repeated every 4 to 5 weeks or every 6 weeks. Boths groups found myelosuppression to be dose-limiting but mild nausea and vomiting were also consistently noted. The MTD for CBDCA was calculated to be in a range of 75 to 100 mg/m^2/day. The plasma half lives of CBDCA in patients were 1-7 min. and 100-233 min. for t½ α and t½ β, respectively.

A number of Pt and Pd complexes with DDTC esters were shown to have _in vitro_ cytotoxicity. Such complexes having the renal protectant linked to the Pt could be a very important class of compounds. Although many cytostatic agents can cross the placenta during the period of organogenesis and represent a serious hazard to the developing fetus, data generated using ^{195m}Pt indicate that cisplatin is not transported during this phase of embryo development but does accumulate later in the gestation period. This latter accumulation correlated well with morphologic lesions noted by microscopy.

A definite circadian rhythm with respect to the protein binding of platinum was observed in humans and rats with the rate of protein binding greatest late in the afternoon. If the nephrotoxicity platinum complexed to protein is less than free platinum one could infer that the potential nephrotoxicity could be reduced by afternoon treatments.

Diethyldithiocarbamate and *cis*-Platinum Toxicity
R.F. Borch, D.L. Bodenner and J.C. Katz

Nephrotoxicity continues to be a major side effect in cis-dichlorodiammineplatinum(II)(DDP) therapy. Numerous strategies have been developed in an attempt to reduce this toxicity. Intravenous prehydration with or without mannitol diuresis is partially effective and has become the mainstay of most clinical protocols (1). A variety of sulfur nucleophiles has been studied as inhibitors of DDP nephrotoxicity, including cysteine, N-acetyl-cysteine, cysteamine, penicillamine (2), methionine, thiourea(3), thiosulfate (4), and diethyldithiocarbamate (DDTC)(5). It is apparent that, for most of these "rescue" agents, the timing of administration is critical. Only thiourea at high doses and DDTC are effective when administered more than one hour after DDP, and of those compounds which reduce toxicity when given before or concurrent with DDP, reduced therapeutic efficacy is frequently observed. Thiosulfate, for example, is effective when given from one hour before to 30 minutes after DDP, but the ILS of mice bearing L1210 leukemia and therapeutic doses of DDP was signif-icantly reduced by simultaneous administration of thiosulfate. Thiourea is very effective in reducing DDP-induced nephrotoxicity; its effect on tumor response to DDP, however, is highly sensitive to dose and time of administration. Thiourea has also been shown to prevent platinum-DNA crosslinks and to reverse the cytotoxicity of DDP in vitro even when administered 4½ hours after DDP treat-ment (6). We have demonstrated that DDTC effectively ameliorates both nephrotoxicity and local gastrointestinal toxicity in the rat at doses as low as 100 mg/kg when administered between 1 and 4 hours after DDP. Although large doses of DDTC (750 mg/kg) do alter the response of rat mammary tumor 13762 to DDP, lower DDTC doses have no effect upon tumor response (5). The results described in this report provide additional evidence for DDTC's promise as a highly selective agent for the inhibition of toxicity induced by cis-platinum.

EFFECT OF DDTC ON L1210 AND P388 RESPONSE TO DDP IN VIVO

The effect of DDTC rescue on the response of L1210 leukemia to DDP was studied in BDF_1 mice inoculated with 10^6 cells ip 24 hours before DDP administration. DDP was given ip at doses of 5 or 10 mg/kg with or without DDTC (250 or 500 mg/kg ip) 1, 2, or 4 hours after DDP; no significant differences in mean survival time (MST) were observed between the DDP and DDP+DDTC groups at any dose or time combination. No long term survivors (>35 days) were noted in any group. Similar experiments with P388 leukemia, however, suggested that DDTC may potentiate the therapeutic effect of DDP. When DDP was administered to P388-bearing BDF_1 mice (6.5 or 10 mg/kg ip) with or without DDTC (250 or 500 mg/kg sc) 2 hours later, mean survival times increased 30-50% in the combined treatment group compared with the corresponding group which received DDP alone. No long term survivors were noted in any group. Similar increases were noted when DDTC was replaced by disulfiram* (250, 500, or 750 mg/kg as an aqueous suspension via gastric tube). The therapeutic efficacy of the DDP+DDTC combination was most apparent when DDP was administered on four successive days (table 1); MST increased almost fourfold and long term survivors exceeded 80% after four successive daily doses of DDP(5 mg/kg ip) followed 2 hours later by DDTC(300 mg/kg sc). Similar results (%T/C=320; survivors=6/8) were obtained when DDTC was replaced by disulfiram (250 mg/kg via gastric tube). In order to assure that this potentiation was not a consequence of cell alteration, new P388 cells were obtained from Mason Research Institute and passed in DBA mice at 7-day intervals. BDF_1 mice were inoculated with cells taken from every 4th passage and treated with DDP with or without DDTC as described above; the results are summarized in table 2. Potentiation appears to be most significant for the early passage cells; although the MST for

---

*Disulfiram is rapidly reduced to DDTC after absorption in vivo and thus represents a clinically available source for oral DDTC.

Table 1. Effect of DDTC on the activity of DDP against P388
leukemia in BDF_1 mice

DDP(mg/kg) ip qd x 4	DDTC(mg/kg) sc 2 hr p̄ DDP	MST Days	% T/C	Survivors Day 41(6)
–	–	9.4	–	0
–	150	9.1	97	0
–	300	9.6	102	0
3	–	21.7	230	1
"	150	28.4	302	2
"	300	31.2	332	3
4	–	24.2	257	1
"	150	32.5	346	4
"	300	29.4	313	3
5	–	26.5	282	2
"	150	30.3	322	3
"	300	36.5	388	5

the control group does not vary with passage, the cells do
become more sensitive to DDP, with the greatest differences seen
in long term survivors. It should be noted that DDP is significantly more toxic to mice weighing less than 20 grams (passage
8 group, table 2) but that DDTC is still effective both in
reducing toxicity and in prolonging survival.

EFFECT OF DDTC ON DDP TOXICITY IN THE MOUSE AND DOG

Both DDTC and disulfiram are effective inhibitors of DDP-
induced nephrotoxicity in mice. Maximum blood urea nitrogen
(BUN) levels after a single DDP dose (10 mg/kg ip) with or
without rescue (250 mg/kg) 2 hours later are 107, 60, and 45 mg/dl
for the DDP alone, oral disulfiram, and ip DDTC groups respectively; maximum BUN levels after 3 successive daily doses of
DDP (4 mg/kg ip) are 103, 69, and 46 mg/dl. Similar protection
is seen when DDTC or disulfiram is combined with hydration. When
BDF_1 mice were pretreated with normal saline (1 cc sc) 2 hours
before DDP and then given DDP (3 mg/kg ip daily x 6) with DDTC or
disulfiram rescue (250 mg/kg) at 2 hours, maximum BUN values were
88, 62, and 41 mg/dl for the DDP alone, disulfiram, and DDTC
groups respectively. Intravenous DDTC is also well tolerated
in the mouse, rat, and dog; the LD10 and LD50 intravenous doses

Table 2. Effect of passage number on the activity of DDP(5 mg/kg qdx4) with or without DDTC(300 mg/kg sc 2 hr p̄ DDP) against P388 leukemia in BDF$_1$ mice

	Control		DDP			DDP + DDTC		
Pass	Wgt,g	MST	MST	%T/C	Survivors Day41(12)	MST	%T/C	Surviv. D41(12)
4	22	9.3	25.4	273	3	30.3	326	7
8	17	9.1	13.8	152	0	20.2	222	4
12	25	9.5	31.9	336	8	40	420	12
16	26	9.7	34.6	357	10	40	420	12

for Swiss Webster mice are 1350 and 1650 mg/kg respectively.

The effect of DDTC rescue in BDF$_1$ mice after four successive day doses of DDP (5 mg/kg) is shown in figure 1. Mice were injected with DDP (5 mg/kg in 0.5 ml saline ip) followed 2 hours later by DDTC (300 mg/kg in 1 ml water sc) or sodium bicarbonate (125 mg/kg in 1 ml water sc) as a rescue control. The combination of hydration and DDTC results in maximum BUN levels just outside the normal range as compared to the significantly elevated levels observed in the absence of DDTC rescue. The wbc nadir is both higher and occurs earlier in the DDTC group (4800/ul on day 8 vs. 3400/ul on day 11; $p < .01$), and wbc recovery also occurs sooner in the rescued group. The initial decrease in L/N ratio characteristic of DDP and most other platinum analogs is also moderated by DDTC, indicating that DDTC may be inhibiting the early lymphopenia induced by DDP.

We have also examined the effect of DDTC on DDP toxicity in the dog. DDP (1.0 mg/kg iv) was administered daily with or without DDTC (200 mg/kg iv 2 hours after DDP) for five successive days (3 dogs/group). Maximum BUN levels were 53, 71, and 125 (mean 83) mg/dl in the DDP group and 21, 26, and 30 (mean 27) mg/dl in the combination group. No significant differences were noted in wbc nadir between the two groups. The dogs were sacrificed, and all major organ systems were evaluated for toxicity. Significant differences between the two groups were found in the kidney, jejunum, and bone marrow (DDP vs. DDP+DDTC):

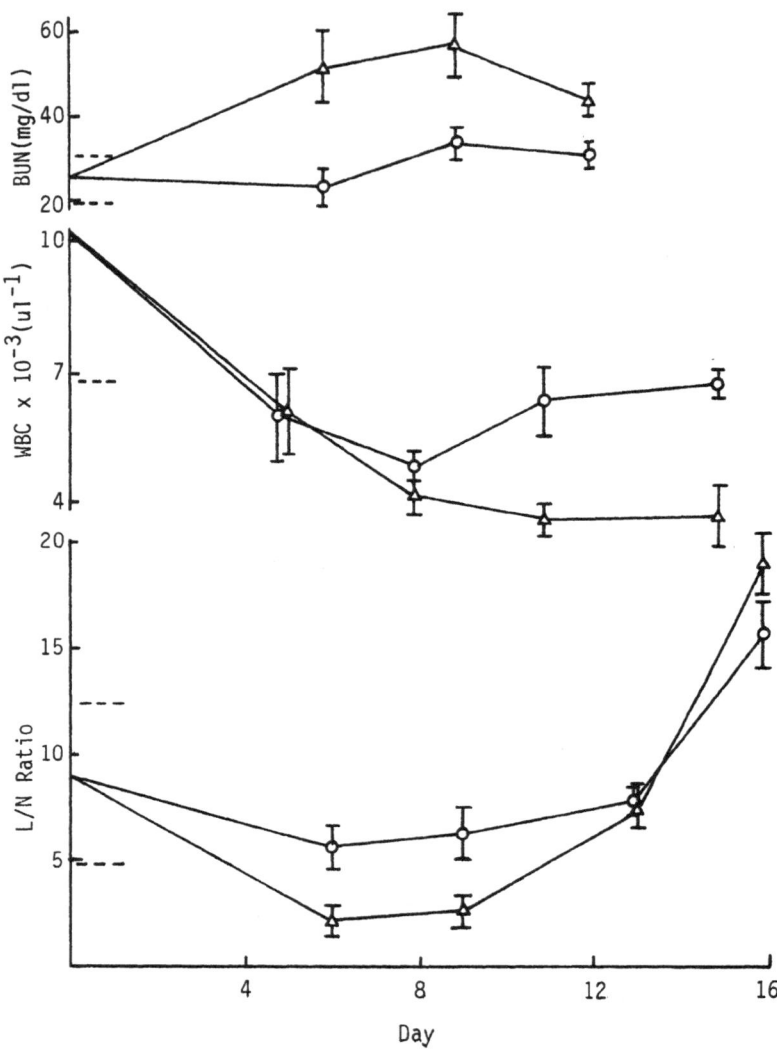

FIGURE 1. Effect of DDTC on BUN, wbc, and lymphocyte/neutrophil ratio in BDF₁ mice after treatment with cis-platinum (5 mg/kg ip qd x 4 days). Dotted lines at left represent the limits of normal values.

△ DDP alone   O   DDP + DDTC (300 mg/kg @ 2 hr)

Kidney: tubular epithelial degeneration and necrosis vs. diffuse
regenerating tubular epithelium; Jejunum: diffuse crypt necrosis
vs. crypt epithelial proliferation; Bone Marrow: hypocellular
with all series present vs. normal. Treatment of a control group
with DDTC alone produced no significant lesions in any organ
system. In a separate experiment, DDP was given as a single dose
(3.0 mg/kg iv) with or without DDTC (100 mg/kg iv 2 hr p̄ DDP).
The group receiving the combination tolerated the treatment
better than the DDP group, with more rapid recovery from nausea,
vomiting, and malaise shortly after DDTC administration.

Thus our in vivo evidence to date indicates that DDTC
ameliorates the nephrotoxicity and local GI toxicity in the mouse,
rat, and dog; it may also have a beneficial effect on DDP-induced
nausea and vomiting. When DDTC is given at therapeutically
beneficial doses, no inhibition of DDP's antitumor effect is seen
in the 13762 rat mammary tumor or the murine L1210 or P388
leukemias, and there is evidence of increased long term survivors
with the addition of DDTC to DDP in P388-bearing BDF_1 mice.
Preliminary evidence also suggests that DDTC may have protective
effects on the bone marrow.

EFFECT OF DDTC ON L1210 CELL SURVIVAL AFTER DDP EXPOSURE IN VITRO
L1210 cells grown in RPMI 1640 supplemented with 10% horse
serum were incubated with DDP (1-20 uM) for 1 hour; the cells were
washed x 3, incubated for 1.5, 2, or 4 hours with normal medium,
and then exposed to medium containing DDTC (0.5 or 1 mM) for 1
hour. Cells were washed, seeded in soft agar, incubated for
approximately 14 days, and the colonies counted. Slopes for the
exponential phase of the dose-response curves were $0.21\pm.02$,
$0.32\pm.03$, and $0.25\pm.06$ uM^{-1} for DDP-DDTC time intervals of 1.5,
2, and 4 hours respectively, corresponding to D_o (dose increment)
values of 4.8, 3.1, and 4.0 uM respectively. None of these values
was significantly different from that for cells treated with DDP
alone ($0.27\pm.05$; $D_o = 3.7$ uM). Thus DDTC does not reverse the
cytotoxic effects of DDP against L1210 cells in culture when
administered after DDP.

EFFECT OF DDTC ON PLATINUM-DNA COMPLEXES

The effect of DDTC on DDP-induced crosslinks in cultured
L1210 cells was examined by the alkaline elution technique (7).
L1210 cells were labelled by growing with either ^{14}C- or ^{3}H-
thymidine. The ^{14}C-labelled cells were divided into four groups
and incubated as follows: normal medium (control); DDP (20 uM,
1 hr); DDTC (1 mM, 1 hr); and DDP (20uM, 1hr), wash x 2, then
DDTC (1 mM, 1 hr) 3 hours later. Each group of cells was then
given 300 rads. The ^{3}H-labelled cells were given 150 rads and
combined with the ^{14}C-labelled cells. The cells were carefully
layered on PVC filters, lysed with SDS, treated for 1 hour with
ProK, and eluted with tetrapropylammonium hydroxide, pH 12. A
total of 10 fractions were collected, each 3-ml fraction collected
over 90 minutes. Fractions and filter were analyzed for ^{14}C and
^{3}H expressed as fraction ^{14}C vs. fraction ^{3}H retained on the
filter. The results plotted on log-log scale are shown in figure
2a. The curve for DDTC alone is essentially identical to the
control, indicating that DDTC has no effect on the DNA elution
profile. The DDP curve is significantly different from control
and shows evidence of substantial interstrand crosslinking.
Subsequent exposure of DDP-treated cells to DDTC gave an elution
profile virtually superimposable on the curve for DDP alone,
indicating that under these conditions DDP-induced DNA crosslinks
were unaffected by DDTC. A modification of the alkaline elution
method was developed which permits direct evaluation of drug
effects on cellular DNA outside the cell. Control and DDP-
treated cells were prepared and irradiated as described above.
The cells were placed on the filter, lysed, and the filters were
washed with EDTA x 2. A solution of the appropriate agent in
buffer was then added, incubated for the desired time, and allowed
to drain. The cells were then treated with ProK and eluted as
described above. Reversal of crosslinks was quantitated by
measuring the fraction ^{14}C retained at 0.6 ^{3}H retention and
expressing the difference in percent from the cells treated with
DDP alone. The data for DDTC (500 mM, 4 hr) is shown in figure
2b; under these conditions <5% reversal of crosslinks has occurred.
The results for DDTC, thiourea, and cyanide reversal under

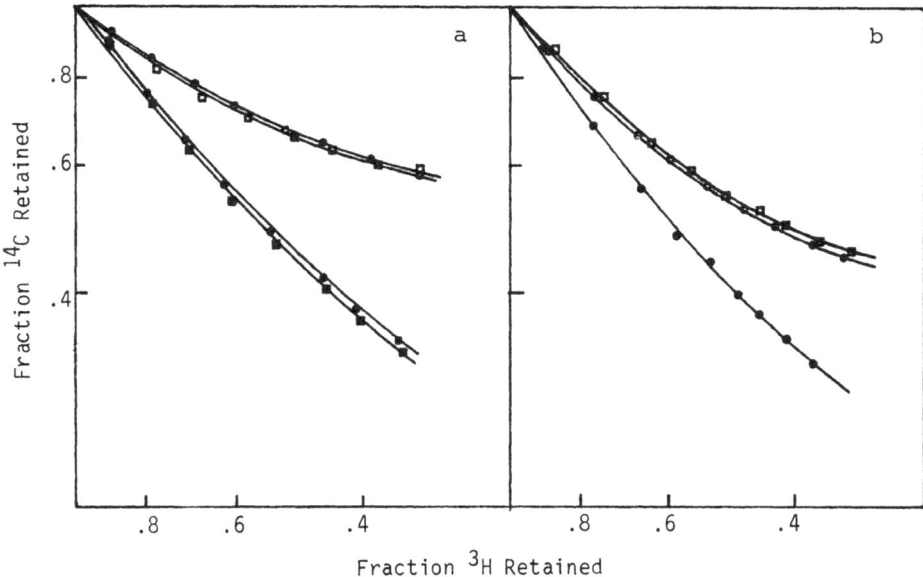

FIGURE 2. Alkaline Elution of L1210 DNA following exposure of cells to cis-platinum. a) ● control; □ cells treated with DDP (20 uM, 1 hr); ■ cells treated with DDTC (1 mM, 1 hr); O cells treated with DDP followed by DDTC 3 hr later. b) ● control; □ cells treated with DDP (20 uM, 1 hr); O cells treated with DDP and the DNA treated with DDTC (500 mM, 4 hr) on the filter.

different conditions are summarized in table 3; it is apparent that the platinum crosslinks are accessible on the filter as indicated by the facile reversal by cyanide. It is interesting to note that thiourea is more effective than DDTC in reversing crosslinks under these conditions. In a separate experiment, labelled cells were irradiated, lysed on the filter, treated with ProK, and exposed to aquated cis-platinum (freshly prepared by reaction of DDP with silver perchlorate) at concentrations from 5-50uM for 2 hours. Subsequent alkaline elution showed that concentration-dependent crosslinking had occurred by exposure of DNA to activated platinum on the filter. These methods have proved to be very useful for evaluating the effects of drugs on the formation and reversal of DNA crosslinks in an extracellular environment.

Table 3. Reversal of DDP-induced crosslinks by reaction with
        L1210 DNA

Agent	Conc (mM)	Time (hr)	Reversal (%)
DDTC	10	1	0
"	10	4	0
"	500	4	<5
Thiourea	2	1	15
"	10	4	23
"	500	4	54
Cyanide	2	1	27
"	10	2	40
"	40	4	75

The effect of DDTC on the reversal of platinum-DNA complexes
was also evaluated using salmon sperm DNA which had been incubated with DDP for 72 hours at various Pt:base ratios r.
The complexes were reacted with DDTC (10 mM, 37°), and aliquots
were removed every 30 minutes for 2 hours. The DNA was separated
by spin dialysis and the filtrate analyzed for the $Pt(DDTC)_2$
complex by HPLC; the results are given in figure 3. When the
Pt:base ratio is < .05, reversal is <1% after 2 hours; at higher
ratios, however, reversal becomes significant. These results
can be explained by examining the effect of DDTC on Pt-guanosine
and Pt-adenosine complexes. Reaction of DDP with guanosine
produces both a mono and bis adduct which can be analyzed (and
preparatively separated if desired) by cation exchange HPLC.
Treatment of either adduct with DDTC (10 mM, 37°) shows no
evidence of reaction after 2 hours. Similar reaction of DDP with
adenosine affords a complex mixture of products by HPLC in which
two adducts of unknown structure predominate. In contrast to the
platinum-guanosine adducts, these two complexes react with DDTC
with half-lives of approximately 30 and 100 minutes (figure 4);
the product of these reactions is $Pt(DDTC)_2$. Thus the platinum-
DNA reversal seen at high Pt:base ratios may represent removal
of platinum coordinated to adenine rather than guanine bases in
DNA; presumably these complexes become frequent only at high
Pt:base ratios.

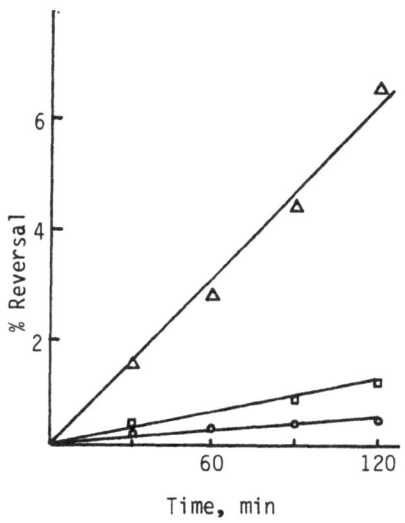

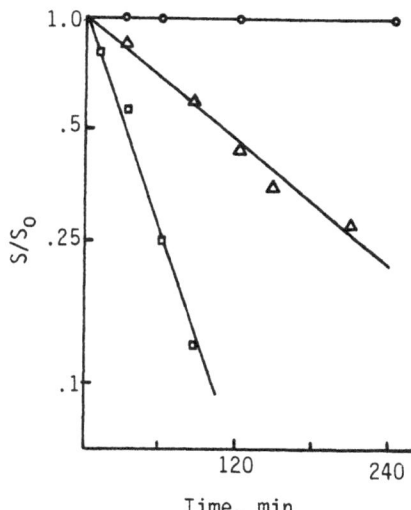

FIGURE 3. Reversal of platinum-DNA complexes by DDTC (10 mM, 37°). **O** r=0.02; **□** r=0.05; **△** r=0.1.

FIGURE 4. Effect of DDTC (10 mM 37°) on the platinum complexes of adenosine and guanosine. **O** Pt-guanosine; **△** Pt-Adenosine A; **□** Pt-Adenosine B.

We have demonstrated that DDTC is essentially unreactive toward platinum-DNA adducts at low platinum:base ratios, that DDTC has no effect on platinum-DNA crosslinks in cells or in isolated DNA, and that it has no effect on L1210 cell survival after DDP treatment in vitro. These results combined with DDTC's demonstrated protective effects in kidney and gut and its possible beneficial effects on nausea and vomiting and bone marrow toxicity indicate that DDTC would be an excellent candidate for clinical trials. The basis for DDTC's selectivity is not entirely obvious at this time and must await the results of experiments currently underway in our laboratory.

ACKNOWLEDGMENT

Financial support from the National Institutes of Health (Grant # CA34620) and the Wilson Foundation is gratefully acknowledged.

REFERENCES

1. a)D. Hayes, E. Cvitkovic, and R. Golby, Cancer, 39:1372 (1977); b)C. Merrin, Proc. Amer. Assoc. Cancer Res., 17:243 (1976).

2. T. F. Slater, M. Ahmed, and S. A. Ibrahim, J. Clin. Hematol. Oncol., 7:534 (1977).

3. J. H. Burchenal, K. Kalaher, K. Dew, L. Lokys, and G. Gale, Biochimie, 60:961 (1978).

4. a)S. B. Howell and R. Taetle, Cancer Treat. Reports, 64:611 (1980); b)S. B. Howell, C. L. Pfeifle, W. E. Wung, et. al., Ann. Int. Med., 97:845 (1982).

5. a)R. F. Borch and M. E. Pleasants, Proc. Natl. Acad. Sci.USA, 76:6611 (1979); b)R. F. Borch, J. C. Katz, P. H. Lieder, and M. E. Pleasants, Proc. Natl. Acad. Sci. USA, 77:5441 (1980).

6. M. O. Bradley, S. Patterson, and L. A. Zwelling, Mutation Research, 96:67 (1982).

7. L. A. Zwelling, T. Anderson, and K. W. Kohn, Cancer Research, 39:365 (1979).

Selected Aspects of Cisplatin Nephrotoxicity
in the Rat and Man
W.J.M. Hrushesky

1. ABSTRACT

Gastrointestinal toxicity, nephrotoxicity, peripheral neuropathy, and progressive anemia are each side effects of high-dose intermittent cisplatin therapy. We have characterized each of these toxicities in a Clinical Research Center setting in about 100 patients, who received 5 to 10 monthly courses of therapy. We have attempted to define the molecular bases for some of them and have begun to use the information generated to design and test methods of lessening these toxicities. Studies in rats first defined the circadian stage dependence of cisplatin pharmacology and nephrotoxicity. Clinical studies have since documented much higher urinary cisplatin concentrations when the drug is given in the morning as compared to the evening. Cisplatin nephrotoxicity can be largely avoided by administering the drug at the time of day associated with highest daily potassium excretion for that individual (usually in the late afternoon). A multivariate analysis of kidney toxicity data further revealed that older patients tolerated cisplatin therapy as well as, or better than, their younger counterparts. Additionally, cisplatin nephrotoxicity was only one-third as great in a subset of 14 patients with a single kidney. The amount of gastrointestinal toxicity also depends to some extent upon what time of day the drug is given. The neurotoxicity of cisplatin was defined and quantitated by serial graded clinical examinations, EMG and nerve conduction studies, and light and EMG studies of sural nerve biopsies. This toxicity is an irreversible predominantly sensory peripheral neuropathy. Although cisplatin binds avidly to B12 in vitro, we find no evidence for blockage of the B12-dependent conversion of malonic acid to malonyl COA or homocysteine to methionine (each necessary for the production of fatty acids and myelin). B12 therapy does not seem to prevent this toxicity. Cisplatin-induced anemia is normochromic and normocytic. Serum B12, B12 binding capacity, serum and red cell folates are normal. There was absolutely no evidence for hemolysis. Reticulocyte counts were low, and the bone marrow examination revealed that red cell precursors were generally decreased. Serum iron concentration, total iron binding capacity, transferrin, and ferritin were each quite high. Liver and bone marrow showed increased iron stores. Erythropoietin values were much lower than they would be expected to be, given the degree of anemia observed. These data point to an interference with iron utilization. Cisplatin effects upon heme and globin synthesis and ferrochetolase activity were also studied. Disulfiram therapy in mice bearing L1210 leukemia decreases cisplatin lethal toxicity and increases antitumor effect. The effect of disulfiram rescue upon cisplatin pharmacokinetics and toxicity was also studied in patients with encouraging results. Selective chemical and temporal modification of various cisplatin toxicities may serve as a model for the manipulation of therapeutic indices of other toxic yet active drugs.

2. INTRODUCTION

While it is undeniably true that the discovery of new and better drugs for the treatment of cancer is an essential goal of cancer research, it is interesting to observe that extensive analog development has seldom resulted in related agents replacing clinically active drugs. Literally tens of thousands of cyclophosphamide, mitomycin, anthracycline, bleomycin, cisplatin and other analogs have been undergoing extensive preclinical and clinical testing for decades. The testing of chemically-related compounds against experimental murine tumors, human tumor stem cells or other model systems is perceived as being more cost-effective than the support of research striving to understand how agents of proven utility induce their toxic and therapeutic effects. Recent conversations with research directors from two large drug companies with major cancer drug programs have brought this "silver bullet" philosophy very clearly into focus. There is little incentive for a drug company to investigate methods of improving anticancer drug therapeutic index if that proprietary drug has unique clinical utility. The development of related or new drugs on the other hand might gain the company new or larger shares of the current market.

While not denigrating the overall importance of new drug discovery and analog development, it seems as though investigation of ways of dissociating the toxic and therapeutic effects of drugs with established clinically important antitumor activity is also an area which should yield returns. This is demonstrated quite effectively by Ozols, who finds a 50 percent objective response rate in ovarian cancer patients to high doses of cisplatin after these patients failed lower doses of the drug.[1] No analog so far discovered can hope to match this performance in failed patients. It is true that the toxicities of cisplatin are impressive and worrisome. As these toxicities have become more fully understood at the clinical and basic levels, however, practices have evolved that allow the clinician to decrease or avoid certain of them.

This symposium has correctly emphasized promising cisplatin analogs, each of which may be anticipated to have differing but nonetheless present dose-limiting toxicities. It is my purpose to describe the preclinical-clinical cisplatin nephrotoxicity in order that this outline may serve as a basis for the investigation of methods permitting the more precise use of this very important drug with established antitumor activity. This paper reviews the consideration of the circadian timing of cisplatin therapy and how varying this affects the drug's therapeutic index.

2.1. The Murine Basis for Temporal Modification of Cisplatin Toxicity and Therapeutic Effectiveness.

The timing of drug administration relative to the endogenous time structure of the individual on the circadian time scale has been demonstrated to be of extreme importance in predicting the amount of toxicity resulting from a given dose of drug for every agent studied in an adequate chronobiologic fashion.[2] In principle, this predictable variability in drug toxicity is especially important for drugs with a narrow therapeutic index, such as anticancer agents.[3] We have studied seven anticancer agents for time-dependent toxicity and have found time variant toxicity for each of them (see Table 1).

Table 1. Animal results for each of seven anticancer agents tested for circadian rhythms in lethal toxicity.

Drug tested[2]	Animal (only females used)	P[1]	Predictable[3] range of survival[4]	Timing of least drug toxicity[5]
Cis-diammine-dichloroplatinum	Fischer 344 rat	.002	76% to 124%	19 hrs, 16 min.
Doxorubicin	Mouse	<.001	66% to 133%	8 hrs, 16 min.
Daunorubicin	Mouse	.021	71% to 129%	4 hrs, 28 min.
Cytosine Arabinoside	Mouse	<.001	44% to 156%	8 hrs, 24 min.
L Phenylalamine Mustard	Mouse	.015	69% to 131%	9 hrs, 11 min.
Cyclophosphamide	Mouse	.027	68% to 132%	12 hrs, 20 min.
Vincristine	Mouse	.007	54% to 146%	12 hrs, 52 min.

[1] Results from least-squares fitting of 24-hour cosine curve.
[2] i.p., all drugs, except cis-diamminedichloroplatinum, were tested in mice kept in LD 12:12; cis-diamminedichloroplatinum was tested in rats kept in LD 8:16. Light on 0000. Each drug was tested in a mean of 5 experiments using a mean of 750 animals per drug tested.
[3] Extent of predictable circadian variation in survival.
[4] Expressed as % of 24-hour mean survival.
[5] Timing expressed in hours after lighting onset. Usually light onset signals the beginning of the murine sleep or rest phase.

It is clear that the time structure of circadian drug toxicity is different for each agent studied so that no overall rule about the safest or most dangerous time for cancer chemotherapy may be formulated.

The mechanisms by which each anticancer drug is rendered time dependently toxic are complex and may be considered more clearly by their categorization. The exposure of an animal to a drug at any given circadian stage results in the presentation of that drug to rhythmically modulating: drug uptake, activation, metabolism and excretion; hormonally affected cellular and subcellular target-drug interaction; immune-host interaction; and host and tumor cytokinetics. The time-dependent susceptibility of host and tumor to the toxicity and therapeutic effectiveness of the anticancer drug in question results from the sum of all these time-dependent interactions.

2.2. Lethal Cisplatin Toxicity.

During 1979, in anticipation of clinical studies of circadian drug timing, eleven experiments investigating the circadian time dependence of cisplatin lethality were performed upon 1503 female Fischer rats.

Each rat received 11 mg/kg of cisplatin at one of six equispaced circadian stages.[4] Both percent survival censoring at 50 percent overall mortality in each study and overall mean survival time censoring when the last drug death occurred (12 days) were highly dependent upon when the cisplatin had been given (See Table 2).

Table 2. Time dependence of cisplatin lethality.

Time of cisplatin hrs after lights on	%Surviving at 50% mortality mean $\pm$ S.E.*	Survival time in hours mean $\pm$ S.E.**
1	50.8 $\pm$ 4.7	155 $\pm$ 5
5	40.5 $\pm$ 4.4	151 $\pm$ 6
9	36.9 $\pm$ 5.7	149 $\pm$ 6
13	47.6 $\pm$ 5.8	152 $\pm$ 4
17	64.4 $\pm$ 7.1	186 $\pm$ 6
21	54.2 $\pm$ 3.8	168 $\pm$ 6
***ANOVA	f = 3.4, p < 0.01	f = 7, p < 0.001
****Cosinor	p < 0.002	

*Mean of 11 separate experiments upon 1503 8 to 12-week-old female Fischer rats.
**No deaths occurred after day 12 288 hrs. Survival time assigned to each long-term survivor, truncating for analysis at day 12.
***Analysis of variance.
****Results from least-squares fitting of 24-hour cosine curve.

The most favorable time for cisplatin administration was late in the animal's active span, 16-19 hours after lights were turned on when the animals were synchronized on a schedule of 8 hours of light (rest or sleep) alternating with 16 hours of darkness (activity). This time corresponds to the usual time of peak in core temperature of these rats, which occurs about 4-5 hours after the daily peak of urine volume in a subset of rats in which the 24-hour rhythm in urine production was measured. β-N-Acetylglucosaminidase, a renal tubular brush border enzyme which reflects the metabolic activity of these tubular cells, is also excreted rhythmically within the circadian time scale. The circadian rhythm in the excretion of this enzyme, expressed in units per mg of excreted creatinine, peaks about 4 hours after lights or roughly 12 hours away from the time of highest cisplatin lethal toxicity.[5] The relationship of each of these rhythms in the female Fischer 344 rat is summarized in Table 3.

Table 3. Relationship of certain circadian rhythms in the Fischer 344 female rat to the circadian rhythms in cisplatin (11 mg/kg) lethal toxicity.

Endpoint	Mean + SE	*Amplitude + SE	Timing of peak HALO	p value**
Rectal temperature degrees Centigrade	37.4+0.02	0.6+0.1	16 hrs, 44 min.	0.001
Urine production ml/hr	0.2+.02	0.17+0.03	12 hrs, 20 min.	0.007
Urinary βNAG units per mg/ creat per hr	66+4	72+10	3 hrs, 56 min.	0.001
Cisplatin lethality***	50%	12%	19 hrs, 16 min.	0.002

*Amplitude is one-half of the predictable circadian variation
**Determined by probability of rejecting the zero amplitude hypothesis after least-squares fitting of a 24-hr cosine curve to the data
***Expressed in relationship to mean survival for animals treated at one of six circadian stages.

Since hydration protocols were said to modulate cisplatin nephrotoxicity, we investigated whether the circadian stage dependence of cisplatin nephrotoxicity could be overcome by an intraperitoneally delivered 3 percent body weight saline flush.[4,6] In three successive experiments this "hydration regimen" prolonged life, time dependently. When saline was administered at the worst circadian stages a small increase in mean survival resulted. However, when it was given to animals at the best circadian stages a proportionately greater increase in survival time resulted. It is interesting to question whether the ability of other drugs or methods of protecting individuals from certain drug toxicities might also be dependent in part upon when these drugs are used or the methods are applied (See Table 4).

Table 4. The survival benefit of a 3 percent body weight "saline flush" is dependent upon the circadian stage of saline treatment.

	Time of saline flush in hours after lights on					
Increase in survival time conferred by "saline flush"	Time	01	05	09	13	17	21
	%	69	45	49	38	78	55

Each percentage value is the mean of 3 experiments and represents the percentage increase in survival time when animals receiving cisplatin (11 mg/kg) and 3 percent body weight saline are compared with animals receiving cisplatin alone.

2.3. Cisplatin Nephrotoxicity.

The dose of 11 mg/kg used in our lethality experiments killed about 80 percent of the rats injected. Since we do not give chemotherapy to human beings in such overwhelming dosages, we thought it important to define the organ-specific kidney toxicity of a dose of drug which resulted in no animal deaths, but which was of therapeutic benefit. In our hands, cisplatin at a dose of 5 mg/kg demonstrated marked antitumor effects in a transplantable immunocytoma and resulted in no deaths. When rats were given 5 mg/kg of cisplatin at the most favorable circadian stage, they lost less weight, ate more, had lower BUNs, excreted less NAG in their urine and had less severely damaged kidney tubules when the kidneys were examined histologically than when the same dose was given at the opposite circadian stage.[7]

Pharmacokinetic studies done in rats receiving cisplatin at different circadian stages revealed that administration of 5 mg/kg of cisplatin at the least favorable circadian stage resulted in statistically significantly greater nephrotoxicity and higher peak urinary cisplatin concentrations.[4,5,7,8] Area under the curve of concentration of cisplatin excreted was also greater in these animals. It is not clear whether this association of high urinary cisplatin concentration with a greater amount of nephrotoxicity represents a cause-and-effect relationship but it can be hypothesized that urinary concentration may reflect the amount of exposure of the kidney tubular cells to cisplatin.

2.4. Cisplatin Pharmacokinetics in Man.

Cisplatin urinary excretion kinetics after a 30-minute infusion of 60 mg/m^2 i.v. were studied in 51 treatment courses in 11 patients suffering from advanced genitourinary cancers. Each patient received one half the treatment courses at 6 a.m. and 6 p.m., respectively. Initial treatment time was randomly assigned, and subsequent treatment times were then alternated. 4100 cc of 5 per cent Dextrose mixed in 0.45 normal saline solution were given in the 6-9 hour periplatinum infusion span. No diuretics were used. Evening cisplatin infusion resulted in statistically significantly greater urine output, lower peak cisplatin concentrations and lower areas under the curve of cisplatin concentration (see Table 5).[9]

Table 5. Cisplatin pharmacokinetics as reflected by free platinum urinary excretion.

Time of therapy	No. of patients	No. of courses	Urine volume 4.5 hr post-cisplatin ml $\pm$ SE	Free platinum peak. Urinary concentration mg/ml $\pm$ SE	Free platinum area of con-centration over 4.5 hr post-cisplatin mg/hr/ml
6 a.m.	11	25	900 $\pm$ 80	43.8 $\pm$ 2	71 $\pm$ 5
6 p.m.	11	26	1140 $\pm$ 102	29.6 $\pm$ 1.7	40 $\pm$ 4
f-test; p-value			f=12.7,p<.001	f=6.7,p<0.01	f=7.4,p<0.01

2.5. Cisplatin Toxicity in Man.

Patients bearing cancer or with other serious illnesses may not be precisely enough synchronized with regard to circadian rhythms important in determining the amount of drug toxicity the patient might experience. In order to investigate this finding more thoroughly the circadian rhythm characteristics of body temperature, neutrophil count, lymphocyte count, heart rate, blood pressure, urinary volume, urinary sodium, urinary potassium and urinary cortisol excretion were studied. The populations studied differed substantially in tumor burden, performance status, response characteristics and survival. The group of patients with greater tumor burden had a greater degree of circadian dyssynchrony. Cortisol excretion was much higher and peaked substantially later in the day in poor prognosis cancer patients than in good prognosis patients or normal volunteers. On the other hand, urinary potassium excretion patterns were statistically quite indistinguishable from one another.[10]

Forty-three patients were subsequently studied prior to 295 separate treatment courses, which were administered randomly at either 6 a.m. or 6 p.m. Creatinine clearance fall after each treatment was then inspected. Somewhat less nephrotoxicity was seen when the drug was given at 6 p.m. as compared to 6 a.m. Twenty-four to 48 hours prior to each treatment urine was collected every two hours and potassium excretion was determined. That individual's circadian rhythm in urinary potassium excretion expressed as millequivalents per hour was calculated for each course. The amount of subsequent renal damage was represented by the creatinine clearance determination done in the Clinical Research Center prior to the next course of treatment. Creatinine clearance results were then compared according to how far from the daily potassium peak the patient had, in fact, received the cisplatin. Creatinine clearance results were compared according to whether cisplatin was received 0 to 6 hours, 6 to 12, 12 to 18 or 18 to 24 hours after the daily peak in potassium excretion. This procedure compared treatment time as gauged by a measure of internal rather than external time. Patients who were treated within six hours on either side of the span during which their rate of potassium excretion was highest (in mEq/hr) suffered absolutely no loss of renal function, while those patients receiving cisplatin farthest away from the time of highest potassium excretion had an average of 8 cc loss in creatinine clearance per treatment course. Since the standard treatment course of cisplatin for this group of patients included nine courses of therapy, inopportune timing of repeated cisplatin administration resulted in a substantial and unnecessary loss of kidney function (FIGURE 1).[10-11]

Comparison of Kidney Function Loss in Patients Receiving Cisplatin Close To or Far From Daily Peak Potassium Excretion

2.6. Effect of Patient Age and Pre-treatment Renal Function on Subsequent Cisplatin-induced Nephrotoxicity.

A priori downward dose modification is often performed in elderly patients. Many of the patients in which cisplatin is a clinically indicated drug have an absent kidney because of the surgery they have undergone as primary therapy for their testicular, bladder, cervical, or ovarian carcinomas. In order to rationally guide cisplatin therapy, we therefore asked whether urinary cisplatin kinetics or nephrotoxicity are affected by advancing age or having a single kidney. This problem was addressed using a multivariate approach analyzing cisplatin concentration and creatinine clearance change as a function of: disease type, disease stage, patient age, circadian stage of drug administration, season of drug administration, pre-treatment kidney number, pre-treatment creatinine clearance and patient sex. Fourteen patients had a single kidney and 29 had two kidneys. Four age groups were considered and an analysis for random distribution of kidney status across age groups showed this to be the case. Older patients and patients with a single kidney had significantly lower pre-treatment creatinine clearances when compared to younger people and patients with two kidneys. Urinary cisplatin concentrations were statistically significantly lower in patients with one kidney and were the same in older patients and younger patients. Older and younger patients with two kidneys had equal, progressive, total cisplatin dose-related deterioration of renal function. Surprisingly, renal function did not decline in people with a single kidney regardless of age, but did so markedly in those with two kidneys.[12] A summary of the age-related toxicity data may be seen in Table 6.

Table 6. Relationship of age to change in renal function before and after cisplatin (60 mg/m^2 per month).

Age	No. of Patients	Doses/pt	Pre-Rx CrCl Mean	Post-Rx CrCl Mean	Overall % Decrease CrCl
≤ 50	9	7.2	82 cc/min	53 cc/min	32%
51-60	10	6.3	91 cc/min	71 cc/min	17%
61-70	16	7.3	72 cc/min	50 cc/min	27%
> 70	8	6.2	70 cc/min	54 cc/min	20%

Cisplatin dose or schedule modification is not indicated on the basis of advancing age or decreased renal function secondary to surgical loss or total ureteral obstruction of one kidney.

Other manifestations of cisplatin nephrotoxicity that were also worse in patients receiving cisplatin at times of day associated with low potassium excretion include hypomagnesemia, a loss of urinary concentrating ability, as well as severe diuretic sensitivity and exaggerated diuretic-induced potassium and sometimes sodium loss. Hypomagnesemia occurred in conjunction with creatinine clearance fall and the two were correlated ($p < 0.01$). This problem did not usually become clinically manifest until the third or fourth course of therapy. Magnesiums often fell to levels of 1 mg. Symptoms included irritability, weakness, protracted nausea, anorexia and a very interesting coarse tremor. All of these symptoms were improved by replacement magnesium therapy. Hypomagnesemia responded to oral magnesium glutonate in doses of 1500 mg three times daily. Hypo-magnesemia often continued for 6 to 12 months after discontinuation of cisplatin therapy. Magnesium replacement therapy could eventually be discontinued in these patients although their creatinine clearance loss was permanent.

Both thiazide and especially loop diuretics were associated with substantial urinary potassium losses in all patients who received them. Hypokalemia induced by these agents in the face of cisplatin renal damage was extremely difficult to replete. When diuretic therapy was stopped, hypokalemia in patients with even a 50 percent loss of renal function secondary to cisplatin therapy was easily managed with oral KCl supplements.

Sodium wasting was virtually never a clinical concern in patients who were not also receiving diuretics. Three of the initial 43 patients studied in our Clinical Research Center, however, developed severe and symptomatic hyponatremia (110-120 mEq/l) with very high urinary sodium losses. Each of these patients was in mild congestive heart failure and was receiving Lasix when the problem occurred. Each patient responded to withdrawal of Lasix, sodium repletion, and fluid restriction. Chronic management of these patients with platinum damaged kidneys and congestive heart failure is a challenging task. Each patient suffering from hyponatremia has also had hypokalemia and hypomagnesemia necessitating careful balance of repletion therapy, diuresis and cardiotonic therapy. The problem has been solved in these patients by replacing Lasix with thiazide with or without the addition of spironolactone accompanied by digoxin and very careful monitoring of the electrolyte status, renal and cardiac function. It is fortunate that over a period of months the renal lesion responsible for potassium leak usually stabilizes or gradually improves. Reinstitution of loop diuretics in these patients, however, is often accompanied by a recurrence of electrolyte difficulties. See summary in Table 7.

Table 7. Electrolyte abnormalities associated with cisplatin renal damage.

Problem	Incidence	Cause	Range of values	Onset in relation to amount of renal damage	Symptoms or signs	Association with diuretic therapy	Duration	Therapy
Hypo- magnesemia	very common 75%	renal secondary to tubular damage.	0.7-1.3 usually ~1.0	predictable association with CrCl fall after 3 or 4 treatments.	weakness anorexia irritability coarse tremor tetany hyperreflexia	weak	usually continues for 3-12 mo after cisplatin discontin- uation.	Magnesium gluconate 1500 mg po tid and/or Mg sulfate im or iv.
Hypokalemia	not uncommon 30%	(same)	2.5-3.5 usually > 2.8.	less predict- able relation- to CrCl fall.	weakness	strong	continues as long as diuretic used & for some time after.	oral or i.v. KCl.
Hyponatremia	uncommon <10%	renal tubular cisplatin damage combined with effect of diuretic- induced naturesis.	can be <115.	always occurs in severely damaged kidneys (creatinine clearance < 50 cc/min).	confusion lethargy weakness	very strong	continues as long as the diuretic is continued.	restrict fluid intake & liberalize Na intake; discontinue Lasix and replace with thiazide and/or spirono- lactone and monitor closely.

2.7. <u>New Avenues for Attenuating Cisplatin Nephrotoxicity</u>.

The work of Borch in decreasing cisplatin nephrotoxicity in the mouse, rat and dog by subsequent administration of oral disulfiram or i.v. or i.p. Diethyl Dithio Carbamate is being followed up within a chronobiologic framework at the University of Minnesota. Preliminary results indicate that treating patients with very high doses of cisplatin at the time of day associated with the peak daily potassium excretion and following this by a single large dose of orally administered disulfiram results in total elimination of both the gastrointestinal and the nephrotoxicity of this drug. Additional cases are required before we will be able to determine if this protocol also effects the incidence or severity of cisplatin-induced neurotoxicity or anemia.

2.7.1. <u>Cisplatin-induced Anemia</u>. Protracted single agent cisplatin therapy results in a progressive anemia and thrombocytopenia without concomitant leukopenia. Intermittent moderate dose doxorubicin therapy does not result in progressive anemia. Nephrotoxicity is the most prominent cisplatin side effect. Since erythropoietin is synthesized in the kidney we characterized this anemia and its relationship to serum erythropoietin concentrations. Twenty-one patients each receiving 9 monthly courses of cisplatin (60 mg/m^2) and doxorubicin (60 mg/m^2) were studied in our Clinical Research Center prior to each treatment. During therapy creatinine clearance fell 40 percent from 81 ± 3 to 49 ± 4 cc/minute. Prior to any transfusion, the mean hemoglobin fell about 20 percent from 12 to 9.5 gram percent throughout the remaining months of treatment. The cisplatin-induced anemia is normochromic, normocytic, nonhemolytic with disproportionately low reticulocyte counts, normal B_{12}, B_{12} binding, serum folate, red cell folate, serum iron, and total iron binding capacity. Following minimal transfusion, percent transferrin saturation, and serum ferritin rose promptly and markedly. By the final treatment liver and bone marrow iron stores were high with normal numbers of marrow sideroblasts while bone marrows were hypocellular. The fall in hemoglobin was correlated with the creatinine clearance fall ($r=0.44$, $p<.01$), hemoglobin falling $.3$ gram percent for every 10 cc fall in creatinine clearance. In the presence of progressing anemia, erythropoietin concentrations failed to

rise and actually fell in association with creatinine clearance
(r=.3,p<.05). The hypoproliferative picture and aberrant behavior of
erythropoietin in response to anemia support the hypothesis that
erythropoetin deficiency secondary to renal toxicity is a primary
mechanism of cisplatin-induced anemia. A greater degree of anemia, when
measured by hemoglobin fall and transfusion requirement, occurred in
patients treated with cisplatin in the morning than those treated in the
evening (f=11,p<.001). Patients receiving morning cisplatin required an
average of 10 units of red blood cells to keep their hemoglobins above
10 gram percent during the 9 months of therapy while those receiving
evening cisplatin required less than 6 units of cells.[13]

2.7.2. Neurotoxicity. Thirty patients with advanced cancer,
previously untreated, receiving monthly courses of cisplatin (60
mg/m^2)-Adriamycin (60 mg/m^2) chemotherapy, were studied by clinical
examination, electromyography/nerve conduction velocity (EMG/NCV)
studies, and sural nerve biopsies. Baseline clinical and EMG/NCV
studies were performed on 19/30 patients. Mild peripheral neuropathy
was present at time of initial examination in 8 patients; 3 had
concurrent diagnoses of alcohol abuse (1), severe nutritional deficiency
(1), and poorly controlled diabetes (1). During chemotherapy, 2
patients dropped out of the study; 11/17 patients have had repeat
examinations done to date; 10/11 (91 percent) showed progression of
peripheral neuropathy clinically and by EMG/NCV. An additional 7
patients were examined 6-24 months after completion of treatment;
peripheral neuropathy was present in 6 (86 percent). Clinical
characteristics of the neuropathy were progressive loss of vibratory
sense, diminution/loss of deep tendon reflexes, and mild distal sensory
loss to pin and light touch. Mild progressive weakness was seen in 3
patients. Prolongation of sural nerve conduction velocities, increased
distal latencies, and development of fibrillations in scattered muscles
were seen by EMG/NCV. Sural nerve biopsies, performed on 7 patients
with clinical neuropathy after 9 courses of treatment, revealed loss of
large diameter nerve fibers and axonal degeneration. This nearly
universal complication of cisplatin therapy was symptomatic in nearly
all affected individuals and a cause of significant disability in 3 of
the 30 patients studied quantitatively. Those patients who received

morning cisplatin had statistically significantly less abnormality of pin prick, light touch sensation and less depression of reflexes than did those who received evening cisplatin. Position sense, vibration sense, motor function and EMG and nerve conduction studies were not different depending upon the circadian stage of cisplatin treatment.[14]

3. DISCUSSION

The processes by which anticancer drugs kill or injure normal and malignant cells are exceedingly complex. Many toxic effects may be chemically or temporally eliminated without interference with the majority of antitumor effectiveness. We must not be trapped by useful but overly simplistic working hypotheses of drug mechanism. The relative importance of normal immune function, endogenous hormonal effects, drug distribution and metabolism need to be thought of as important aspects of the overall balance between host and tumor. Direct cytotoxic effects, which can be observed in vitro and in vivo and which generally furnish the working hypothesis with which we view antitumor drug activity, cannot be considered adequately apart from these other variables.

For example, anthracycline quinone chemistry is becoming more well understood daily. The original observation of anthracycline-DNA intercolation set up a working hypothesis that these drugs must react with nuclear DNA in order to be effective. The work of Tritton, however showed that the exposure of the surface of tumor cells to doxorubicin bound to sepharose beads is adequate for cytotoxicity.[14] Work by Bachur, Meyers, Doroshow, Pietronigro, Hochstein, Daugherty, Israel, Kohn, and others reveal a growing understanding of the free radical chemistry of anthracycline drugs.[15-30] Their work supports the possibility of chemically dissociating some of the free radical mediated host toxicities from the antitumor effects of these drugs. Similar approaches modulate the therapeutic index for other quinone drugs with antitumor activity such as mitomycin and bleomycin.[31-34]

It has been noted for over 25 years that the alkylating agents cyclophosphamide and melphalan are able to kill tumor cells somewhat selectively for unclear reasons. Bocian has recently demonstrated that in certain in vivo systems much of this antitumor selectivity may be based upon the antisuppressor cell activity of these alkylating agents rather than direct antitumor cytotoxicity.[35] This kind of an observation has strategic implications which differ substantially from those engendered by a hypothesis based solely upon direct tumor cell toxicity.

It may be unfortunate that the phenotypic abnormality associated with Vinca alkaloid treatment, mitotic arrest, was so easily observed. The interactions of these agents with normal and malignant cells are undoubtedly extremely complex, but almost all Vinca research has centered around this visible and quantifiable phenomenon. Much has been learned about tubulin function, but little has been learned about how to increase the therapeutic index of these critically important drugs. The relationship between neurohumoral networks and normal and malignant cellular function growth and reproduction is just now becoming appreciated. The interesting work of Noble delineating hormone-Vinca interaction opens up the possibility of highly selective modulation of Vinca toxicity and antitumor effectiveness.[36]

The circadian stage dependence of cisplatin-induced nephrotoxicity anemia, neurotoxicity and gastrointestinal toxicity has already been documented in our Clinical Research Center. The most effective use of this drug must presently entail consideration of optimal drug timing, as well as chemical ways of increasing its antitumor selectivity.

It is time for both the drug houses and the National Institutes of Health to support studies attempting to sharpen our ability to use chemotherapeutic agents already proven to be highly effective in addition to the massive support already allocated for analog, new drug screening and development. If this entails reconsideration of patent policies and also the subsequent proprietary marketing of procedures, methods and chemicals to accomplish this goal, then this possibility should be explored.

4. REFERENCES

1. Ozols RF, Corden BJ, Collins J, Young RC. 1983. Renal effects and clinical pharmacokinetics of high-dose (HD) cisplatin (P) (40 mg/m QD x 5) in hypertonic saline. 4th Intl. Symp. Platinum Coord. Complexes Cancer Chemother. C-II, p. 75.
2. Hrushesky W, Cornelissen G, Halberg F, De Prins J, Nesbitt M, Kennedy BJ. 1978. Rhythm parameters of experimental data on carcinostatics potentially applicable to clinical chronotherapy. Proc. MN Academy Science 46:22.
3. Hrushesky WJM. 1983, in press. Chemotherapy timing: an important variable in toxicity and response. In: M Perry and J Yarbro (eds), Toxicity of Chemotherapy. New York, Grune & Stratton, Inc.
4. Hrushesky WJ, Levi FA, Halberg F, Kennedy BJ. 1982. Circadian stage dependence of cis-diamminedichloroplatinum lethal toxicity in rats. Cancer Res. 42:945-949.
5. Levi F, Hrushesky W, Borch R, Pleasants M, Kennedy BJ, Halberg F. 1982. Cisplatin urinary pharmacokinetics and nephrotoxicity: a common circadian mechanism. Cancer Treat. Rep. 66(#11):1933-1938.
6. Levi FA, Hrushesky WJ, Kennedy BJ. 1981. Perspectives en chronochimiotherapie anticancereuse. Le Quotidien Du Medecin Chronobiologie Supplement 2546, pp. 46-51.
7. Levi FA, Hrushesky WJ, Blomquist CH, Lakatua DJ, Haus E, Halberg F, Kennedy BJ. 1982. Reduction of cis-diamminedichloroplatinum nephrotoxicity in rats by optimal circadian timing. Cancer Res. 42:950-955.
8. Levi F, Hrushesky W, Halberg F, Haus E, Langevin T, Kennedy BJ. 1982. Lethal nephrotoxicity and hematologic toxicity of cisdiamminedichloroplatinum ameliorated by optimal circadian timing. Eur. J. Cancer Clin. Oncol. 18(#5):471-477.
9. Hrushesky WJM, Borch R, Levi F. 1982. A circadian time dependence of cisplatin urinary pharmacokinetics. Clin. Pharm. Ther. 32:330-339.
10. Hrushesky WJM, Lakatua DJ, Haus E, Langevin T, Halberg F, Kennedy BJ. 1983, submitted. Chemotherapy timing: is clock hour a sufficient reference?
11. Levi F, Pleasants M, Hrushesky W, Borch R, Halberg F, Kennedy BJ. 1983, in press. Urinary chronopharmacokinetics of cisdiamminedichloroplatinum (II) in the rat. In: Proc. XIVth Conf. Int. Soc. Chronobiol.
12. Hrushesky WJM, Shimp W, Kennedy BJ. 1983, in press. Lack of age-dependent cisplatin nephrotoxicity. Am. J. Med.
13. Wood P, Hrushesky WJM. 1983, submitted. Characterization of cisplatin-induced anemia: an erythropoietin deficiency syndrome.
14. Tritton TR, Yee G. 1982. The anticancer agent adriamycin can be actively cytotoxic without entering cells. Science 217:248-250.
15. Hrushesky WJM, Wood P, Eaton J, Meshnik S. 1983, submitted. Methylene blue prevents anthracycline toxicity.
16. Bachur NR, Gordon SL, Gee MV. 1978. A general mechanism for microsomal activation of quinone anticancer agents to free radicals. Cancer Res. 38:43-47.
17. Meyer CD, McGuire WP, Liss RH, Ifrim I, Grotzinger K, Young RC. 1977. Adriamycin: the role of lipid peroxidation in cardiac toxicity and tumor response. Science 197:165-167.

18. Doroshow J. 1982. Role of NADH dehydrogenase in oxygen radical formation by anthracycline (a) antibiotics. Proc. Am. Assoc. Clin. Res. 23:172.
19. Doroshow J. 1983. Effect of anthracycline antibiotics on oxygen radical formation in rat heart. Cancer Res. 43:460-472.
20. Goodman J, Hochstein P. 1977. Generation of free radicals and lipid peroxidations by redox cycling of adriamycin and daunomycin. Biophysical Res. Communications 77(#2).
21. Daugherty JP, Ng TC, Digerness SB, Evanochko WT, Durant JR, Glickson JD. 1983. Detection of acute adriamycin (ADR)-induced alterations in phosphate metabolites of perfused rat hearts by ^{31}P nuclear magnetic resonance (NMR). AACR 24(#1022):259.
22. Mimnaugh EG, Trush MA, Ginsberg E, Gram TE. 1982. Differential effects of anthracycline drugs on rat heart and liver microsomal reduced nicotinamide adenine dinucleotide phosphate-dependent lipid peroxidation. Cancer Res. 42:3574-3582.
23. Doroshow JH, Locker GY, Myers CE. 1980. Enzymatic defenses of the mouse heart against reactive oxygen metabolites. J. Clin. Invest. 65:128-135.
24. Doroshow JH, Locker GY, Ifrim I, Myers CE. 1981. Prevention of doxorubicin cardiac toxicity in the mouse by N-acetylcysteine. J. Clin. Invest. 68:1053-1064.
25. Bachur NR, Gordon SL, Gee MV. 1977. Anthracycline antibiotic augmentation of microsomal electron transport and free radical formation. Mol. Pharmacol. 13:901-910.
26. Handa K, Santo S. 1975. Generation of free radicals of quinone containing anticancer chemicals in NADPH-microsome systems as evidenced by initiation of sulfite oxidation. Japan S. Cancer Res. (Tokyo). 66:43-47.
27. Gianni L, Muindi J, Myers CE. 1983. Iron binding by anthracyclines: structural determinants and mechanism of redox catalysis. AACR 24(#1002):254.
28. Pietronigro D, Levin M, Hovsepian M, Demopoulos H, Silber R. 1983. Tetrazolium salts (TS) stimulate adriamycin (ADM) toxicity in L1210 cells. AACR 24(#1010):256.
29. Doroshow J. 1983. Anthracycline (A)-stimulated hydroxyl radical (OH-) production in the heart. AACR 24(#1005):255.
30. Yamanaka N, Kato T, Nishida K, Shimizu S, Fukushima M, Ota K. 1980. Increase of antitumor effect of bleomycin by reduced nicotinamide adenine dinucleotide phosphate and microsomes in vitro and in vivo. Cancer Res. 40:2051-2053.
31. Kowal CD, Diven WF, Kozikowski AP. 1983. Mitomycin-nucleotide interactions: formation of a covalently linked mitomycin C (MMC) and fluorodeoxyuridylate (FdUMP) molecule, and kinetics of aziridine ring opening. AACR 24(#983):249.
32. Fracasso PM, Keyes SR, Rockwell S, Sartorelli AC. 1983. Biotransformation of mitomycin C by NADPH-cytochrome P-450 reductase and DT-diaphorase in cultured cell lines. AACR 24(#982):249.
33. Andrews PA, Pan S, Glover CJ, Bachur NR. 1983. Electrochemical reduction of mitomycin C to alkylating intermediates. AACR 24(#971):246.

34. Pan S, Glover CJ, Andrews PA, Aisner J, Bachur NR. 1983. Kinetics of activation of mitomycin C and its metabolites by NADPH cytochrome P450 reductase and xanthine oxidase. AACR 24(#977):248.
35. Bocian RC, Ben-Efraim B, Mokyr MB, Dray S. 1983. Increase in the efficacy of low-dose melphalan therapy with progression of MOPC-315 plasmacytoma growth. AACR 24(#808):205.
36. Noble RL, Gout PW, Beer CT. 1983. The chemotherapeutic effectiveness of vinca alkaloids against transplanted t-cell lymphomas in Nb rats is directly related to the hormonal status of the host. AACR 24(#1126):285.

Evaluation of Platinum Complexes for Emetic Potential
J.E. Schurig, A.P. Florczyk and W.T. Bradner

1. INTRODUCTION

Many anticancer drugs cause some degree of nausea and vomiting in the cancer patient. Prolonged nausea and vomiting can become a serious hindrance to effective cancer chemotherapy because of the undesirable effects on nutrition, quality of life and compliance of the patient. The problem of anticancer drug-induced nausea and vomiting and the search for effective treatment have been the subject of several reviews recently (1-7).

Cisplatin is considered to be one of the most emetogenic anticancer drugs (8). One of the objectives of our platinum analog program is to identify compounds that have potential for being less emetic than cisplatin. This report reviews the development of a ferret emesis model and its application in the screening of platinum analogs for emetic activity.

2. CONTROL OF EMESIS

This subject has been reviewed in detail recently by Borison and McCarthy (9). The following represents a brief overview. The control mechanism for emesis consists of two distinct units in the medulla: the emetic center and the chemoreceptor trigger zone (CTZ). A simplified schematic diagram (10) of the interactions involved in the induction of emesis by cancer chemotherapeutic agents is shown in Figure 1. The emetic center lies in the reticular formation in the floor of the fourth ventricle and is the final common pathway for all emetic stimulii. The CTZ is also located in the fourth ventricle in the area postrema and appears to be activated by chemical stimuli in the blood or cerebrospinal fluid. When stimulated, the CTZ activates the emetic center and emesis results. The emetic center is also activated by stimulii from the GI tract via the vagal and sympathetic afferent nerves. A fourth source of input to the emetic center comes from the cortex and may be involved in anticipatory vomiting (11).

The specific mechanism(s) of the emetic effects of anticancer drugs are not well understood. There is evidence, based on CTZ-ablation studies in cats (12,13), that stimulation of the visceral afferent nerves and the CTZ can be involved. The emetic effect of most anticancer drugs is delayed in onset which further complicates determination of the mechanism of emesis.

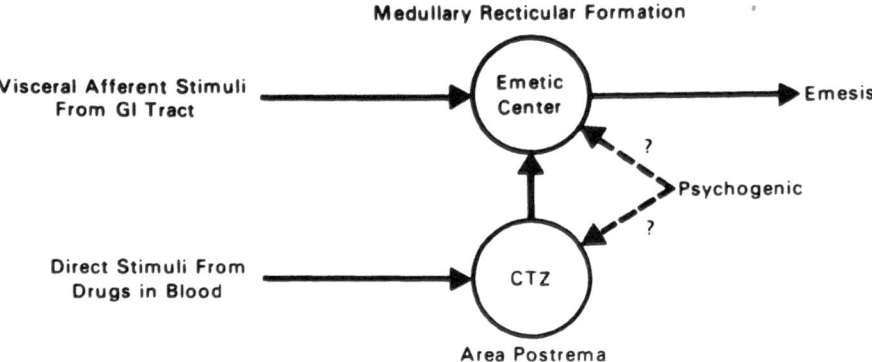

Figure 1.   Mechanism of cancer chemotherapy-induced vomiting. [From Penta, et al. (ref. 10) with permission from Masson Publishing USA, Inc.].

3. ANIMAL MODELS FOR EMESIS TESTING

It is known that many animal species such as mice, rats, guinea pigs and rabbits do not vomit. Dogs and cats have been described as useful for emesis testing whereas the monkey is reported to be unreliable (14). Gylys, et al. (15), quantitated the emetic effects of cisplatin in beagle dogs and used this animal model to test antiemetics, most notably metoclopramide, against cisplatin. There are also reports on apomorphine-induced emesis in dogs and use of this model to evaluate dopamine antagonists as potential antiemetics (16, 17).

The use of the cat as a model of emesis induced by anticancer drugs and pharmacological agents has been reported on extensively by Dr. Herbert Borison and his colleagues (see reference 9 for a recent review). Their studies in cats formed the basis for describing the neuropharmacology and physiology of the emetic process. They have also used cisplatin-induced emesis in cats as a test system for evaluating potential new antiemetics (18-20).

It was apparent to us that the effective animal models available to screen platinum analogs for emesis were limited to the dog or cat. However, these animals are not readily adaptable to a screening program for a number of reasons: 1) they are expensive to procure and house, 2) availability is often limited, especially cats, based on our experience, and 3) these are large animals and thus require large quantities of test drug which is usually in limited supply early in the developmental process. Therefore, the initial challenge we faced in screening platinum analogs for emesis was to develop an animal model that was cost effective for use as a screening test and required small quantities of drug.

4. THE FERRET EMESIS MODEL

Our discovery of the ability of the ferret to vomit was rather serendipitous. Another research group had received some ferrets and we noted the animals were small (∿1 kg) and inexpensive ($25 each) relative to cats and dogs. We discovered that the ferret would vomit after apomorphine, 5 mg/kg sc, which suggested that it has an emetic CTZ. Therefore, we decided to evaluate the ferret in more detail as a potential model for determining the emetic effects of anticancer drugs.

The specific methods used for emesis testing in ferrets have been described previously (21,22). The test drugs are administered as an iv bolus via an indwelling jugular catheter and the ferrets are observed for 6 hours. During the observation period the time to the first emetic episode and the number of episodes are recorded. An emetic episode is characterized by retching and expulsion of vomitus. If there is less than 1 minute between two episodes, they are considered a single event.

4.1 Emetic effects of anticancer drugs in the ferret

The initial objective was to test cisplatin in the ferret and compare the results qualitatively with its emetic effects in other animals. The emetic effects of cisplatin in ferrets are summarized in Table 1. Cisplatin caused emesis at 10, 8 and 6 mg/kg but not at 4 mg/kg. The emetic episodes began 60-100 minutes after administration and continued for about 2 hours.

The number of episodes increased with the dose while the onset time tended to decrease with increasing doses. Cisplatin caused an average of about 7 emetic episodes at 8 mg/kg and this dose was selected as the standard for comparison. Gylys and coworkers (15) reported cisplatin caused emesis in dogs at 3 mg/kg with about 15 emetic episodes beginning 90-120 minutes after

Table 1. Emetic Effect of Cisplatin in Ferrets

Dose[a] (mg/kg iv)	No. With Emesis No. Tested	No. of Episodes	Emesis Onset in Responding Animals(min)
4	0/3	0	-
6	4/4	2.5 ± 1.3	99 ± 4
8	4/4	6.8 ± 0.5	75 ± 4
10	2/2	10.5 ± 2.5	60 ± 2

[a] All doses of cisplatin caused death in 3-7 days.
Values are Mean ± S.E.

administration. McCarthy and Borison (20) reported cisplatin caused emesis in cats at 7.5 mg/kg with an average of 3.7 episodes beginning about 70 minutes after dosing. Therefore, the ferret appeared similar to the cat in its sensitivity to the emetic effects of cisplatin.

As indicated in the footnote in Table 1, all of the doses of cisplatin caused lethality in 3-7 days. We were unable to produce emesis with cisplatin in the ferret at non-lethal doses. This is somewhat similar to the situation in the cat where cisplatin, 7.5 mg/kg, causes lethality several days after dosing (L.E. McCarthy, personal communication). In the dog, however, the 3 mg/kg dose of cisplatin is an approximate LD_{10} (J.A. Gylys, personal communication).

We have evaluated additional known emetic anticancer drugs in the ferret model to determine its spectrum of sensitivity. The results obtained using Adriamycin, cyclophosphamide and combinations of cisplatin + Adriamycin and Adriamycin + cyclophosphamide are summarized in Table 2. Adriamycin was not emetic at 4 mg/kg but caused an average of 6 episodes at 8 mg/kg beginning about 80 minutes after administration. This latency in onset was similar to that observed with cisplatin. Cyclophosphamide caused emesis at 100 and 150 mg/kg with 3 and 11 episodes, respectively. The average onset time cyclophosphamide was shorter than with cisplatin or Adriamycin.

Table 2. Emetic Effects of Anticancer Drugs in Ferrets

Drug	Dose (mg/kg iv)	No. With Emesis No. Tested	No. of Episodes	Emesis Onset in Responding Animals (min)
Adriamycin	4*	0/2	-	-
	8*	4/4	6 ± 2	84 ± 6
Cyclophosphamide	100*	3/3	3 ± 1	39 ± 18
	150*	3/3	11 ± 5	21 ± 10
Cisplatin + Adriamycin	4* 4	4/4	6 ± 2	101 ± 6
Adriamycin + Cyclophosphamide	4* 100	4/4	12 ± 2	30 ± 8

*
Lethal dose or combination in 3-10 days
Values are Mean ± S.E.

The combination of cisplatin, 4 mg/kg, plus Adriamycin, 4 mg/kg, caused an average of 6 emetic episodes beginning about 100 minutes after dosing (Adriamycin was given immediately after cisplatin). Individually cisplatin and Adriamycin were not emetic at 4 mg/kg (Tables 1 and 2, respectively). The combination of Adriamycin at 4 mg/kg with cyclophosphamide at 100 mg/kg was also emetic, causing 12 episodes beginning 30 minutes after adminstration. The onset time was similar to that seen with cyclophosphamide alone. Again, the emetic effect of the combination was greater than either drug alone at the same dose.

The results of these studies indicated the ferret was responsive to the emetic effects of cisplatin, Adriamycin and cyclophosphamide alone and in combination. These results were in good agreement, qualitatively, with the clinical experience with these drugs (9) and suggested the ferret was an effective alternative to the cat and dog.

5. EVALUATION OF THE EMETIC EFFECTS OF PLATINUM ANALOGS IN THE FERRET

5.1 Platinum analogs in clinical trials

The platinum analogs currently in Phase I clinical trials, JM-8 (cis-diammine-1,1-cyclobutane dicarboxylate platinum II; CBDCA), JM-9 (cis-di-chloro-trans-dihydroxy-bis-isopropylamine platinum IV; CHIP), JM-82 (cis-1,2-diaminocyclohexane carboxyphthalato platinum II) and TNO-6 (cis-1,1-diamino-methylcyclohexane platinum II sulfate) were evaluated for emetic effects in the ferret. The initial test dose of each analog was selected by determining its approximate potency relative to cisplatin, based on murine LD_{50} values (single dose ip), and multiplying that factor by 6 mg/kg, the lowest emetic dose of cisplatin. Subsequent doses were selected based on the emetic response and lethality of the initial dose. Generally, our objective was to achieve a dose causing lethality or emesis in all animals.

The results of these studies are summarized in Table 3. JM-8 caused emesis in 1 of 3 ferrets at 72 mg/kg (4 episodes in that ferret) and no emesis at lower doses. JM-9, JM-82 and TNO-6 caused emesis at all doses tested. The incidence and number of episodes tended to increase with the dose with JM-9 and JM-82 whereas the effects of TNO-6 were not dose-related over the range tested. The latency in onset of emesis with JM-8, JM-9 and the lower doses of JM-82 was similar to that of cisplatin. The highest dose of JM-82 and both doses of TNO-6 caused emesis with a shorter latency than cisplatin.

In Table 4 the emetic effects of these platinum analogs in ferrets are compared with the emetic effects reported in the Phase I clinical trials (23-26). As was found in the ferrets, all of the analogs caused emesis in man. JM-8 was less emetic than cisplatin in the ferrets based on incidence and number of episodes. In the clinical studies JM-8 caused emesis in most patients but the drug was reported to be less emetic than cisplatin (23) in terms of number of episodes and severity. JM-82 caused emesis in man which was considered less severe than with cisplatin (25); however, in ferrets JM-82 was comparable to cisplatin based on incidence and number of episodes.

Table 3. Emetic Effects of the Phase I Platinum Analogs in Ferrets

Analog	Dose (mg/kg iv)	No. With Emesis / No. Tested	No. of Episodes	Emesis onset in Responding Animals (min)
Cisplatin	6*	4/4	2.5 ± 0.5	99 ± 4
	8*	9/9	8.0 ± 1.4	68 ± 6
JM-8	48*	0/2	0	-
	60*	0/3	0	-
	72*	1/3	1.3 ± 1.3 (4)	52
JM-9	8	1/4	2.0 ± 1.0 (8)	73
	12*	3/4	5.5 ± 2.5 (7)	69 ± 9
JM-82	12	1/2	1 (2)	71
	18	3/3	3.7 ± 2.1	78 ± 29
	36	3/3	8.3 ± 5.0	13 ± 9
TNO-6	2	3/3	12.7 ± 1.9	14 ± 1
	4*	3/3	12.3 ± 1.5	11 ± 1

* Lethal dose in 3-10 days
Values are Mean ± S.E.
Values in parenthesis = No. of episodes in responding animals.

Table 4. Emetic Effects of the Phase I Platinum Analogs in Ferrets and Man

Drug	Emetic Effects Ferret	Man
Cisplatin	+	+
JM-8	±	+*
JM-9	+	+
JM-82	+	+*
TNO-6	+	+

+ = Emesis in the majority of ferrets or patients.
± = Emesis in <50% at highest dose tested.
* Emesis reported to be less severe than with cisplatin.

5.2 Screening new platinum analogs

Analogs which pass the murine antitumor and nephrotoxicity screens are candidates for emesis testing in ferrets if solubility is adequate. The analogs we have screened to date for emetic effects are listed in Table 5 along with their structures.

Table 5. Platinum Analog Structures

$$
\begin{array}{ccc}
 & X & \\
A\diagdown & | & \diagup L \\
 & Pt & \\
A\diagup & | & \diagdown L \\
 & X &
\end{array}
$$

| Analog | Ligand | | |
	Amine	Leaving	Axial
JM-10	Ammine	2-ethylmalonate	-
JM-40	Ethylenediamine	Malonate	-
TNO-4	1,1-diaminomethylcyclobutane	Cl	Cl
TNO-5	1,1-diaminomethylcyclopentane	Cl	Cl
TNO-18Na	1,1-diaminomethycyclohexane	2-hydroxymalonate	-
TNO-21	2,2-diethyl 1,3 propanediamine	2-ethylmalonate	-
TNO-23	2,2-diethyl 1,3 propanediamine	1,1-CBDCA	-
TNO-24	2,2-diethyl 1,3 propanediamine	Cl	OH
TNO-26	1,1-diaminomethylcyclobutane	Cl	OH
TNO-27	1,1-diaminomethylcyclohexane	SO_4	Cl
TNO-31	Hydroxo bridged dimer of TNO-32		-
TNO-32	1,1-diaminomethylcyclohexane	NO_3	-
TNO-37	Hydroxo bridged trimer of TNO-6		
	(1,1-diaminomethylcyclohexane	SO_4	-)

The emetic effects of these analogs in ferrets are summarized in Table 6. The selection of the test doses was according to the criteria described in the previous section. Most of the analogs caused emesis in the ferrets

Table 6.   Emetic Effects of Platinum Analogs in the Ferret

Analog	Dose mg/kg iv	No. with emesis / No. tested	No. of Episodes	Emesis onset in Responding Animals (min)
Cisplatin	8*	9/9	8.0 ± 1.4	68 ± 6
JM-10	48	0/3	0	-
	60*	0/3	0	-
	72*	0/3	0	-
JM-40	48	0/3	0	-
	72*	2/3	6.3 ± 3.3 (9.5)	84
TNO-4	4*	3/3	9.7 ± 1.3	24 ± 2
TNO-5	8*	3/3	9.0 ± 3.1	25 ± 5
TNO-18Na	6	1/3	2.3 ± 2.3 (7)	27
	12	3/3	7.7 ± 0.9	26 ± 2
TNO-21	60	2/3	7.0 ± 3.5 (10)	89
	72	3/3	5.3 ± 1.8	118 ± 10
TNO-23	60	0/3	0	-
	72*	2/3	3.0 ± 2.5 (4.5)	142
TNO-24	24*	3/3	12.0 ± 1.0	53 ± 5
TNO-26	12	3/3	10.7 ± 2.3	27 ± 3
TNO-27	4	3/3	9.7 ± 2.7	18 ± 1
TNO-31	4	3/3	13.0 ± 1.2	30 ± 4
TNO-32	4*	3/3	11.7 ± 1.8	12 ± 1
TNO-37	4	3/3	13.7 ± 3.0	19 ± 3

* Lethal dose in 3-10 days
Values are Mean ± SE
Values in parenthesis = No. of episodes in responding animals

with the incidence and number of episodes at the highest dose (or only dose) tested being comparable to the effect of cisplatin at 8 mg/kg. The exceptions included JM-10, JM-40 and TNO-23. JM-10 had no emetic effect at any dose tested. JM-40 and TNO-23 did not cause emesis in all of the ferrets emesis in all of the ferrets at the high dose. The ferrets responding to TNO-23 had fewer episodes than with cisplatin whereas the ferrets responding to JM-40 had essentially the same number of episodes as cisplatin treated animals.

The time of onset of emesis in responding animals was quite variable among the analogs. Ferrets responding to JM-40, TNO-21, TNO-23 and TNO-24 had emesis onset times that were generally comparable to or greater than the cisplatin-treated ferrets. The onset times in the ferrets treated with the other emetic analogs were shorter than with cisplatin.

6. DISCUSSION

The search for a better platinum analog should include an evaluation of the antitumor active compounds for emetic effects relative to cisplatin. However, this evaluation should not be placed in a strict pass (less emetic than cisplatin) or fail (comparable to cisplatin) position in a decision network. Rather the results of an emesis screen should be used to identify platinum analogs which are potentially less emetic than cisplatin so that these analogs can be given high priority in advanced test systems.

Previous test systems for evaluating the emetic effects of anticancer drugs utilized cats or dogs (15, 18). These animals are not suitable for use in emesis screening because of their high cost and large size. We investigated the ferret as a smaller, more cost efficient test system that could be used in an emesis screening program. Cisplatin, Adriamycin and cyclophosphamide, known emetic anticancer drugs (8,9), caused emesis in the ferret suggesting the ferret can predict for the emetic effects of anticancer drugs. With each of these drugs the onset of emesis was delayed in the ferret as it is in humans. However, the ability of this parameter to predict relative latency is unclear since cyclophosphamide does not have a shorter latency than cisplatin in man (9) as it did in the ferret.

The emetic doses of cisplatin, Adriamycin and cyclophosphamide caused death in 3-10 days after administration. This lack of separation between the emetic dose and the lethal dose is an undesirable characteristic of the ferret

emesis model. However, considering the available alternative test systems, we
do not believe this diminishes the usefulness of the ferret in emesis testirg.

The ferret provided good qualitative prediction of the emetic effects
observed with JM-8, JM-9, JM-82 and TNO-6 in the initial Phase I trials. Tre
results from the clinical evaluation of JM-8 (23) indicate this analog was
less emetic than cisplatin which is in agreement with the results from the
ferret studies. We were not able to predict, based on the ferret data, that
in man JM-82 would cause emesis that was less severe than with cisplatin
because we cannot obtain a subjective assessment of the severity of emesis in
the ferret. It should be possible to make more quantitative comparisons of
the emetic effects of each analog in ferrets and man as additional results
from the clinical evaluations become available.

We have screened thirteen new platinum analogs for emetic effects in the
ferret. Eleven of these compounds caused emesis which was comparable, in
terms of incidence and number of episodes, to cisplatin. TNO-23 (2,2-diethyl
1,3-propanediamine CBDCA platinum II) was less emetic than cisplatin and
JM-10 (diammine 2-ethylmalonate platinum II) had no emetic effect.
Therefore, the ferret emesis model has identified three platinum analogs
(including JM-8) which have the potential for being less emetic than cisplatin.

The results obtained thus far in the ferret emesis model do not demonstrate a clear relationship between the structure of a platinum analog and
the magnitude of its emetic effect. The only compounds considered less
emetic than cisplatin (JM-8, JM-10 and TNO-23) have bidentate leaving
ligands. This suggests that analogs with bidentate leaving ligands have the
potential for being less emetic than cisplatin, whereas analogs with monodentate leaving ligands are very likely to be comparable to cisplatin.
However, the analogs with bidentate leaving ligands usually have low milli-
gram potency relative to cisplatin. We have not yet identified a potent
platinum analog with low emetic potential.

ACKNOWLEDGEMENTS

The authors acknowledge the expert technical assistance of Ms. Suzanne
Spencer and thank Mrs. Rita Sutliff for preparation of the manuscript.

REFERENCES

1. Frytak, S., and Moertel, C.G.: Management of nausea and vomiting in the cancer patient. JAMA 245:393-396, 1981.
2. Siegel, L.J. and Longo, D.L.: The control of chemotherapy-induced emesis. Ann. Intern. Med. 95:352-359, 1981.
3. Treatment of Cancer Chemotherapy Induced Nausea and Vomiting, edited by D.S. Poster, J.S. Penta and S. Bruno. Masson Publishing, New York, 1981.
4. Supplement, J. Clin. Pharmacol. 21:1981.
5. Supplement, Cancer Treat. Rev. 9:1982.
6. Supplement, Drugs 25:1983.
7. Antiemetics and Cancer Chemotherapy, edited by J. Lazlo. Williams and Wilkins, Baltimore, 1983.
8. Lazlo, J.: Treatment of nausea and vomiting caused by cancer chemotherapy. Cancer Treat. Rev. 9:3-9, 1982.
9. Borison, H.L. and McCarthy, L.E.: Neuropharmacology of chemotherapy-induced emesis. Drugs 25:8-17, 1983.
10. Penta, J.S., Poster, D.S., Bruno, S., Pinna, K. and Macdonald, J.S.: Cancer chemotherapy-induced nausea and vomiting: a review. In Treatment of Cancer Chemotherapy-Induced Nausea and Vomiting, edited by D.S. Poster, J.S. Penta and S. Bruno. Masson Publishing, New York, 1981, pp. 1-32.
11. Morrow, G.R.: Prevalence and correlates of anticipatory nausea and vomiting in chemotherapy patients. J. Nat. Cancer Inst. 68:585-588, 1982.
12. McCarthy, L.E. and Borison, H.L.: Cisplatin emesis and cannabinoids in cats. Pharmacologist 22:241, 1980.
13. Borison, H.L, Brand, E.D. and Orkand, R.K.: Emetic action of nitrogen mustard (mechlorethanmine hydrochloride) in dogs and cats. Am. J. Physiol. 192:410-416, 1958.
14. McCarthy, L.E. and Borison, H.L.: Animal models for predicting antemetic drug activity. In Antiemetics and Cancer Chemotherapy, edited by J. Lazlo. Williams and Wilkins, Baltimore, 1983, pp. 21-33.
15. Gylys, J.A., Doran, K.M. and Buyniski, J.P.: Antagonism of cisplatin-induced emesis in the dog. Res. Comm. Chem. Path. Pharmacol. 23:6-68, 1979.
16. Niemegeers, C.J.E., Schellekens, K.H.L. and Janssen, P.A.J.: The antiemetic effects of domperidone, a novel potent gastrokinetic. Arch. Int. Pharmacodyn 244:130-140, 1980.
17. Perrot, J., Nahas, G., Laville, C. and Debay, A.: Substituted benzamides as antiemetics. In Treatment of Cancer Chemotherapy-Induced Nausea and Vomiting, edited by D.S. Poster, J.S. Penta and S. Bruno. Masson Publishing, New York, 1981, pp. 195-208.
18. London, S.W., McCarthy, L.E. and Borison, H.L.: Suppression of cancer chemotherapy-induced vomiting in the cat by nabilone, a synthetic cannabinoid (40465). Proc. Soc. Exp. Biol. and Med. 160:437-440, 1979.
19. McCarthy, L.E. and Borison, H.L.: Cisplatin emesis and cannabinoids in cats. Pharmacologist 22:241, 1980.
20. McCarthy, L.E. and Borison, H.L.: Antiemetic activity of N-methyl-levonantradol and nabilone in cisplatin-treated cats. J. Clin. Pharmacol. 21:30S-37S, 1981.
21. Florczyk, A.P. and Schurig, J.E.: A technique for chronic jugular catherization in the ferret. Pharmacol. Biochem. Behav. 14:255-257, 1981.

22. Florczyk, A.P., Schurig, J.E. and Bradner, W.T.: Cisplatin-induced emesis in the ferret: a new animal model. Cancer Treat. Rep. 66: 187-189, 1982.
23. Calvert, A.H., Harland, S.J., Newel, D.R., Siddik, Z.H., Jones, A.C., McElvain, T.J., Raju, S., Wiltshaw, E., Smith, I.E., Baker, J.M., Peckham, M.J. and Harrap, K.R.: Early clinical stludies with cis-diammine-2,2-cyclobutane dicarboxylate platinum II. Cancer Chemother. Pharmacol. 9:140-147, 1982.
24. Creaven, P.J., Mittelman, A., Pendyla, L., Tseng, M., Pontes, E., Spaulding, M., Moayeri, H., Madajewicz, S., Cowens, J.W., Soloman, J.:Phase I study of a new antineoplastic platinum analog cis-dichloro-trans-dihydroxy-bis-isopropylamine platinum IV (CHIP). Proc. Amer. Soc. Clin. Oncol. 1:22, 1982.
25. Kelsen, D.P., Scher, H., Alcock, N., Leyland-Jones, B., Donner, A., Williams, L., Greene, G., Burchenal, J.H., Tan, C., Phillips, F.S. and Young, C.W.: Phase I clinical trial and pharmacokinetics of 4'-carboxyphthalato-(1,2-diamino-cyclohexane) platinum (II). Cancer Res. 42:4831-3835, 1982.
26. Pinedo, H., Ten Bokkel Huinink, W., Simonetti, G., Gail, H., Van der Vijgh, W., Canetta, R., Van Putten, L., Vermorken, J. and McVie, G.: Phase I study and pharmacokinetics of cis-1,1-di(aminomethyl)-cyclo-hexane Pt. II sulfate (TNO-6). Proc. Amer. Soc. Clin. Oncol. 1:26, 1982.

POSTER PRESENTATIONS

III-1 PHARMACOKINETICS OF THE TRANSPLACENTAL PASSAGE OF cis-PLATINUM IN MICE.
P. Köpf-Maier.

III-2 EFFECT OF RHODIUM COMPLEXES ON EXPERIMENTAL CARCINOGENESIS IN LIVER OF RATS TREATED WITH THIOACETAMIDE (TAM).
C. Cascales, D.G. Craciunescu, P. Martin-Sanz and M. Cascales.

III-3 ACUTE EFFECTS OF INFUSION OF cis-DIAMMINEDICHLOROPLATINUM (CDDP) ON RENAL FUNCTION.
S. Meijer, J.J.G. Offerman, D.T. Sleijfer, A.J.M. Donker, N.H. Mulder and H.S. Koops.

III-4 PHASE I TRIAL OF CHIP.
B.S. Yap, D.M. Tenney, H.Y. Yap, C. Plager, N.E. Papadopoulos, F.H. Lee, B.F. Issell and G.P. Bodey.

III-5 A PHASE I STUDY OF cis-DICHLORO-trans-DIHYDROXY-bis (ISOPROPYLAMINE)-PLATINUM IV (CHIP) ADMINISTERED BY INTRAVENOUS BOLUS DAILY FOR 5 DAYS.
S.J. Ginsberg, F.H. Lee, B.F. Issell, B.J. Poiesz, A.R. Rudolph, A.C. Louie, E.C. Bradley, R.W. Tinsley, S.M. DiFino, A.J. Scalzo, J.J. Gullo, M.D. Lerner, N.N. Palmer, A.V. Fitzpatrick and R.L. Comis.

III-6 PLATINUM AND IRON CONCENTRATION AS A FUNCTION OF TIME IN KIDNEYS OF RATS TREATED WITH CISPLATIN.
A.F. Le Roy, J.P. Berry, P. Brille, Y. Gouveia, P. Ribaud, P. Galle and G. Mathe.

III-7 THE RENAL TUBULAR TRANSPORT OF PLATINUM ANTITUMOUR DRUGS IN RELATION TO THEIR NEPHROTOXICITY.
P.T. Daley-Yates and D.C.H. McBrien.

III-8 PHASE I CLINICAL TRIAL OF 1,2-DIAMINOCYCLOHEXANE (ISOCITRATO) Pt (II)-(PHIC).
J.P. Armand, C. Picard, R.L. De Jager, J.P. Macquet and P.R. Combes.

III-9 SYNTHESIS AND IN VITRO CYTOSTATIC ACTIVITY OF PALLADIUM (II) AND PLATINUM (II) COMPLEXES WITH DITHIOCARBAMIC ESTERS.
L. Sindellari, G. Faraglia, M. Nicolini, A. Furlani and V. Scarcia.

III-10 PLATINUM (P) TREATMENT AND ELECTROLYTE IMBALANCE.
M.V. Fiorentino, M. Scalabrin and E. Ventrelli.

III-11 PHASE I STUDY AND CLINICAL PHARMACOKINETICS OF CARBOPLATIN (CBDCA) (NSC 241240) IN PATIENTS WITH AND WITHOUT RENAL FAILURE.
M.J. Egorin, D.A. Van Echo, M.Y. Whitacre, E.A. Olman and J. Aisner.

III-12 cis-DIAMINODICHLOROPLATINUM ULTRA HIGH DOSE (DDP-HD) IN TESTICULAR CARCINOMA: TOXICITY AND ACTIVITY.
H.J. Schmoll, J. Weiss and V. Diehl.

III-13 COMPARATIVE NEPHROTOXICITY OF PHIC AND CISPLATIN IN BABOONS.
B. Remandet, P. Richez, P. Vic, D. Gouy, J. Berthe and G. Mazue.

III-1 PHARMACOKINETICS OF THE TRANSPLACENTAL PASSAGE OF CIS-PLATINUM IN MICE. Petra Köpf-Maier. Institut für Anatomie der Freien Universität Berlin, Königin-Luise-Straße 15, D-1000 Berlin 33, Germany

In the present study we intended to gain information on the passage behavior of cis-platinum at the placental barrier and on the teratogenic action of this cytostatic drug at various stages of pregnancy.

Pregnant NMRI mice received a single i.p. application of ^{195m}Pt-labeled cis-platinum (10 mg/kg; 0.25 µCi/g mouse) on day 10, 11, 12, ..., or 17 of gestation. At various intervals after application, the embryos were removed and analyzed with respect to the content of radioactivity per g embryo. For morphologic purposes, the embryonic neocortex, which is very sensitive to the action of cytostatics, was removed and prepared for light and electron microscopy.

The tracer studies revealed the following results: (i) After treatment on day 10, 11, and 12 of pregnancy, only minimum amounts (less than 1 % of the per g-radioactivity) of ^{195m}Pt were detectable in the embryos. (ii) Between day 13 and day 17 of the murine pregnancy, increasing amounts of ^{195m}Pt passed the placenta; after treatment on day 17, even an effect of accumulation within the fetal compartment was observable.

The morphologic studies demonstrated analogous characteristics for the induction of structural alterations by cis-platinum: (i) After treatment on day 10 or 11 of gestation, no pathologic alterations were detectable in proliferating embryonal tissues, such as the neuroepithelium. (ii) After treatment on day 13, severe morphologic lesions occurred: The mitotic index in the neuroepithelium (control value 6.4 %) decreased significantly to less than 1 %; moreover, numerous cells in the neuroepithelial layer became necrotic within 24 h (maximum value 55 % of all cells). (iii) After treatment on day 14, 15, or 16, the appearance of necroses was also observable; because of the decreasing proliferation activity, however, the number of necrotic cells was smaller than the number on day 13.

Compared to other cytostatic drugs, the inability of cis-platinum to pass the placenta during organogenesis is quite uncommon. It may be supposed that the inorganic character and the unionized, but dipolar nature of the cis-platinum molecule are responsible for the inability to pass the placenta during organogenesis. When placental maturation, however, is accomplished, the noble metal complex is obviously transferred by a carrier-mediated transport.

III-2 EFFECT OF RHODIUM COMPLEXES ON EXPERIMENTAL CARCINOGENESIS IN LIVER OF RATS TREATED WITH THIOACETAMIDE (TAM). Carmen Cascales, Dan G.Craciunescu, Paloma Martín-Sanz and María Cascales. Departamento de Bioquímica y Química Inorgánica. Facultad de Farmacia. Universidad Complutense. Madrid-3. Spain.

Resently, Rh(III) complexes belonging to the $|Rh(L)_4X_2|X^-$ structure (where L=Pyridine, thiazole, sulphonamide derivatives, $X^- = Cl^-$ or Br^-) have been found effective against P_{388} tumours and also very effective against Gram positive bacteria. Among them, we prepared a $|Rh(L)_4Cl_2|^+Cl^-$ complex, where L=sulphaquinoxaline (acting as monodentate ligand), a mild antitumour compound with $LD_{50} > 300$ mg/Kg.

Since Fitzhugh & Nelson(Science 108,626-631,1948) showed thioacetamide to be a weak hepatocarcinogen the liver, rats treated with TAM have been studied from several points of view. Changes in the urea cycle enzymes and aminotransferases have been recently studied (Cascales et al.,J.Clin.Chem.Clin.Biochem.17,129-132,1979) in liver of TAM-treated rats. TAM was administered i.p. to male Wistar rats at a dose level of 100 mg/Kg/day for eight weeks. Two weeks before the end of treatment five doses of 50 mg/Kg of Rhodium complex were also i.p. administered. Liver homogenates were obtained from control TAM-treated and TAM + antitumoral-treated rats (1 g of liver: 4 ml 0.25M sucrose, 0.02M Tris-buffer pH 7.6 and 0.1 mM dithioerithritol) In the soluble and mitochondrial fractions aminotransferases GOT and GPT and glutamate dehydrogenase (GDH) were determined as described by Bergmeyer (Methoden der enzymatischen Analyse. ed.Bergmeyer H.U. 1974. Verlag-Chemie, Weinheim). Protein levels were also determined (Lowry et al., J.B.C. 193,265-275,1951).

Enzyme	EC	Fraction	TAM	TAM + Rh(III)
GOT	2.6.1.1.	Soluble	49 ± 0.8***	88 ± 11***
"		Mitochondrial	135 ± 2.6**	82 ± 1.4***
GPT	2.6.2.2.	Soluble	51 ± 4.9***	43 ± 4.2*
"		Mitochondrial	63 ± 8.2***	73 ± 14
GDH	1.4.1.3.	Mitochondrial	71 ± 6.1***	92 ± 4.1**
Protein		Soluble	78 ± 7.2*	95 ± 11*
"		Mitochondrial	143 ± 18***	87 ± 9***

Results, expressed as percentage of the control values, are the means±SEM of six experimental observations.***p<0.001;**p<0.01;*p< 0.05. Soluble and mitochondrial GOT elicit a significant restoration of their activities by the effect of Rh(III) complexes and also GDH and protein levels exhibit a marked positive change when antitumoral were administered. However, GPT activities remain practically un changed both in the mitochondrial and soluble fractions.

III-3 ACUTE EFFECTS OF INFUSION OF CIS-DIAMMINE-DICHLOROPLATINUM (CDDP) ON RENAL FUNCTION. S.Meijer, J.J.G.Offerman, D.Th. Sleijfer, A.J.M.Donker, N.H.Mulder and H.Schraffordt Koops, Department of Medical Oncology, Nephrology and Surgical Oncology, University Hospital, Oostersingel 59, 9713 EZ Groningen, the Netherlands.

In order to evaluate the pathogenetic mechanism of CDDP induced nephrotoxicity we studied the immediate changes in renal function during CDDP infusion in six consecutive patients. Furthermore, the study was repeated on day 21 after completion of the first course in the regimen according to Einhorn (1). CDDP was administered after prehydration with 2 l NaCl 0.9%. In the 24 hours after the start of CDDP an additional 4 l NaCl 0.9% were given. No mannitol or diuretics were added.

Renal function studies included direct measurement of glomerular filtration rate (GFR) and effective renal plasma flow (ERPF) by determination of ^{125}I iothalamate and ^{131}I hippuran clearances. The method is based on simultaneous and constant infusion of the radio-pharmaceuticals and corrects for incomplete urine voiding (2).

Results: During administration of CDDP (20 mg/m^2) over a 4 hour period, we found in all 6 patients a significant decrease in ERPF: mean 14%, range 2-26%, p < 0.05, starting within 1-6 hours after the start of the CDDP infusion. GFR in this period varied from 87-109%, mean 96% of the pretreatment values. On day 21 mean ERPF was 86% with a range of 68-110% of the pretreatment values. Mean GFR was decreased significantly to 88%, with a range of 76-97%, p < 0.05.

In conclusion, cisplatinum-induced disturbance in renal function appeared already a few hours after the first CDDP exposition. It consisted of a decrease in ERPF. This suggests a change in renal perfusion. It is tempting to speculate on methods to prevent these initial changes, as they might possibly influence the decrease in GFR found on day 21.

1. Einhorn LH, Donohue J. Ann.Intern.Med. 1977; 87: 293-298.
2. Donker AJM, Hem GK van der, Sluiter WJ, et al. Neth.J.Med. 1977; 20: 97-103.

III-4 PHASE I TRIAL OF CHIP. B.S. Yap, D.M. Tenney, H.Y. Yap, C. Plager, N. E. Papadopoulos, F.H. Lee, B. F. Issell, G.P. Bodey. The University of Texas System Cancer Center M. D. Anderson Hospital & Tumor Institute, Houston, Texas 77030 and Bristol Laboratories, Syracuse, New York 13201.

Cis-Dichloro-Transdihydroxy-Bis-Isopropylamine Platinum IV (CHIP, JM9), is one of several new platinum analogs, which was developed because it was more water soluble than cisplatin and showed minimal nephrotoxicity in animal toxicological testing. Its spectrum of activity is similar to that of cisplatin against L1210 leukemia, P-388 leukemia, B-16 melanoma, Lewis lung, carcinoma, Walker carcinosarcoma, Murphy-Sturm lymphosarcoma, colon CX-1 and lung LX-1 xerographs. Sixteen patients with a variety of refractory metastatic solid tumors have been treated on this study. These included 7 patients with sarcoma, 5 melanoma, 2 colon and 2 breast. There were 9 male and 7 female patients; median age was 45 years (range 23 to 58 years); median performance status 1 (range 0 to 2); and median number of prior chemotherapeutic regimens 2 (range 1 to 6). CHIP was given as a single intravenous infusion in 100 cc 5% dextrose over 30 mins. This was repeated every week for 4 weeks followed by a 2 week observation period. No pre- or post-treatment hydration or diuresis was given. Treatment courses were given in escalating doses from 40 mg/M^2 to 95 mg/M^2/week x 4 and dose levels studied included 40,60,75 and 95 mg/M^2/week. In this continuing study, 19 treatment courses are evaluable for toxicity. The dose-limiting toxicity was thrombocytopenia, first seen at 60 mg/M^2. At this dose level, the median lowest platelet count was 130,000/mm^3 (range 24,000 to 275,000/mm^3); at 75 mg/M^2, 144,000/mm^3 (range 58,000 to 229,000/mm^3), and at 95 mg/M^2, 80,000/mm^3 (range 41,000 to 223,000/mm^3). Leukopenia was minimal. All patients had mild to moderate nausea and vomiting and 3 patients had diarrhea. There was no nephrotoxicity, ototoxicity or alopecia. No antitumor activity was seen in this heavily pretreated group of patients. The maximal tolerated dose of CHIP appears to be 95 mg/M^2/week x 4, with the dose-limiting toxicity being thrombocytopenia.

III-5 A PHASE I STUDY OF CIS-DICHLORO-TRANS-DIHYDROXY-BIS
(ISOPROPYLAMINE)-PLATINUM IV (CHIP) ADMINISTERED BY
INTRAVENOUS BOLUS DAILY FOR 5 DAYS. Sandra J. Ginsberg*, Francis
H. Lee, Brian F. Issell, Bernard J. Poiesz*, Alfred R. Rudolph,
Arthur C. Louie, Edward C. Bradley, Roger W. Tinsley*, Santo M.
DiFino*, Anthony J. Scalzo*, John J. Gullo*, Mary D. Lerner*, Nancy
N. Palmer*, Alicia V. Fitzpatrick*, Robert L. Comis*. *Upstate
Medical Center, 750 E. Adams St., Syracuse, NY, 13210, USA and
Bristol Laboratories, P.O. Box 657, Syracuse, NY, 13201, USA.

CHIP is a cisplatin analogue which has exhibited less nephrotoxicity than cisplatin in animal models. In this study CHIP was
administered over 30 minutes daily x 5 consecutive days q 3 wks
without pretreatment hydration or diuresis. Thirty-four patients
(pts) were studied at doses of 20 mg/M^2/d (7 pts), 30 mg/M^2/d
(4 pts), 45 mg/M^2/d (15 pts), 65 mg/M^2/d (8 pts). Eighteen of the
34 pts had received prior chemotherapy and/or radiotherapy, while
16 pts had been previously untreated. Non-hematologic toxicities
included: mild-to-moderate nausea and vomiting at all dose levels;
decreased creatinine clearance in 3 pts receiving 45 mg/M^2/d
(2 pts) and 65 mg/M^2/d (1 pt); a fixed drug eruption in 1 pt
receiving 65 mg/M^2/d; and, diarrhea in 2 pts receiving 45 and
65 mg/M^2/d. Mild to moderate anemia (hemoglobin nadir - 9-12
g/dl) was observed at all dose levels. Non-dose-limiting
leukopenia (WBC nadir - 2.0-3.9 x 10^3/μl) occurred at all dose
levels; 1 pt had severe leukopenia (WBC nadir - 900/μl) at 45
mg/M^2/d. Pts who had received prior chemotherapy and/or
radiotherapy experienced thrombocytopenia (TCP) at all dose levels.
Four of 7 previously treated pts receiving 45 mg/M^2/d had
dose-limiting TCP (mean platelet nadir - 22 x 10^3/μl; range -
9 x 10^3 - 44 x 10^3/μl). TCP (mean platelet nadir - 60 x 10^3/μl)
occurred in 2 of 9 and 1 of 6 previously untreated pts at 45 and
65 mg/M^2/d, respectively. Of the 34 pts treated, 2 achieved
partial responses (PR). The PRs occurred in pts with adenocarcinoma of the lung and colon carcinoma metastatic to the lung.
In addition, another patient with adenocarcinoma of the lung had
stable disease lasting 9+ months. We conclude that: (1) The
dose-limiting toxicity of CHIP is thrombocytopenia; (2) The maximum
tolerated dose of CHIP in previously treated pts is 45 mg/M^2/d;
(3) Therapeutic responses to CHIP occur.

III-6 PLATINUM AND IRON CONCENTRATION AS A FUNCTION
OF TIME IN KIDNEYS OF RATS TREATED WITH CISPLATIN.
A. F. Le Roy*, J.P. Berry**, P. Brille***, Y. Gouveia***, P.
Ribaud***, P. Galle**, and G. Mathe*** *National Institutes of Health,
U.S. Department of Health and Human Services Bethesda, MD 20205, USA.
**Laboratoire de Biophysique -Centre de Microanalyse S.C.R 7 INSERM,
Faculte de Medecine 94000 Creteil, France ***Institut de Cancerologie et
Immunogenetique INSERM U 50 -Hopital Paul Brousse 94804 Villejuif,
France

Cisplatin has been shown to be an effective therapeutic agent in the
treatment of a number of types of cancers, but its use has been limited by
its toxicity especially in the kidney.

Using methods of electron-probe microanalysis with wavelength dispersive
spectrometry, we have established the presence of iron and platinum in
intra-cellular organelles of kidney cells of rats treated with successive
weekly doses of cis-platin. Based on these findings, the concentrations of
iron and platinum in kidney tissue were measured by means of flameless
atomic absorption spectrophotometry (FAAS) after each successive dose of
cisplatin administered over a period of six weeks to provide quantitative
measures of these elemental concentrations in the tissues with time.

The results obtained by FAAS confirm those obtained qualitatively with the
microprobe and provide quantitative data on the elemental concentrations
of iron and platinum in the tissue. They show that while the platinum level
in this tissue undergoes a small increase in concentration during the period
studied, there is a marked steady increase in concentration of iron with time
reaching a level about five times that found in controls. The renal toxicity
observed in subjects treated with cis-platin could thus be due in part to the
accumulation of relatively large quantities of insoluble iron compounds in
the tissue.

III-7 THE RENAL TUBULAR TRANSPORT OF PLATINUM ANTITUMOUR DRUGS IN RELATION TO THEIR NEPHROTOXICITY. Peter T. Daley-Yates and David C.H. McBrien. Biochemistry Department, Brunel University, Uxbridge, Middlesex UB8 3PH, United Kingdom.

The fractional renal clearance with respect to inulin of total** platinum derived from cisplatin (cis-dichlorodiammine PtII), trans-DDP (trans-dichlorodiammine PtII), CBDCA (cis-diammine-1,1-cyclo-butanedicarboxylate PtII) and CHIP (cis-dichloro trans-dihydroxy-isopropylamine PtIV) has been measured <u>in vivo</u> in rats with ureters cannulated to permit simultaneous collection of urine and blood from concious animals. The effects on clearance of total platinum** from cisplatin of several agents which can inhibit either cation or anion transport in the kidney have also been determined.

Platinum compound (doses shown in mg/kg)	Fractional Clearance in vivo 1h post dose with respect to GFR as measured using inulin	Nephrotoxicity (assessed by BUN after 5 mg/kg dose of Pt
transDDP(15)	3.28 ± 1.45	-
CHIP (15)	4.04 ± 1.43	-*
CBDCA (15)	3.35 ± 1.56	-*
cisplatin (15)	3.08 ± 0.77	+++
" + Furosemide (15 + 200)	2.07 ± 0.77	++++
" + Probenecid (15 + 200)	5.05 ± 1.4	++++
" + Choline Cl (15 + 200)	5.67 ± 1.9	+
" + Triethanolamine(15 + 200)	4.69 ± 1.7	+++

*not our data   **total=total ultrafilterable (MW<25,000)

Metabolites of cisplatin in urine and plasma were separated by HPLC (Biochem.Pharmacol. 32 181-184, 1983) and their individual fractional clearances determined. One hour post dosing the principal Pt compound is the parent complex and this is itself actively secreted with a fractional clearance of 3.5. Active tubular secretion is not <u>per se</u> responsible for nephrotoxicity since it is evident from the Table above that platinum from non-nephrotoxic platinum compounds is also actively transported into the urine.
(this work was supported by a grant from Bristol-Myers).

III-8 PHASE I CLINICAL TRIAL OF 1,2 - DIAMINOCYCLOHEXANE (ISO-CITRATO) Pt (II) - (PHIC). J.P. Armand, C. Picard, R.L. de Jager, J.P. Macquet, P.R. Combes. Centre Claudius Regaud, Laboratoire de Pharmacologie et de Toxicologie Fondamentales and Sanofi Research, Toulouse, France.

PHIC is a more soluble analog of Cisplatin (DDP) that is less nephrotoxic in animal model and has a higher therapeutic index in experimental tumor systems. It is active against L1210/DDP. PHIC was given to 12 pts. (22 cycles) with advanced solid tumors as an intravenous solution in 250 ml of D5W over 1 hour and without additional hydration. Treatment was administered daily x 5 and repeated at 4 weeks interval. Cumulative dose levels over 5 days were : 300, 600, 900 and 1200 mg/m2. The maximum tolerated dose (MTD) is 1200 mg/m2 in heavily pretreated patients. Dose limiting toxicity was thrombocytopenia reversible in 4 weeks with platelet nadirs < 30.000/mm3 in 4/6 courses at the MTD. Leukopenia was minimal. Nausea and vomiting less severe than with DDP were present at 900 and 1200 mg/m2.
   Except for fever (3 pts.) and phlebitis (2 pts.) no other toxicity was seen. Weekly serum creatinine determinations were normal in all pts. There was no objective tumor regression. One patient with renal impairment (crea > 180) received 4 cycles at 1200 mg/m2 without renal toxicity. A prolonged stabilization of the disease was noted.
   Total Pt plasma and urine pharmacokinetics at 300, 600, 900 mg/m2 showed V_d : 10 l. ; t 1/2 α : 15 min.; t 1/2 β : 34 hr. Urinary excretion/24 hr.: 60 %. PHIC plasma concentrations were dose dependent and protein binding : 80 - 90 %.
   Further studies are recommended.

III-9

SYNTHESIS AND IN VITRO CYTOSTATIC ACTIVITY OF PALLADIUM(II) AND PLATINUM(II) COMPLEXES WITH DITHIOCARBAMIC ESTERS.

Livia Sindellari*, Giuseppina Faraglia and Marino Nicolini, Istituto di Chimica Generale, Università di Padova, Via Loredan 4, 35100 Padova, Italy; Ariella Furlani and Vito Scarcia, Istituto di Farmacologia e Farmacognosia, Università di Trieste, via A. Valerio 32, 34100 Trieste, Italy.

The diethyldithiocarbamate (DTC) and its analogues are widely used in view of its chelating properties in the treatment of patients with acute nickel carbonyl, arsenic and thallium poisoning (1). Recently new interesting biological DTC properties have been emphasized. It has been suggested that DTC may be a potentially powerful sensitizing agent in tumour therapy in lowering the cell defense against O_2^- toxicity (2). The DTC has shown also to exert a protective effect against a variety of chemically-induced malignant tumours and a unique immunopotentiating activity (3). A further interest in this compound arose from observation that DTC was an effective agent in attempts to reduce the dose-limiting toxicity of mechloretamine (4) and nephrotoxicity of cis-platin(5), whereas it did not alter appreciably the therapeutic efficacy of this antineoplastic agent (6).

The present communication reports the synthesis, characterization and preliminary data of the "in vitro" screening on KB cells of the new synthesized compounds MLX_2 and ML_2X_2 (M=Pd or Pt; L=N,N'-dialkyl S-alkyldithiocarbamate; X=Cl, Br,I).

Some of the compounds show significant cytostatic activity. Particularly $Pd(TEDT)Cl_2$, $Pd(DMDTE)_2Br_2$ and $Pt(DMDTE)_2Cl_2$ have ID_{50} values in the 0.1 - 1 μg/ml range.

"In vivo" studies are in progress.*

* Bressa G., Carrara M., Cima L., Zampiron S., Institute of Pharmacology, Padova, Italy.

1) M.A.Zemaitis and F.E.Greene, Toxicol.Appl.Pharmacol.,1979,48,343.
2) P.S.Lin,L.Kwock,P.Lui and K. Hefter, Int.J.Radiation Oncology Biol. Phys., 1979,5, 1699.
3) G. Renaux, Trends Pharmacol. Sci., 1981, 2, 248.
4) M. Sossai,F. Pozza, L.Cima, F. Calzavara and C.E. Tòth, Progr.Bioch Pharmacol., 1965, 1, 720.
5) R.F.Barch and M.E.Pleasants, Proc.Natl.Acad.Sci,1979,76,6611.
6) G.R.Gale,L.M.Atkins,E.M.WalkerJr., Ann.Clin.Lab.Sci.,1982,12,345.

III-10 **PLATINUM (P) TREATMENT AND ELECTROLYTE IMBALANCE.**

Fiorentino M.V., Scalabrin M. and Venturelli E. - Division of Medical Oncology, Padova Medical Center, 35100 PADOVA, ITALY.

Serum (S) Mg imbalance after P is: (I) non relevant or ephemere (J.Exp.Clin.Cancer Res 1;139,1982) or (II) regular and cumulative (Chemioterapia 2-3;118,1982) or even long-standing (CTR 9;1767, 1982); little attention being paid to K and Ca and to correlations between electrolyte changes and BUN, Creatinine (C) and C Clearance (C Cl). We have studied:

A) General behaviour of Mg,K,Ca,BUN,C Cl in 100 miscellaneous pts over 2 hundred courses of P: S Mg decreases in 22% of courses and recovers to near normal levels in a few weeks. Pts already hypocalcaemic may undergo tetany. BUN and C Cl are modified only on short term. S K decreases for a few days only (effect of diuretics ?).

B) Sequential study of 34 testicular cancer pts treated with Einhorn's PVB regimen for 6 courses. Decrease of S K is always transient even after the last course; BUN and C Cl recover in weeks in 32/34 pts. Decrease in S Mg affects progressively 21/34 (62%) and is related to: 1) concomitant increase of Urinary Mg; 2) number of courses (P 0.001).

See table for mean Mg values studied in sequence. Late recovery of Mg kidney retention , as suggested in (III) is under study here.

	Course	I	III	VI
Mean S Mg values prae/post P in 34 patients of group B		150/155	157/146	177/116
Difference prae/post		.05	.09	.11

C) Sequential study with isotope renography in 21 miscellaneous pts; 9 pertain to group B previously described: of 5 with normal initial test (T 1/2 shorter than 10") 2 had no changes; 3 had a slowered elimination phase; of 4 initially abnormal, 2 improved (obstruction reduced ?). Among 12 other miscellaneous pts, of 6 initially abnormal 2 improved, 3 deteriorated; of 6 initially normal 4 deteriorated. No correlation between Mg changes and renogram is apparent by now.

III-11 PHASE I STUDY AND CLINICAL PHARMACOKINETICS OF CARBOPLATIN (CBDCA) (NSC 241240) IN PATIENTS WITH AND WITHOUT RENAL FAILURE. M.J. Egorin, D.A. Van Echo, M.Y. Whitacre, E. A. Olman, and J. Aisner. U. of Md Cancer Center, Balto., MD 21201

21 patients (pts) with refractory tumors were treated with iv bolus CBDCA qd x 5, every 4-5 weeks. Starting dose was 11 mg/m^2 with escalation to 99 mg/m^2. 57 courses were given to 11 females & 10 males with median age of 55 (range 40-71) & median Karnofsky performance status of 80% (range 60-100%). 18 pts were treated previously with: chemotherapy alone (6), chemotherapy + radiation (6), radiation alone (4), interferon + chemotherapy (1), or chemotherapy plus hyperthermia (1). 3 pts were previously untreated. CBC, BUN, creatinine and creatinine clearance were obtained weekly. Myelosuppression was dose limiting at 77 mg/m^2 in previously treated pts & 99 mg/m^2 in untreated pts. In previously treated pts, median WBC nadirs at 55, 77 & 99 mg/m^2 were 4.5, 3.5 & 3.1 x 10^3/μl & occurred on median days 18, 30, and 31. In previously untreated pts 99 mg/m^2 CBDCA produced a median WBC nadir of 3.4 x 10^3 μl on median day 26. In previously treated pts, platelet nadirs for 55, 77 & 99 mg/m^2 dosages were 124, 89, and 64 x 10^3 μl, with nadirs on days 24, 23, & 24. In previously untreated pts 99 mg/m^2 CBDCA produced a median platelet nadir of 125 x 10^3 μl on median day 23. 6/11 pts receiving 77 mg/m^2 had WBC nadirs occurring > 32 days after therapy, delaying their second course by 7-14 days. Nonhematologic toxicity of grade 1-2 nausea & vomiting, occurred in 9/12 pts receiving 77 mg/m^2 & grade I to III nausea & vomiting occurred in 7/10 patients at 99 mg/m^2. 2/10 pts at 99 mg/m^2 developed lower extremity musculo-skeletal pain. No renal, hepatic, cardiac or CNS toxicities were noted. Objective responses were noted in 1 pts with melanoma, renal cell carcinoma & colorecal carcinoma. One complete response was noted in 1 pt with head and neck cancer. Pharmacokinetics did not vary systematically with dose. Ultrafilterable platinum plasma t 1/2 α ranged from 1-7 min & t 1/2 β from 100-233 min. Ultrafilterable platinum represented 70-80% of total plasma platinum for the first 2 hrs & then declined to 45% by 6 hrs. Repeated dosing produced no accumulation of platinum in plasma on days 2-5. Urinary excretion of platinum was greatest during the first 4 hrs and 24 hrs cumulative excretion was 45-60% of the administered dose. The recommended dose for phase II studies for pts with good performance status & minimal prior therapy is 99 mg/m^2 q d x 5 & for heavily pretreated pts or pts with poor performance status is 77 mg/m^2 q d x 5. 18 additional courses utilizing single iv CBDCA have been administered to 13 pts with creatinine clearances ranging from 5.6-73 cc/min. Urinary excretion of platinum & area under the plasma concentration curve of ultrafilterable platinum varied directly with creatinine clearance. Platelet nadirs varied inversely with AUC. From these relationships it possible to tailor individual doses of CBDCA for each patient based on their creatinine clearance.

III-12 CISDIAMINODICHLORO-PLATINUM ULTRA HIGH DOSE (DDP-HD) IN TESTICULAR CARCINOMA: TOXICITY AND ACTIVITY

+) Schmoll,[+] Hans-Joachim, Weiß, Johannes, Diehl, Volker. Medical School Hannover Div, of Hematology and Oncology, Department of Medicine, Konstanty-Gutschow-Str., 3000 Hannover, FRG

In a prospective study 16 patients (pts.) with disseminated testicular carcinoma have been treated with ultra high doses of Cis-platinum (DDP); 5 pts. have been pretreated with Vinblastin/ Bleomycin/DDP conventional dose and recieved DDP-HD in combination with VP 16 (group a); 11 pts. with bylky abdominal or/and lung disease were treated with VP 16/Bleomycin/DDP-HD as first line therapy for poor prognosis.

Dosage of DDP was 30-40 mg/m^2 day 1 - 5, dissolved in 250 ml hypertonic 3% saline, with prehydration and posthydration period of 24 hours including 2500 ml/m^2 0.9% NaCl, alternating with Ringer solution; 20 mg furosemide were given i.v. directly before and after DDP-infusion, which lasted 60 minutes. VP 16 was given in 250 ml/ 0.9% NaCl over 60 minutes, directly before DDP-infusion, in the dose of 120 - 140 mg/m^2 day 1 - 5. Bleomycin dosage was 15 mg/m^2 day 1, 8, 15. Cycles were repeated in 21 day intervals, with a minimum of 2 cycles for evaluation of response, and to a maximum of 4 cycles.

Toxicity: Most prominent and dose limiting was thrombocytopenia and granulocytopenia responsible for dose reduction in 60% of the 38 evaluable cycles. 2/16 pts. had transient raise of serum creatinin to 2.0 mg%; one of them was pretreated with 800 mg DDP. Nausea and vomiting were markedly increased but manageable and tolerable. Diarrhea is a problematic DDP-related toxicity which occured in 8/38 cycles. 1 drug related death after the first cycle with diarrhea septicemia and oedema of the brain in the phase of bone marrow aplasia was seen.

Response: group a) 1/5 CR, 4/5 PR; group b) all pts. responded dramatically with fast and massive shrinkage of the tumor burden; it is too early for final destination of response.

Conclusion: Ultra high dose DDP is manageable with hypertonic NaCl-infusion without increased renal toxicity. In combination with VP 16 +/- Bleomycin the toxicity is high and requires supportive care comparable to treatment of acute leucemia.

COMPARATIVE NEPHROTOXICITY OF PHIC AND CISPLATIN IN BABOONS
III-13 B. Remandet, P. Richez, P. Vic, D. Gouy, J. Berthe & G. Mazue.

Nephrotoxicity of PHIC (Cis-isocitrato (1.2-diaminocyclohexane)
was studied in baboons (Papio papio) receiving repeated weekly intravenous administrations at dose levels of 25, 50, 100 or 150 mg/kg.
Baboons receiving Cisplatin at 5 or 10 mg/kg at 6-weekly intervals
were used as positive controls. Animals underwent regular clinical
and biochemical examinations as well as renal biopsies (after hetero-
topic transposition of the left kidney) ending with necropsic examinations (macroscopy, photon and electron microscopy).
    Timing of death was dose-related for both compounds: the first
cases occurred after 1 injection with Cisplatin at 10 mg/kg and with
PHIC at 150 mg/kg; after 2 injections with Cisplatin at 5 mg/kg and
with PHIC at 100 mg/kg; after 3 injections with PHIC at 50 mg/kg and
after 11 injections with PHIC at 25 mg/kg. Death was preceded by
weakness, loss of appetite and bodyweight decrease. Increases in
BUN and creatinemia were observed with PHIC at 150 mg/kg and with
Cisplatin at both dose levels used (5 and 10 mg/kg).
    Anatomopathological examinations revealed proximal tubular necro-
sis with dystrophic regeneration. After the first injection, lesions
induced by Cisplatin at 5 and 10 mg/kg were comparable with those
induced by PHIC at 100 and 150 mg/kg respectively. Only discrete
and cyclic renal lesions were observed at 25 and 50 mg/kg with PHIC.
    No primary glomerular lesions were observed with either compound.
    On this basis, the dose level of 100 mg/kg of PHIC should be con-
sidered to be at least equinephrotoxic with the dose level of
5 mg/kg of Cisplatin.

III-14 CIRCADIAN CHANGES OF THE CIS PLATIN BINDING ON PLASMATIC
PROTEINS. B. Hecquet, J. Meynadier, L. Adenis. Centre
Oscar Lambret, BP 307 - 59020 LILLE Cedex France.

    Circadian dependence of cis-platinum toxicity have now been shown
in the rat and man. The nephrotoxicity is correlated with the circadian rhythm of the cis-platin urinary excretion. The mechanism
of the rhythm of excretion is not know but a circadian change of a
tubular enzyme activity has been postulated.
    The protein binding is another important parameter of the pharma-
cokinetic of cis-platin which can affect the urinary excretion of the
free molecule. We studied in vitro the rate of cis-platin binding
on proteins in plasma collected at several hours of the day. The
binding seems to be dependent on the time of the day when plasma is
collected with a maximum of binding in the afternoon and a minimum
early in the morning.
    The amplitude of the variation depends on the patients. The vari-
ation in cis-platin binding is probably due to a weak fluctuation of
plasmatic protein concentration, the fluctuation having long been
recognized.
    Consequently the variation of the plasmatic binding ov cis-platin
is a pharmacokinetic parameter which can alter the amount of "free"
circulating cis-platin.
    When cis-platin is injected in the afternoon the level of free
cis-platin is probably lower than when cis-platin is injected in the
morning.
    Nephrotoxicity is correlated with the concentration of plasmatic
"free" cis-platin so that the minimum of toxicity will occur when
cis-platin is injected in the afternoon.

III-15 PHASE I STUDY OF CARBOPLATIN GIVEN ON A 5-DAY SCHEDULE.
C. Nicaise, M. Rozencweig, N. Crespeigne, L. Lenaz, Y.
Kenis. Institut Jules Bordet, Brussels, Belgium and Bristol-Myers
International Division, New York, NY 10154.

Carboplatin is a new platinum derivative which was proposed for
clinical trials on the basis of experimental data suggesting a lower potential for nephrotoxicity as compared to cisplatin. This phase I study was designed to determine the maximum tolerated dose of
carboplatin given on a 5-day i.v. schedule. The drug was dissolved
in 150 cc of D5W and infused over 15 min without pre- or posthydration. No routine antiemetics were administered. Twenty-six adult
patients with advanced solid tumors were entered. There were 17 men
and 9 women with a median age of 58 years (29 - 73) and a median
performance status (WHO) of 2 (0 - 3). All but three patients were
previously treated; fourteen had prior chemotherapy and four of
these were previously treated with cisplatin. A total of 40 courses
of carboplatin were given. The starting daily dose of 40 mg/sq m
was based on available clinical data and doses were escalated up to
125 mg/sq/dx5. Hematologic toxicity, especially thrombocytopenia appeared to be dose-related and dose-limiting. The maximum tolerated
dose was 125 mg/sq m/dx5 with a median WBC, PMN and platelet nadirs
$(x10^3/\mu l)$ of 1.5 (1.1 - 1.8), 0.4 (0.2 - 0.6) and 19 (12 - 26) respectively. At this dose level, one patient died from septic shock
and two required platelet transfusions. At 100 mg/sq m/dx5, the
corresponding figures were 3.1 (0.9 - 6.7), 1.2 (0.2 - 5.3) and 79
(25 - 155) respectively. Myelosuppression was generally delayed and
prolonged. At 100 mg/sq m/dx5, leukopenia occurred on day 18 (8 -
34) with a nadir on day 36 (12 - 38) and recovery on day 41 (18 -
50). Nausea and vomiting were generally mild and experienced by
nearly all patients. However, severe emesis was observed in two patients only. A mild and transient raise in the serum creatinine level was observed in a single patient. Mild albuminuria and increase
in the urinary level of β_2 microglobulin were observed in eight patients each. These abnormalities were apparently dose-independent.
Four patients had a drop in their creatinine clearance < 60 ml/min.
The other side effects were rare and negligible. They included fa-
tigue, paresthesia, local pain, stomatitis, headache and alopecia.
Antitumor response was strongly suggested in two patients, one with
thyroid carcinoma and one with cervix carcinoma. With this schedule
carboplatin demonstrated reduced nonhematological toxic effects as
compared to cisplatin. The drug appears to be an attractive compound for phase II trials. A dose of 100 mg/sq m daily for 5 consecutive days every 5-6 weeks may be proposed for these trials.

III-16 TOXICOLOGICAL AND ANTITUMOR ACTIVITY STUDIES ON A NEW CLASS
OF WATER SOLUBLE DIAMINOCYCLOHEXANE·PT (II) COMPLEXES.
A.R. Khokhar, D.B. Brown, M.P. Hacker, and J.J. McCormack. Vermont
Regional Cancer Center and Departments of Chemistry and Pharma-
cology, University of Vermont, Burlington, VT 05405 U.S.A.

Diaminocyclohexane·Pt·Cl$_2$ (DACH·Pt·Cl$_2$) is a highly effective
platinum complex with significantly less nephrotoxicity than cisplatin. The complex is unfortunately quite insoluble in water. We
have synthesized a number of new water soluble DACH·Pt·X complexes
where X is either a bidentate or monodentate ligand. These complexes have been tested for cytotoxicity in vitro against L1210/o
and L1210 resistant to cisplatin. Each complex has marked cytotoxic
activity (ID$_{50}$ values between 0.5 and 5 μg/ml) and is not cross
resistant with cisplatin. Several of these complexes have been
tested against L1210 in vivo and good antitumor activity (% ILS in
excess of 165%) noted with most. The number of long-term survivors
(alive 30 days past tumor inoculation) was markedly enhanced when
these complexes were administered daily x 5. One complex, DACH·
Pt·(Ascorbate)$_2$ was shown to be non cross resistant with cisplatin
when tested in vivo against L1210 resistant to cisplatin. The
nephrotoxicity was measured by elevation of BUN values 4 days after
a single i.p. injection of the calculated LD$_{10}$ or LD$_{50}$ dose. Each
complex proved significantly less renal toxic than cisplatin. Our
results suggest that this series of DACH·Pt complexes are:
1) highly water soluble; 2) effective antitumor agents; 3) non cross
resistant with cisplatin; 4) relatively non nephrotoxic, and that
at least one of this series should prove to be a very likely
candidate for clinical evaluation.

These studies were supported by NCI grants CA32244 and CA24543.

Section IV
Development of New Platinum Coordination Complexes

Chaired by M.J. Cleare

Overview
M.J. Cleare

1. INTRODUCTION

The Chairman opened the session with some comments on targets for new platinum drugs. Although the field of platinum based anti-cancer drugs has developed enormously since the pioneering work of Dr. Barnett Rosenberg, it is important to keep a sense of perspective. Cisplatin is very toxic, not well tolerated and is active against a limited number of tumour types, being only regularly curative in one (testicular). The classification produced by Durant at the Atlanta meeting (Table 1) still represents the clinical contribution of cisplatin today. The need to search for more tumour specific platinum and other metal based drugs is as strong now as it was in 1970 when structure activity studies first got underway.

TABLE 1 - CLINICAL CONTRIBUTIONS OF CISPLATIN

Change		Major Indications
Unresponsive	→ Resistant	Cervix, Prostate
Resistant	→ Responsive	Bladder, Head & Neck
Responsive	→ Sensitive	Ovary
Sensitive	→ Curable	Testicular

J.R. Durant - Atlanta Conference

Targets for successful second generation platinum drugs remain one of the following and preferably all three:

(i) Reduced toxic side effects with activity at least comparable to that of cisplatin.

(ii) Improved spectrum of activity - with high potency and long term duration response.

(iii) Activity against cisplatin resistant tumours.

The first objective seems to have been achieved in preclinical testing with several analogues and in the case of Carboplatin (JM8) also in the clinic (see paper by Calvert et al). The link between toxicity and chemical reactivity of the drug seems clear. The major question is whether the current approach to changing the simple organic and inorganic around the platinum centre would enable the other goals (particularly (ii)) to be achieved. The real need was to define means of proceeding towards more tumour specific metal based drugs. The participants were commended to study the papers and posters with this in mind.

After three papers reviewing current activity in the synthesis and development of analogues, the animal testing of analogues, and the development of one analogue (Carboplatin-JM8) from laboratory to clinic, there followed the viewing of 20 posters.

2. DISCUSSION

The discussion covered three main areas: (a) Screening methods especially to determine superior drugs to those currently on trial; (b) New approaches to drug design; (c) Clinical data.

2.1 Screening Methods

There was considerable interest in the human tumour stem cell assay system as a means of evaluating Pt drugs, particularly in comparison to cisplatin. A poster describing the use of the test, again cisplatin and 3 analogues, was presented by Rossof et al (IV-10). Besides the obvious problems of the low percentage of successful control takes there seemed to be little differentiation between the analogues. This may be reflecting the actual situation. Mary Wolpert (NCI) described the extensive studies commissioned by the NCI to develop the technique, although the results to date were somewhat disappointing.

Dr. Das Sarma referred to his poster (IV-7) concerning the use of bacteriophage lambda induction as a speedy screen. However, it was thought that data obtained to date suggested bacterial methods to be a very coarse screen.

Animal tests as indicated in the paper by Rose et al have proved to be fairly successful if carried out against several transplanted tumour types. These are relatively expensive and not routinely available to all researchers. This particularly applies to the xenograft testing which seems likely to give the best results on spectrum of action.

It was concluded that selective screening techniques which are available to synthetic chemists would make a major contribution to the development of Pt analogues and the search for more selective drugs. This is, of course, a common problem for all classes of anti-tumour drugs but will be particularly severe in metal drugs when many combinations of ligands can be readily synthesised and a high proportion are likely to show activity.

2.2 New Approaches to Drug Design

Discussion centred around the incorporation of ligands designed to introduce some biological specificity to the Pt centre, particularly tumour targeting. Richmond summarised the approach discussed in poster IV-15. This involves the use of a ligand which binds to estrogen receptors in an attempt to make Pt drugs for selective breast tumours. Concern was expressed about this and targeting of Pt drugs in general as to whether sufficient Pt centres (the lethal factor) could be introduced into cells this way.

The other approach mentioned was the use of Pt drugs in combination with radiation therapy (i.e. as radiosensitisers). A poster (IV-12) on this was submitted by Farrell et al and the subject had been discussed in an earlier session. The conclusion was that this was a promising approach as shown by results to date, but it was not obvious that the same Pt complexes showing good activity in their own right would be optimum for radiosensitisation. This approach has good potential for broadening the spectrum of tumours which could be treated by metal-based drugs.

Posters describing the synthesis of Pt analogues closely related to those currently on clinical trials showed the wide range of active species which can be obtained. Of particular interest were the series of [Pt(1,2-diaminocyclohexane)X_2] complexes where X is a series of organic acids (Poster IV-4, Craciunescu et al, and Poster IV-9, Andrulis et al). Optical resolution of the amine ligand can also result in higher activity scores for the Pt complexes in animal models (IV-14, Kidani et al). [Pt(oxalato)(1,2-diaminocyclohexane)] showed very high activity with the amine in the IR, 2R chiral form, especially against the cisplatin resistant L.1210 tumour.

2.3 Clinical Data

Khan summarised data in Poster IV-2 on the Phase I Clinical trial with 1,2-diaminocyclohexanebis(pyruvato)platinum(II). This analogue had been chosen for clinical trial due to high activity scores against L.1210 and B.16 mouse tumours. The trial is at an early stage but some responses had been observed. The MTD was 540-600 mg/m^2. A proposed Phase II trial on 1,1-diaminomethylcyclohexane(sulphato)platinum(II) was the subject of Poster IV-5 (Franks et al).

3. SUMMARY

Although some of the current analogues appear to represent a significant improvement in toxicity terms on cisplatin, there is much scope for the design of metal-based drugs with some degree of tumour specificity. Screening techniques remain a problem and in vitro human cell systems are required. Combination of metal drugs with radiation therapy is an exciting area worthy of greater attention.

Synthesis and Testing of Platinum Analogues — An Overview
P.C. Hydes

1. INTRODUCTION

   This paper is intended as a review of the major developments in the
synthesis and screening of platinum complexes since the Third International
Symposium on this subject, held in Dallas in 1976. It is not comprehensive
and relies heavily on the publications from two major conferences during the
intervening years(1,2), in addition to a major review paper at the recent
Dutch workshop on anti-tumour agent structure activity relationships (SAR)(3).
The data presented here was selected to illustrate the major trends in SAR's
for complexes of the type $[PtX_2A_2]$ and their Pt(IV) analogues. It obviously
reflects the primary sources of new compounds and the work of the international
screening centres. Omission of any published data is therefore primarily a
function of the scale of the subject, rather than a reflection of the potential
merit of the compounds themselves.

2. STRUCTURE ACTIVITY STUDIES

2.1. A. Groups

   Major papers at the last symposium highlighted the structure activity
relationships for platinum complexes with aliphatic and alicyclic amines(4)
and, in the case of the 1,2-diaminocyclohexane (1,2-dac) ligand, complexes
with a wide range of anionic leaving groups(5). These studies have been
extended by research teams at Johnson Matthey and Bristol-Myers to evaluate
90 complexes of the type cis-[PtX$_2$(aliphatic amine)$_2$] against the L1210
tumour, with subsequent studies on Lewis Lung and B16 tumours for active
complexes from the primary screen(6). Seventeen of these complexes were
comparable in activity to cis-[PtCl$_2$(NH$_3$)$_2$] (T/C >164%) including several
isopropylamine and malonato complexes (see Table 1). Publication of this
data and earlier NCI studies on selected compounds(7) represents a continuing
trend in the evaluation of platinum complexes. Early studies relied on
evaluation against single tumour lines such as the S180, ADJ/PC6A, P388 etc,

generally using a single dose administration schedule. However, tnere is
now an increased awareness among synthetic chemists of the sensitivity of
anti-tumour scores to the details of test methodology, especially the dose
schedule and the number of cells transplanted in the L1210 protocols.

Table 1. Variation of activity for platinum isopropylamine complexes
$[PtX_2Y_2(i-C_3H_7NH_2)_2]$

| Leaving groups | | Optimum dose | L1210 [a] |
X_2	Y_2	$(mg.kg^{-1})$	% T/C
Cl_2	-	32	171
$(NO_3)_2$	-	64	171
$(SO_4)(H_2O)$	-	23	150
$(ClCH_2CO_2^-)_2$	-	32,64	179
$(BrCH_2CO_2^-)_2$	-	3	117
Oxalate	-	68	193
Malonate	-	256	121
Cl_2	Cl_2	24	129
Cl_2	$(OH)_2$	32	171
Malonate	$(OH)_2$	256	107

a) 10^6 cells, i.p. Schedule d1, BDF_1 mice. Data of Bradner et al(6)

FIGURE 1. Structures of bidentate amine groups (A) in $[PtX_2(A)]$ complexes

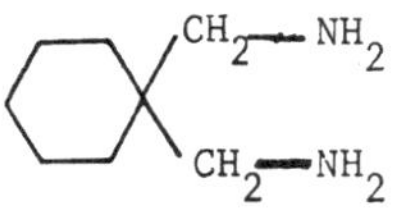

1,1-Diaminomethylcyclohexane
(1,1-damch)

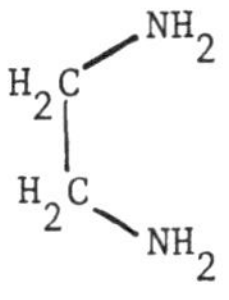

1,2-Diaminoethane
(en)

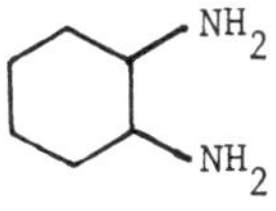

1,2-Diaminocyclohexane
(1,2-dac)

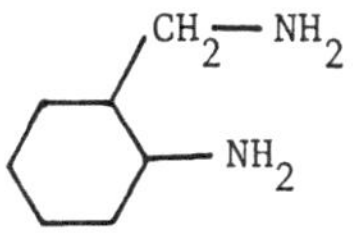

1-Amino-2-Aminomethylcyclohexane
(1,2-aamch)

The discovery of the high activity and water solubility for
[PtX$_2$(1,2-dac)] complexes(5) has resulted in extensive studies in Japan(8),
the USA(9) and Holland(10) on substituted diaminoalkane ligands (Figure 1),
where the parent compound [PtCl$_2$(en)] was one of the first active compounds
identified by Rosenberg in 1969. Complexes with exocyclic
2,3-diaminobicyclo(2,2,1) heptane ligands were shown to be active by
Totani(11) while Yoshikumi(12) and Inagaki(13) demonstrated activity for
1,2-diaminoethanes with ester substituents using a multiple dose schedule
(see Table 2). The corresponding carboxylate complexes were inactive and
analogous sulphonated 1,2-diaminobenzene species were only active at higher
doses compared with the neutral ligand, suggesting that cell permeability
is a significant parameter for active complexes.

Table 2. Variation of activity for [PtCl$_2$(1,2-Diaminoethane)] derivatives

R_1	R_2	L1210 [a]		P388 [b]	
		Dose	% T/C	Dose	% T/C
H-	HOOC-	25	117	-	-
H-	C$_2$H$_5$OOC-	25	175	-	-
HOOC-	HOOC-	100	106	50	117
HOOC-	HOOC-	-	-	5	220 [c]
C$_2$H$_5$OOC-	C$_2$H$_5$OOC-	25	195	25	164
CH$_3$OOC-	CH$_3$OOC-	-	-	5	210 [c]

a) 10^5 cells, CDF$_1$ mice, Schedule d1,5, i.p. Data of Inagaki et al(13)
b) 10^6 cells, CDF$_1$ mice, Schedule d1,5,9, i.p.
c) 10^6 cells, CDF$_1$ mice, Schedule d1-5, i.p. Data of Yoshikumi et al(12)

However, while these 5-membered ring diamine chelate complexes are
active, the corresponding 1,3-diaminopropane 6-membered ring systems are
considerably more active on both single and multiple dose schedules(14,15),
Table 3). The compounds from the Institute for Organic Chemistry (TNO),
Utrecht show significantly higher activity than a range of [Pt(malonate)-
(alkylamine)$_2$] complexes in the L1210 system, with comparable activity for
the B16 tumour, albeit at lower dose due to the greater toxicity of the TNO
compounds as measured by their LD$_{50}$ values.

Table 3. Variation of activity for $[PtCl_2(1,3-Diaminopropane)]$ derivatives

1,3-Diaminopropane	Dose mg.kg^{-1}	L1210 [a] % T/C
CH$_3$, CH$_2$—NH$_2$ / C / CH$_3$, CH$_2$—NH$_2$	12.5	323
CH$_3$, CH$_2$—NH$_2$ / C / C$_2$H$_5$, CH$_2$—NH$_2$	12.5	289
C$_2$H$_5$, CH$_2$—NH$_2$ / C / C$_2$H$_5$, CH$_2$—NH$_2$	9	325
(cyclobutane) CH$_2$—NH$_2$ / CH$_2$—NH$_2$	15	208
(cyclopentane) CH$_2$—NH$_2$ / CH$_2$—NH$_2$	12.5	148 [b]
(cyclohexane) CH$_2$—NH$_2$ / CH$_2$—NH$_2$	12.5	234 [b]

a) Schedule, day 1, 10^6 cells, BDF$_1$ mice. Data of Rose et al(14)
b) CDF$_1$ mice. Data of Berg et al(15)

2.2. Chiral A$_2$ groups

The original studies on the absolute configuration of 1,2-dac ligands in
$[PtX_2(1,2-dac)]$ complexes have been continued by Kidani's group using a
variety of diamine ligands e.g. 1,2-aamch (8), 1,2-propanediamine(1,2-pn)(16)
and 2,3-butanediamine(17). The original observation of preferential activity
for the trans-1-(1R,2R) form of the 5-membered 1,2-dac ring in
$[PtCl_2(1,2-dac)]$ was confirmed for the R-1,2-pn analogue but data for the
oxalates and analogous 6-membered ring 1,2-aamch complexes(8) (Table 4),
suggests the correlation is only valid for a limited range of complexes.
Kidani also used complexes of 2 and 3-aminomethylpiperidine(ampip) as models
for the $[PtX_2(1,2-dac)]$ complex conformations and showed significant
activity for $[Pt(oxalate)(2-ampip)](18)$.

Table 4. Variation of activity for platinum complexes of
1-Amino-2-Methylaminocyclohexane [PtX$_2$(1,2-aamch)]

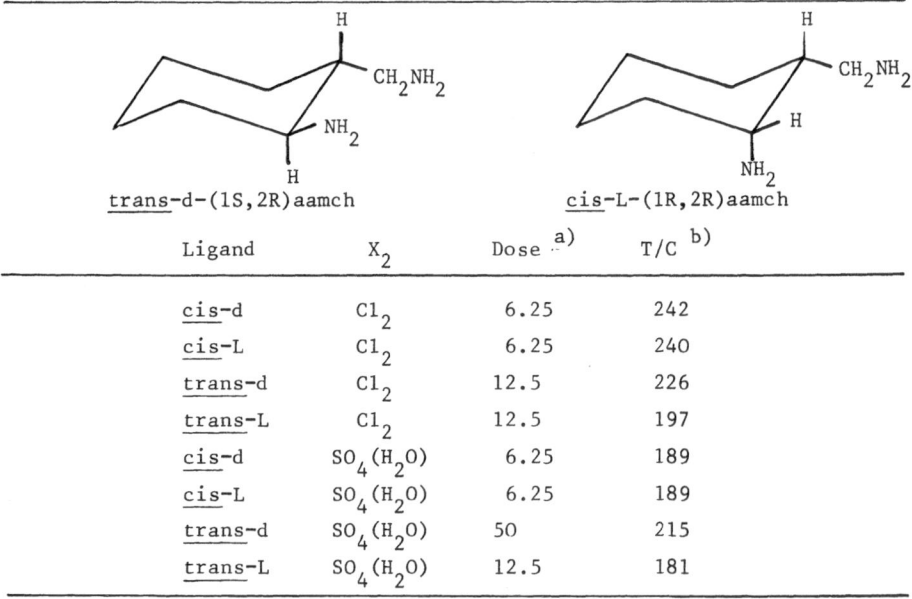

trans-d-(1S,2R)aamch   cis-L-(1R,2R)aamch

Ligand	X$_2$	Dose [a)	T/C [b)
cis-d	Cl$_2$	6.25	242
cis-L	Cl$_2$	6.25	240
trans-d	Cl$_2$	12.5	226
trans-L	Cl$_2$	12.5	197
cis-d	SO$_4$(H$_2$O)	6.25	189
cis-L	SO$_4$(H$_2$O)	6.25	189
trans-d	SO$_4$(H$_2$O)	50	215
trans-L	SO$_4$(H$_2$O)	12.5	181

a) d1,5. Schedule dose mg/kg/day   b) P388, 10^6 cells, CDF$_1$ mice, i.p.
Data of Kidani et al(8)

The influence of chiral diamine ligands has been taken further by
evaluation of the circular dichroism and electrophoretic behaviour of the
complexes formed by interaction of the complexes [PtCl$_2$(chiral diamine)]
with guanosine bases(16) and with DNA(19). The latter group suggested that
interaction of Pt complexes with DNA resulted in loss of essential
conformational character, thus precluding any chiral recognition. It will
be interesting to see if the relatively small difference in activity are
maintained against a broad tumour panel and in the clinic.

2.3. X. Groups

The activity of the [Pt(oxalate)(1,2-diamine)] complexes is in marked
contrast to the pronounced neuromuscular toxicity of the parent compound
[Pt(ox)(en)]. The oxalate group forms a 5-membered chelate ring with
platinum which is very stable, and as with the 6-membered ring malonate
complexes, this suggests the involvement of an in vivo activation mechanism
(20). Several malonates have been shown to be particularly effective against
the B16 melanoma and these compounds are considerably more water soluble
than their [PtCl$_2$A$_2$] precursors, Table 5.

Table 5. Variation of activity for platinum malonate complexes

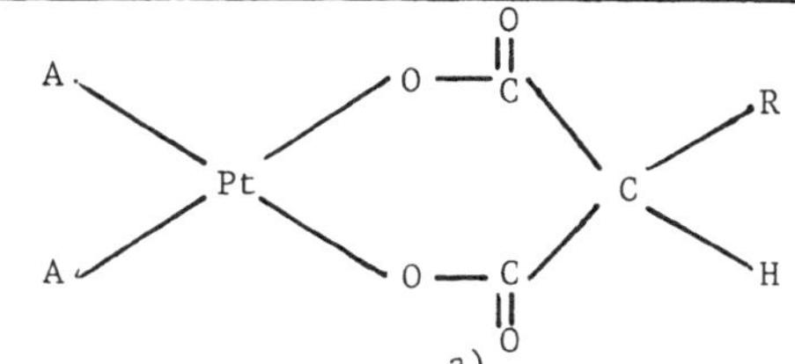

A	R	L1210 a) Dose	% T/C	B16 b) Dose	% T/C
NH_3	C_2H_5	64	186	16	173
NH_3	OH	32	200	32	124 (6/10)
CH_3NH_2	C_2H_5	100	207	65	183 (3/10)
$n-C_3H_7NH_2$	H	8.5	142	-	-
$H_2NC_2H_4NH_2$	H	17	164	25	214

a) 10^6 cells, BDF_1 mice. Schedule d1-9, i.p. Dose; $mg.kg^{-1}.day^{-1}$
b) 0.5ml 10% tumour brei, BDF_1 mice. Schedule d1-9, i.p. Dose; $mg.kg^{-1}.day^{-1}$
Data of Bradner et al(6) and Rose et al(14)

Three groups have also reported data on 1,2-dac complexes with chelating dicarboxylates which form 7-membered rings, as for PALA(21), TMA(22) and isocitrate(23), see Figure 2. These complexes dissociate rapidly in solution to form aquated $[PtX_2(1,2-dac)]_n$ species which, as in the case of the $i-C_3H_7NH_2$ complexes noted earlier, are considerably less toxic than the corresponding ammine (NH_3) species.

FIGURE 2. Structures of bidentate anionic leaving groups (X_2) in $[PtX_2(amine)_2]$ complexes

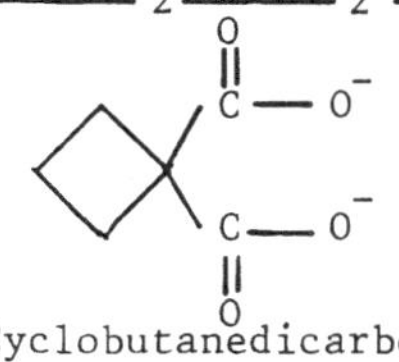

1,1-Cyclobutanedicarboxylate
(1,1-CBDCA)

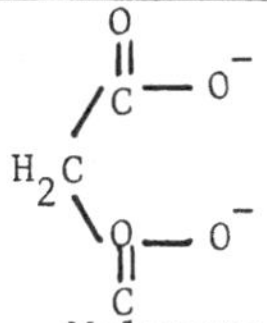

Malonate
(mal)

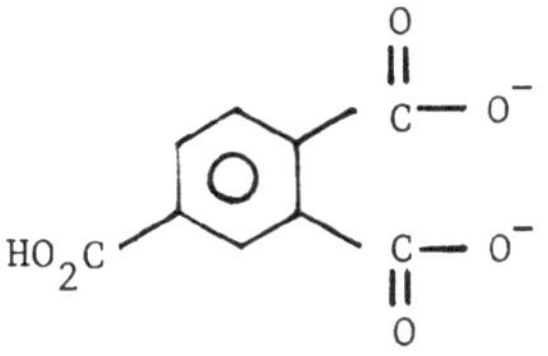

1,2,4-Benzenetricarboxylate
(TMA)

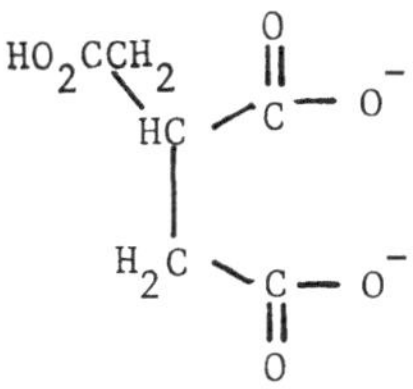

Isocitrate

Table 6.   Anti-tumour activity for [Pt(Pala)(1,2-dac)].H_2O [a)]

Tumour [b)]	Dose mg.kg^{-1}	Schedule (Evaluation Day)	T/C x100	Cures
L1210	3.0	d1-9	285	2/6
	6.0	(30)	357	3/6
	12.0		127	
B16	0.39	d1-9	174	
	0.78	(45)	154	
	1.56		165	
MX-1 Breast xenograft	25.0	d1,5,9	62	
	50.0	(11)	52	
	100.0		12	

a) Approximate formulation
b) Also screened against P388, ADJ/PC6A, Lewis Lung and 5 other tumours
Data of Meischen et al(21)

The [Pt(Pala)(1,2-dac)] complex in particular has been screened against
a wide range of tumours (Table 6) although it must be remembered that the
free ligand (Pala,NSC,224131) has considerable activity in its own right.
The original work of Tobe et al on Pt(IV) complexes(4) has been continued
by several authors and recent work on the 1,1-damch complexes has shown
high activity at low dose for [$PtCl_2(OH)_2$(1,1-damch)] species, (Table 7).
As in the case of the malonates detailed earlier, these complexes are
frequently more soluble than their [$PtCl_2A_2$] precursors and in general
require a higher dose for comparable activity, in line with their probable
reduction to Pt(II) complexes in vivo. It should be noted that purification
of complexes of this type from aqueous solvents can result in adduct formation,
and early studies on CHIP, JM-9, were in fact on the hemiperhydrate(24)
ctc-[$PtCl_2(OH)_2(i-C_3H_7NH_2)_2$]$0.5.H_2O_2$.
The last decade has seen the synthesis and testing of an estimated 1300
analogues of cis-[$PtCl_2(NH_3)_2$] but most attempts at correlating structure and

Table 7. Variation of activity for Pt(II) and Pt(IV) complexes

Amine (A)	cis-[PtCl$_2$A$_2$] [a) b)]		c,t,c-[PtCl$_2$(OH)$_2$A$_2$] [a) b)]	
	Dose	% T/C	Dose	% T/C
NH$_3$	8	200	120	164
i-C$_3$H$_7$NH$_2$	32	171	32	171
i-C$_4$H$_9$NH$_2$	64	171	160	200
1,1-damch	4-6	217 (1/6)	12-15	215 (1/6)

a) Dose; mg.kg^{-1}, i.p. Schedule day 1. b) L1210, 10^6 cells, BDF$_1$ mice
Data of Bradner et al(6) and Rose et al(14)

activity have only been valid for a limited homologous series in a single
tumour screen(4). Cleare classified active species on the basis of kinetic
criteria for the leaving groups(20) i.e.

1) Reactive species which hydrolyse readily in solution e.g. complexes with
PALA, TMA and SO$_4$ ligands, highlighting the significance of the initial
blood uptake phase for active complexes of this type.

2) Species with intermediate hydrolysis activity e.g. complexes with
chloride and chloroacetate ligands.

3) Complexes with bidentate carboxylate ligands e.g. oxalates and malonates
which are inert in vivo to such an extent that an in vivo activation
mechanism has been postulated.

2.4. Toxicity

A recent attempt at quantitative SAR(25) using INDO-SCF methods,
confirmed earlier empiracle studies which suggest that only minor changes in
broad spectrum activity are observed in comparison with a more pronounced
structure toxicity relationship. The toxicity of cis-[PtCl$_2$(NH$_3$)$_2$] analogues
has received increasing attention in recent years, most noticeably by
Prestayko(26) and Schurig(27), (Table 8). Many analogues of cisplatin are
considerably less nephrotoxic as determined by BUN incidence figures but the
majority are equally, if not more toxic e.g. 1,1-damch complexes, when
assessed on the basis of leukopenia in mice(14).

The search for a tumour panel representative of clinical performance
continues with increased data on human tumour xenograft studies at the NCI
and in the major comparitive study by Harrap(28), (Table 9). This trend
is likely to continue and is being supplemented by human tumour stem cell
assays.

Table 8.   Relative toxicity for analogues of cisplatin

Complex	Dose	BUN Incidence	WBC % Decrease (day)
cis-[PtCl$_2$(NH$_3$)$_2$]	17.8	8/10 [a]	38 (5)
	13.4	9/10	53 (3)
	10.0	7/10	47 (3)
c,t,c-[PtCl$_2$(OH)$_2$(i-C$_3$H$_7$NH$_2$)$_2$]	51.5	0/6 [b]	61 (5)
	38.6	1/7	39 (3)
	29.0	0/10	26 (3)
[PtCl$_2$(1,1-damch)]	8.7	2/9 [a]	61 (3)
	6.5	0/10	59 (3
	4.9	0/10	54 (5)

BUN   30mg.100ml^{-1}. Assay day 4,7,11. Max^m day 4(a), day 7(b)
WBC   35% significant. Assay day 3,5,7
Dose; mg.kg^{-1}, i.p. day 1
Data of Shurig et al(27)

Table 9.   Activity of [PtX$_2$A$_2$] complexes against a human epidermoid carcinoma
          (P246) xenograft a)

Complex	Dose [b]	T/C x 100	Deaths (week)
cis-[PtCl$_2$(NH$_3$)$_2$]	6 (2)	1.0	2/6 (3)
	2 (4)	12.0	1/6 (3)
[Pt(1,1-CBDCA)(NH$_3$)$_2$]	48 (4)	1.0	0
	16 (4)	34.0	0
c,t,c-[PtCl$_2$(OH)$_2$(i-C$_3$H$_7$NH$_2$)$_2$]	48 (1)	–	4/6 (1)
	16 (4)	59.0	0
[Pt(SO$_4$)(H$_2$O)(1,2-dac)]	9 (1)	2.0 [c]	2/6 (2,6)
	3 (3)	27.0	0

a) Grown in immune deprived mice   b) mg.kg^{-1} (number of courses)
c) test duration 6 weeks, all others 7 weeks
Data of Harrap et al(24)

Similarly, many complexes are being screened against cisplatin resistant
L1210 tumour models(14), (Table 10), and it will be interesting to correlate
this data with the results of clinical studies (Table 11)(29).   See also
Harrap(29) for the status of clinical trials on all analogues.

Table 10. Cross resistance studies for $[PtX_2A_2]$ complexes against cisplatin resistant L1210

Complex	Dose $(mg.kg^{-1})$	L1210 $^{a)}$ % T/C	L1210/CDDP
cis-$[PtCl_2(NH_3)_2]$	4-8	182	106-121
$[Pt(1,1-CBDCA)(NH_3)_2]$	80-120	146	113
$[Pt(TMA)(1,2-dac)]$	10-20	250	176 (2/6)
$[Pt(SO_4)(H_2O)(1,1-damch)]$	9-12	217	171 (1/6)

a) 10^6 cells, BDF_1 mice, i.p. Data of Rose et al(14)

Table 11. Phase 1 clinical studies

Code	Compound	Centre
JM-8	$[Pt(1,1-CBDCA)(NH_3)_2]$	Royal Marsden Hospital, Sutton
JM-9	$[PtCl_2(OH)_2(i-C_3H_7NH_2)_2]$	Roswell Park Memorial Institute, Buffalo, NY
PHIC	$[Pt(isocitrate)(1,2-dac)]$	Toulouse
JM-82	$[Pt(TMA)(1,2-dac)]$	Memorial Sloan Kettering, NY
TNO-6	$[Pt(SO_4)(H_2O)(1,1-damch)]$	Amsterdam
JM-40	$[Pt(mal)(en)]$	Amsterdam

3. SYNTHETIC DIRECTIONS

Synthesis effort on new platinum complexes is dedicated increasingly towards functionalised amines(30,31) (Table 12) in addition to ligands with potential inherent activity e.g. PALA and triazines(32), (Table 13). However, in the absence of cisplatin analogues with significantly greater unit activity, it seems likely that highly refined 'targeting' and selectivity for the active site will be required for a successor to the second generation analogues with low toxicity discussed above. Complexes of platinum with 'biomolecules' such as peptides(33) and saccharides(34) have been prepared and preliminary studies have confirmed the feasibility of attaching platinum chloride species to polyamine structures with a range of chain lengths(35). Similarly, enhanced inhibition of DNA synthesis has been demonstrated for platinum complexed anti-tumour immunoglobulins in comparison with cis-$[PtCl_2(NH_3)_2]$(36). The majority of the activity data for the above complexes is from in vitro screens and reports on the in vivo studies now in progress are awaited with interest.

226

Table 12. Variation of activity for platinum complexes with aromatic amines

Complex	R	Dose (mg.kg^{-1})	T/C % [a]
cis-[PtCl$_2$(RC$_6$H$_4$NH$_2$)$_2$] (c)	2-F	ND [b]	148
	3-F	ND	167
	3-CF$_3$	ND	111
	4-H	12.5	193
	4-CH$_3$	12.5	171
	4-Cl	25	168
	4-NO$_2$	25	137
	4-OCH$_3$	12.5	144

a) P388 tumour
b) ND - not disclosed
c) Data of Nile et al(30)
d) Data of Kidani et al(31)

Table 13. Cytotoxic activity for platinum complexes with triazine ligands

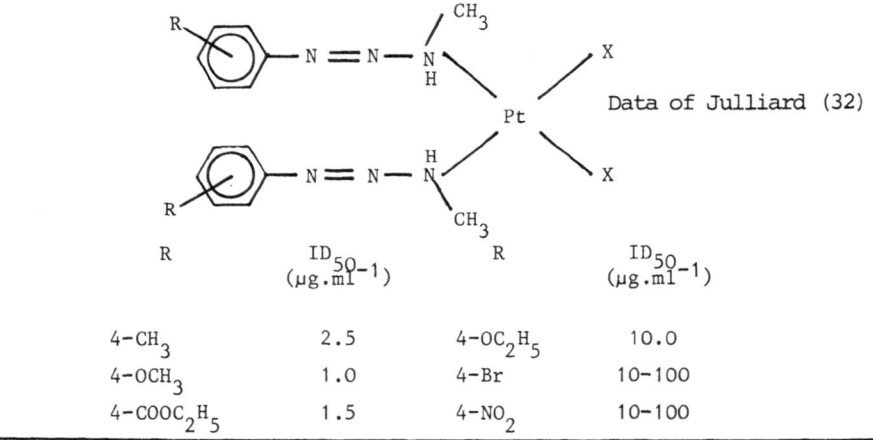

Data of Julliard (32)

R	ID$_{50}$ (µg.ml^{-1})	R	ID$_{50}$ (µg.ml^{-1})
4-CH$_3$	2.5	4-OC$_2$H$_5$	10.0
4-OCH$_3$	1.0	4-Br	10-100
4-COOC$_2$H$_5$	1.5	4-NO$_2$	10-100

REFERENCES
1. Biochimie, 1978, 60, 835-965.
2. 'Cisplatin. Current Status and New Developments', ed. A.W. Prestayko, S.T. Crooke and S.K. Carter, Academic Press, New York, 1980.
3. 'Structure-Activity Relationships of Anti-Tumour Agents', (Developments in Pharmacology; 3) ed. D.N. Reinhoudt, T.A. Connors, H.M. Pinedo and K.W. van de Poll, Martinus Nijhoff, The Hague, 1983.
4. M.L. Tobe and A.R. Khokhar, J.Clin.Haematol.Oncol., 1977, 7, 114.
5. R.J. Speer, H. Ridgway, D.P. Stewart, L.M. Hall, A. Zapata and J.M. Hill, ibid, 1977, 7, 210.
6. W.T. Bradner, W.C. Rose and J.B. Huftalen in Ref 2 p.171.
7. M.J. Cleare, P.C. Hydes, B.W. Malerbi and D.M. Watkins, Biochimie, 1978, 60, 835.

8. M. Noji, K. Okamoto, Y. Kidani and T. Tashiro, J.Med.Chem., 1981, 24, 508.
9. D.P. Stewart, R.J. Speer, H.J. Ridgway and J.M. Hill, J.Clin.Haematol. Oncol., 1979, 9, 175.
10. C.G. van Kralingen and J. Reedijk, Cienc.Biol.(Portugal), 1980, 5, 159.
11. T. Totani and K. Yamaguchi (Shionogi), U.K. Patent Appl. 2074567 (1981) (Chem.Abstr., 1982, 96, 162946).
12. C. Yoshikumi, T. Fujii, K. Saito, M. Fujii and K. Niimura (Kureha) E.P. Appl. 0041729A (1981) (Chem.Abstr., 1982, 96, 174393).
13. K. Inagaki, Y. Kidani, K. Suzuki and T. Tashiro, Chem.Pharm.Bull., 1980, 28, 2286.
14. W.C. Rose, J.E. Schurig, J.B. Huftalen and W.T. Bradner, Cancer.Treat. Rep., 1982, 66, 135.
15. J. Berg, E.J. Bulten and F. Verbeek, U.K. Patent Appl. 2024823A (1979) (Chem.Abstr., 1980, 93, 114040).
16. R. Ugo, M. Gullotti and A. Pasini, Congr.Naz.Chim.Inorg.[Atti] 13th, 1980, 84.
17. M. Gullotti, G. Pacchioni, A. Pasini and R. Ugo, Inorg.Chem., 1982, 21, 2006.
18. K. Inagaki, K. Tajima and Y. Kidani, Inorg.Chim.Acta., 1979, 37, L547.
19. A. Pasini, A. Velcich and A. Mariani, Chem-Biol.Interact., 1982, 42, 311.
20. M.J. Cleare in Ref 3 p.59.
21. S.J. Meischen, G.R. Gale and M.B. Naff, J.Clin.Haematol.Oncol., 1982, 12, 67.
22. P. Schwartz, S.J. Meischen, G.R. Gale, L.M. Atkins, A.B. Smith and E.M. Walker Jr., Cancer.Treat.Rep., 1977, 61, 1519.
23. J-P Macquet, Abs.Eur.Soc.Med.Oncol., 1980, 120.
24. P.C. Hydes and D.R. Hepburn (Johnson Matthey) U.K. Patent Appl. 2085440A (1981) (Chem.Abstr., 1982, 97, 61004).
25. P.G. Abdul-Ahad and G.A. Webb, Int.J.Quantum Chem., 1982, 21, 1105.
26. A.W. Prestayko, W.T. Bradner, J.B. Huftalen, W.C. Rose, J.E. Schurig, M.J. Cleare, P.C. Hydes and S.T. Crooke, Cancer.Treat.Rep., 1979, 63, 1503.
27. J.E. Schurig, W.T. Bradner, J.B. Huftalen, G.J. Doyle and J.A. Gylys in Ref 2 p.227.
28. K.R. Harrap, M. Jones, C.R. Wilkinson, H.McD. Clink, S. Sparrow, B.C.V. Mitchley, S. Clarke and A. Veasey in Ref 2 p.193.
29. K. Harrap in 'Cancer Chemotherapy Vol.1', ed. F.M. Muggia, Martinus Nijhoff, Boston, USA, 1983.
30. T.A. Nile and C.A. Smith, Inorg.Nucl.Chem.Lett., 1979, 15, 183.
31. Y. Kidani, Y. Asano and M. Noji, Chem.Pharm.Bull., 1979, 27, 2577.
32. M. Julliard, G. Vernin and J. Metzger, Synthesis, 1982, 1, 49.
33. W. Beck and M. Girnth, Arch.Pharm (Weinheim) 1981, 314, 955.
34. W. Beck and G. Thiel (BASF) E.P. Appl. 0059911A, (Chem.Abstr., 1983, 98, 34900).
35. C.E. Carraher Jr., W.J. Scott, J.A. Schroeder and D.J. Giron, J. Macromol.Sci.Chem., 1981, A15 (4), 625.
36. E. Hurwitz, R. Kashi and M. Wilchek, J.N.C.I., 1982, 69, 47.

Experimental Antitumor Activity
of Platinum Coordination Complexes
W.C. Rose and W.T. Bradner

INTRODUCTION

The search for a "second-generation" Pt compound to supersede cis-platin has been conducted in many laboratories (1-13). For the past six years, the efforts at Bristol-Myers have been focused on finding analogs with improved antitumor activities and reduced toxicities relative to cisplatin as judged by their effects in animal models (1, 10, 11). The present discussion will be limited to a review of antitumor test results obtained with those Pt compounds now undergoing clinical evaluation, and a few other analogs of potential interest.

Initially, when faced with the task of evaluating a large number of Pt analogs, it was intended that only those clearly superior to cisplatin in our primary screen, L1210 leukemia, would be tested further in our second-ary screen, B16 melanoma. Assuming such analogs passed the toxicity assays, additional antitumor tests were envisioned in order to select the most likely candidates. (Such factors as stability, potency, solubility and ease of synthesis and purification, also enter into any ultimate decisions). After two years of testing, very few compounds were found that were superior to cisplatin versus L1210 leukemia [e.g. JM-20, 1,2-diamino-cyclohexane (DACH) aquasulfato Pt (II), and JM-74, DACH malonato Pt (II)], and only one, JM-5 [diammine 2-hydroxymalonato Pt (II)], that was clearly superior to cisplatin against B16 melanoma. Even after six years of testing, JM-5 remains the only Pt analog that has reproducibly cured mice implanted with B16. The superior activity of JM-5 versus B16 was also found against im implants by Pera et al. (9), who noted the amount of Pt bound to the DNA of B16 cells relative to normal bone marrow cells was greater following administration of JM-5 than cisplatin.

Considering the lack of success in advancing Pt analogs through our screening process, a slightly different approach was tried which allowed for an extended tumor panel evaluation of any analog that yielded increases in lifespan in the L1210 and B16 models that were at least equal to the lower historical limits obtained using cisplatin. These more lenient criteria resulted in more than 70 analogs having been evaluated against such tumors as Lewis lung carcinoma, Madison 109 lung carcinoma (M109), Colon 26 carcinoma (C26),and a line of L1210 leukemia resistant to cisplatin (L1210/cDDP). On a limited basis, these tumors were used as sc or ic implants, in addition to the typical ip implants.

Using the murine tumors named above, no Pt analog has yet been found which has clear superiority to cisplatin in more than one of them (not including L1210/cDDP). It is debatable whether even overall "comparability" can be claimed for any analog, yet it may be useful to review the experimental activity profiles of each Pt analog presently being evaluated clinically. Should any of these Pt analogs prove to be superior to cisplatin in some clinical situation, we can determine if the advantage was reflected in any experimental tumor model.

MATERIALS AND METHODS

Mice and tumors

The mice and tumors have been described previously (11).

Drugs

Cisplatin [cis-diamminedichloro Pt (II)], Na^+-JM-5 [sodium salt of diammine 2-hydroxymalonato Pt (II)], JM-8 [cis-diammine 1,1-cyclobutane dicarboxylato Pt (II)], JM-9 [cis-dichloro-trans-dihydroxy-bis-isopropylamine Pt (IV)], JM-40 [ethylenediamine malonato Pt (II)], JM-82 [DACH 4-carboxyphthalato Pt (II)], TNO-6 [1,1-diaminomethylcyclohexane (DAMCH) aquasulfato Pt (II)], TNO-7 [DAMCH trans-dihydroxy-cis-dichloro Pt (IV)], TNO-8 [1-amino-2- aminomethyl 3,3-5-trimethylcyclohexane dichloro Pt (II)], TNO-10 [2,2-diethyl 1,3-propanediamine dichloro Pt (II)], TNO-18 [DAMCH 2-hydroxymalonato Pt (II)] and TNO-38 [DAMCH oxalato Pt (II)] were supplied for testing by either Johnson Matthey, Inc. of Malvern PA (cisplatin and the JM compounds) or the Institute for Organic Chemistry, TNO, of Utrecht in The Netherlands (TNO compounds).

Cisplatin was dissolved in 0.9% NaCl, JM-8 and JM-9 were dissolved in water or 0.9% NaCl, TNO-7, TNO-8 and TNO-10 were suspended in saline plus carboxymethylcellulose (CMC), TNO-18 and JM-40 were suspended in water plus CMC, TNO-38 and Na^+-JM-5 were dissolved in water, JM-20 and TNO-6 were dissolved in 5% dextrose in water, and JM-82 was dissolved in 1% $NaHCO_3$. All drugs were administered ip.

JM-8, JM-9, JM-40, JM-82 and TNO-6 were all undergoing Phase I or II clinical trials at the time of this writing.

Drug evaluation

Pt analogs were compared to cisplatin on the basis of maximum extensions in lifespan calculated in terms of % T/C values. Such values were determined by dividing the median survival time (MST) of a drug-treated group (T) by the MST of the parallel, control group (C), x 100. An analog's activity in a given tumor model was judged on the basis of the maximum % T/C value achieved relative to both cisplatin's historical and concomitant effects in the same model and experiment, respectively. When cures were obtained, these are shown separately and the % T/C value determined for the dying mice only. Therapeutic effects were generally not reported if more than 17% of the treated mice were judged to have died due to drug toxicity.

RESULTS

Detailed descriptions of the maximum antitumor effects observed in each experiment by each Pt analog relative to the concomitant result obtained using cisplatin are provided in Tables 1-3. To aid in the evaluation of these data, a mean % T/C ratio has been included in Tables 1 and 2 comparing the maximum effects of each analog versus cisplatin.

Against L1210 leukemia (Table 1), each analog was evaluated using both a single injection and multiple injection treatment schedule. Of the five analogs presently being evaluated clinically, only JM-82 and TNO-6 demonstrated an advantage over cisplatin using either single or multiple treatment regimens; the other three, JM-8, JM-9 and JM-40, were generally inferior to cisplatin in this model with the exception of JM-9 given on a single injection basis. Among the newly introduced analogs, Na^+-JM-5 was comparable to cisplatin on a multiple but not single injection treatment schedule, the situation for TNO-8 was just the reverse, and the four other compounds proved to be comparable to superior to cisplatin on either schedule. The extensions in lifespan caused by JM-82, TNO-6, TNO-7, TNO-10 and TNO-18 were occasionally greater than those typically observed using cisplatin, and included the presence of a few cured mice for some of these analogs.

Against B16 melanoma (Table 1), none of the analogs were clearly superior to cisplatin. JM-8 and TNO-38 achieved results in two or three experiments that were essentially equivalent to cisplatin, as did Na^+-JM-5 in a single experiment. JM-40 had a mean maximum T/C ratio of 0.86 based on two studies, but the presence of two cured mice in one of them caused the % T/C value calculated for dying mice only to be depressed. Overall, JM-40 was considered to be comparable to cisplatin in the B16 model. With the exception of both experiments involving JM-9, all the analogs caused extensions in lifespan that fell within the historical range of effects observed using cisplatin.

Using the M109 model (Table 2), three of the clinical candidates, JM-8, JM-9 and TNO-6, failed to achieve an active result (T/C of $\geq 125\%$) based on two or three experiments. JM-40 displayed minimal activity in one of two studies and JM-82 yielded similar activity in two of three experiments. Of the newer analogs, TNO-10 was devoid of activity but each of the others achieved consistent if not convincing levels of activity. TNO-8 was only evaluated once in this model, but it proved to be comparable to cisplatin. Na^+-JM-5 and TNO-38 both achieved % T/C values in excess of 170% but this degree of activity was not repeated in subsequent tests.

Against C26 carcinoma (Table 2), many analogs including the parent compound, caused mice to be cured in our initial experiments which necessitated staging the disease prior to treatment in subsequent testing. Because of the presence of cured mice, the calculation of maximum T/C ratios was not deemed appropriate unless the cure rate was similar for both analog and cisplatin. Also, in the majority of instances, only one experiment was available for evaluation. In the one experiment performed involving JM-8, the analog cured 50% of the treated mice whereas cisplatin

Table 1. Summary of Experimental Antitumor Activities of Cisplatin Analogs:L1210 Leukemia and B16 Melanoma

Max % T/C - cures/total (opt. dose) of analog/cisplatin Vs IP[a]:

Analog code No.	L1210				B16	
	1x	Mean % T/C values; ratio	Multiple[b]	Mean % T/C values; ratio	Multiple[b]	Mean % T/C values; ratio
JM-8	150(128)/186(8) 150(40)/208(8)	150/197 .76	157(64)/214(2) 192(40)/208(8̲)	175/211 .83	174(16)/174(0.8)[b] 172(32)[b]/190(4)[b]	173/182 .95
JM-9	171(32)/186(8) 167(30)/183(8) 165(80)/153(8) 143(40)/171(6) 179(36)/171(8)	165/173 .95	207(16)/214(2) 157(12)/257(3̲)	182/236 .77	145(16)/157(0.8)[b] 144(20)[b]/190(4)[b]	145/174 .83
JM-40	129(69)/177(8) 129(80)/179(8) 146(80)/185(8) 143(60)/164(8)	137/176 .78	164(17)/221(2)	164/221 .74	167-2/10(6.3)/237(2.4) 188(16)/176-2/10(1.6)	178/207 .86
JM-82	243(20)/207(10) 250(20)/183(8) 221(30)/179(10) 200(30)/179(6) 192(10)/167(6)	221/183 1.21	250(4.8)/250(2) 279-2/6(6)/171(3) 243(8̲)/179(2̲)	157/200 1.29	168(0.8)/180(1.6) 167(4.8)/237(2.4)	168/209 .80
TNO-6	233(18)/167(4) 217(12)/183(4) 215(18)/177(8) 208(6)/217(8) 214/(16)/186(8)	217/186 1.17	267(12)[b]/217(4)[b] 217(4)[b]/183(2)[b] 277(8-2x)/231(6-2x) 237(12-2x)/186(3̲)	249/204 1.22	154(1.6)/163(0.8) 165(8)[b]/205-1/10(2.4) 147(8)[b]/189(4)[b]	155/186 .83
Na[+]-JM-5	143(100)/150(8) 143(90)/214(10) 143(120)/193(8)	143/186 .77	207(24)/214(2.4)	207/214 .97	185(16)/173(1.6)	185/173 1.07

TNO-7	214-3/6(16)/179(8) 283(12)/167(4) 225-1/6(15)/183(4) 176(12)/153(8) 186(20)/157(8)	217/168 1.29	236-2/6(6)/243(2.4)[b] 417(12)[b]/217(4)[b] 206(4)/147(2.4) 229(6)/214(2.4)	272/205 1.33	191(12)[b]/237(2.4) 169(6)/200(1.6) 183(16)[b]/211(4)[b]	181/216 .84
TNO-8	214(120)/179(8) 217(40)/217(10)	216/198 1.09	200(15)/257(2.4)	200/257 .78	155(4)/179(1.6)	155/179 .87
TNO-10	283-2/6(9)/167(4) 175-2/6(8)/183(4)	229/175 1.31	242(1.5)/200(1.6)	242/200 1.21	168(2.4)/205-1/10(2.4)	168/205 .82
TNO-18	246(36)/185(8) 186(24)/186(8) 233(24)/275(10)	222/215 1.03	269(8)/177(2.4)	269/177 1.52	179(10)/234(6)[b]	179/234 .76
TNO-38	156(4)/150(6) 200(6)/183(8) 200(8)/171(10)	185/168 1.10	206(1)/144(2.4)	206/144 1.43	155(3)/152(1.6) 169(2.4)/172(0,8) 174(4)[b]/190(4)[b]	166/171 .97

a % T/C values are shown for dying mice only with cures indicated separately when present. Each line of data represents the maximum effects obtained (and the optimal dose, ip) for the given analog and cisplatin in an experiment.

b If not otherwise indicated, "multiple" refers to once daily treatments administered on Days 1 → 9 post-implant; a dose shown underlined was given once daily on Days 1 → 5; a dose followed by a superscript "b" was administered on Days 1, 5 and 9 post-implant.

234

Table 2. Summary of Experimental Antitumor Activities of Cisplatin
Analogs:Madison 109 Lung Carcinoma and Colon 26 Carcinoma

	Max. % T/C - cures/total (opt. dose) of analog/cisplatin Vs IP[a]:			
	M109		C26	
Analog code No.	2x or 4x[b]	Mean % T/C values; ratio	4x[b]	Mean % T/C values; ratio
JM-8	114(40)/150(4) 100(40)/142(6) 120(<u>80</u>)/153(<u>6</u>)	111/148 .75	136-4/8(40)/159(2)	-[c]
JM-9	121(<u>45</u>)/153(3) 103(<u>25</u>)/153(6)	111/153 .73	160-1/8(20)/229-4/8(2) 154-2/8(20)/156-7/8(3)	-
JM-40	128(36)/169(6) 123(<u>36</u>)/153(<u>6</u>)	126/161 .78	220-4/8(40)/194-4/8(3)	220/194 1.13
JM-82	126(8)/147(3) 134(9)/141(6) 117(2)/153(<u>6</u>)	126/147 .86	128(6)/159(2)	128/159 .81
TNO-6	97(<u>12</u>)/172(6) 105(<u>3</u>)/142(<u>6</u>) 107(<u>2</u>)/153(<u>6</u>)	103/156 .66	185-1/8(6)/224-3/8(3) 131(4)/181-2/8(2)	-
Na+-JM-5	172(<u>80</u>)/252(6) 125(<u>75</u>)/141(<u>6</u>)	149/197 .76	204-1/8(30)/216-2/8(2)	204/216 .94
TNO-7	150(3.5)/172(6) 131(10)/200(<u>6</u>)	141/186 .76	166-1/8(3.5)/159-5/8(3)	-
TNO-8	147(<u>25</u>)/147(3)	147/147 1.0	157(25)/128-4/8(2)	-
TNO-10	119(<u>8</u>)/172(<u>6</u>)	119/172 .69	132-5/8(3)/224-3/8(3)	-
TNO-18	133(10)/194(<u>6</u>)	133/194 .69	322-1/8(16)/187-4/8(3)	-
TNO-38	175(5)/175(6) 129(3.2)/15<u>3</u>(6) 137(3)/153(<u>6</u>)	147/160 .92	126(4)/163(3)	126/163 .77

[a] See footnote "a" in Table 1.

[b] If the dose is underlined it was given on Days 1 and 4 post-implant, if not underlined, the dose shown was given once daily on Days 1→4 post-implant.

[c] When the disparity in cure rates obtained using an analog and cisplatin was great, no calculation of a mean % T/C ratio was performed.

failed to cure any mice and achieved only a modest extension in lifespan. Although JM-8 clearly was superior to cisplatin in this experiment, the level of activity achieved was not beyond that observed historically for the parent compound, and one would prefer to see this difference in activity levels confirmed before concluding that JM-8 was indeed superior in the C26 model. Among the other clinical candidates, JM-9 and TNO-6 were active but inferior to cisplatin in two studies, JM-40 was comparable to cisplatin, and JM-82 demonstrated only borderline activity. Of the remaining compounds, TNO-10 and TNO-18, both of which had done rather poorly versus M109, did quite well against C26, whereas TNO-8 and TNO-38 achieved only borderline or modest levels of activity despite their having done well against both M109 and B16. TNO-7 did less well than cisplatin in this model and Na^+-JM-5 was comparable to the parent drug.

Each analog was also evaluated simultaneously against a line of L1210 leukemia resistant to cisplatin (L1210/cDDP) and the parent line of L1210 (Table 3). The L1210/cDDP line was judged to be cross-resistant to an analog if the extent of cell killing (estimated from parallel cell titrations in untreated mice) versus that line was ≥ 1.5 log_{10} less than that obtained against the parent line, or the analog failed to achieve a T/C $\geq$ 125%.

Na^+-JM-5, JM-8, JM-9 and JM-40 all failed to achieve a T/C $\geq 125\%$ versus L1210/cDDP. TNO-38 was active against the resistant line but the degree of cell killing was diminished compared to that observed against the parent line. Although the leukemic cell titrations included in the experiment were inadequate to determine an exact difference in cell kill achieved against each leukemia, the extensions in lifespan compared to control mice were sufficiently different to assign a label of "partial cross-resistance" to the sensitivity of L1210/cDDP to TNO-38. This characterization of TNO-38 was unexpected considering the sensitivity, even perhaps occasional collateral sensitivity, shown by L1210/cDDP for each of the other analogs (e.g. TNO-6, TNO-7 and TNO-18) sharing the DAMCH moiety with TNO-38. Each of the other analogs showed good activity against L1210/cDDP, including a few that cured mice of this leukemia but not the parent line treated in parallel.

DISCUSSION

The L1210 leukemia model was used as the primary screening test for Pt analogs. At the time these analogs were evaluated, any compound achieving a T/C value, using either treatment regimen, that was at least as good as the lowest historical value obtained using cisplatin, proceeded to the next tumor screen. Had the criteria for proceeding been more stringent (for example, a maximum T/C value of at least 90% that obtained concomitantly using cisplatin), neither JM-8 nor JM-40 would have been further evaluated. If one abides by the thesis that compounds which are active in a number of screening systems may have more likelihood of being active clinically, and the higher the experimental activities the greater the possibility of demonstrating clinical activity, then it would appear reasonable to ask that an analog be at least comparable to cisplatin in a tumor model that was fairly sensitive to the parent compound. Of course, should it be determined following clinical evaluations that relative activity levels in L1210 bore no relationship to clinical outcome, then that model would have been a poor primary screen to have used these many years. Wolpert-DeFillippes (13) has reported, and the present data confirm, that the B16 and L1210 tumors rank Pt analogs differently. But the logistics of screening many analogs against B16 places a heavy burden on resources, without any better guarantee as to clinical correlation.

Of the analogs described which are not involved in clinical trials, Na^+-JM-5 represented a salt of an analog reported previously to be one of the few ever found to be clearly and reproducibly superior to cisplatin versus B16 melanoma (1). Unfortunately, improving the solubility of JM-5 resulted in a decrease in anti-B16 activity to the point where it was only comparable to cisplatin. Both TNO-7 and TNO-18 performed quite well compared to the parent compound, but they too suffer from poor solubility and thus far attempts to develop a soluble formulation have resulted in materials not quite as active as their insoluble counterparts. Of the remaining new analogs mentioned, only TNO-38 had adequate solubility.

The ip tumor models described herein were not the only models used to evaluate Pt analogs. However, ic and sc implants of those same tumors

Table 3. Antitumor Activity of Pt Analogs Against a Line of L1210
          Leukemia Resistant to Cisplatin (L1210/cDDP)

Analog code No.	Max. % T/C-cures/total (approx. log cell kill)[a] Vs: L1210	L1210/cDDP	Cross-resistance?
Cisplatin	164-193(≥3)	94-131(0-1.5)	-
JM-8	146(1.5)	113(<1)	Yes
JM-9	167(2)	118(1)	Yes
JM-40	129(2 est.)[b] 143(2.5)	109(<1 est.) 106(<1)	Yes
JM-82	250(>4) 192(>3) 171(>3)	188-2/6(>4) 294(>3) 169(≥3)	No
TNO-6	217(>3)	171-1/6(>3)	No
Na$^+$-JM-5	143(1.5)	100(0)	Yes
TNO-7	225-1/6(>3)	229(>3)	No
TNO-8	217(>3 est.)	159-2/6(>3 est.)	No
TNO-10	175-2/6(>3)	229-2/6(>3)	No
TNO-18	186(≥3 est.) 233(≥4)	133-3/6(>3 est.) 269(>4)	No
TNO-38	200(>3) 200(>3)	156(3) 163(>3)	Partial

[a] % T/C values shown are for dying mice only with cures indicated
separately when present. All drugs were administered as a single ip
injection one day post-implant of 10^6 leukemic cells. Each line of data
within an analog's listing was derived from a separate experiment.

[b] Estimated log cell kill based on historical data because no titration
was performed concurrently or none that was technically acceptable.

used in the ip setting were not more susceptible to any analog than they
were to cisplatin. In fact, even those analogs found comparable to cisplatin in a given ip tumor model usually did relatively less well when
compared in the sc models (iv dosing was used when possible).

With respect to activity against the L1210/cDDP leukemia, the ligands
associated with lack of cross-resistance can be expanded from the DACH,
DAMCH, and 2,2-diethyl 1,3-propanediamine moieties previously reported

238

(1,2, 11), to now include 1-amino-2-aminomethyl 3,3,5-trimethylcyclohexane
(e.g. TNO-8). It should become apparent soon whether this particular
murine model of cisplatin resistance has any predictability for a parallel
clinical situation. It is also conceivable that there could be a good
positive correlation for effectiveness but a poor negative correlation for
predicting resistance, or vice versa.

Neither the analogs currently being evaluated clinically nor the
others described herein surpassed cisplatin with respect to overall
experimental antitumor activity. Yet we are fortunate that clinical
feedback will be forthcoming for several analogs and perhaps we will be
able to discern some relationship between clinical activity and that
observed in one or more experimental screening models.

REFERENCES

1. Bradner WT, Rose WC, Huftalen JB. 1980. Antitumor activity of
   platinum analogs. In Cisplatin: Current Status and New Developments
   (Prestayko AW, Crooke ST, and Carter SK, eds.), Academic Press, Inc.,
   New York, pp. 171-182.
2. Burchenal JH, Kalaher K, Dew K, Lokys L, Gale G. 1978. Studies of
   cross-resistance, synergistic combinations and blocking of activity of
   platinum derivatives. Biochime 60:961-965.
3. Cleare MJ, Hydes PC, Malerbi BW, Watkins DM. 1978. Anti-tumour
   platinum complexes: relationships between chemical properties and
   activity. Biochimie 60:835-850.
4. Connors TA, Cleare MJ, Harrap KR. 1979. Structure-activity relationships of the antitumor platinum coordination complexes. Cancer Treat.
   63:1499-1502.
5. Craciunescu DG, Doadrio A, Furlani A, Scarcia V. 1982.
   Structure-antitumor activity relationships for new platinum complexes.
   Chem.-Biol. Interactions 42:153-164.
6. Hall LM, Speer RJ, Ridgway HJ, Norton SJ. 1979. Unsymmetrical
   C-substituted ethylenediamine platinum coordination complexes:
   synthesis and activity against mouse leukemia L1210. J. Inorg. Biochem.
   11:139-149.
7. Kidani Y, Okamoto K, Noji M, Tashiro T. 1978. Antitumor activity
   of platinum (II) complexes of 1-amino-2-amino-methylcyclohexane
   isomers. Gann 69:863-864.
8. Meishen SJ, Gale GR, Lake LM, Frangakis CJ, Rosenblum MG, Walker Jr.,
   EM, Atkins LM, Smith AB. 1976. Antileukemic properties of
   organoplatinum complexes. J. Natl. Cancer Inst. 57:841-845.
9. Pera Jr., MF, Sessford D, Roberts JJ. 1982. Toxicity of cisplatin
   and hydroxymalonatodiammine platinum (II) towards mouse bone marrow and
   B16 melanoma in relation to DNA binding in vivo. Biochem. Pharmacol.
   31:2273-2278.

10. Prestayko AW, Bradner WT, Huftalen JB, Rose WC, Schurig JE, Clear MJ, Hydes PC, Crooke ST. 1979. Antileukemic (L1210) activity and toxicity of cis-dichlorodiammineplatinum (II) analogs. Cancer Treat. Rep. 63:1503-1508.
11. Rose WC, Schurig JE, Huftalen JB, Bradner WT. 1982. Antitumor activity and toxicity of cisplatin analogs. Cancer Treat. Rep. 66:135-146.
12. Sheperd R, Kusnierczyk H, Jones M, Harrap KR. 1980. Critera for the selection of second-generation platinum compounds. Br. J. Cancer 42:668-676.
13. Wolpert-DeFillippes MK. 1980. Antitumor activity of cisplatin analogs. In Cisplatin: Current Status and New Developments (Prestayko AW, Crooke ST and Carter SK, eds.), Academic Press, Inc., New York, pp. 183-191.

JM8 Development and Clinical Projects

A.H. Calvert, S.J. Harland, K.R. Harrap,
E. Wiltshaw and I.E. Smith

INTRODUCTION

Since its introduction in the early 1970's cisplatin has become
established as one of the major cytotoxic drugs used in the treatment of
cancer. Of particular note are its application in combination therapy to
the treatment of testicular cancer (1) and in the treatment of ovarian
cancer (2). The majority of patients with testicular teratoma are probably
cured of their disease. Cisplatin is probably the most active single agent
in the treatment of ovarian cancer producing an overall response rate in
excess of 50% and a complete response rate of 20-30% (2). In our hands a
group of 27 patients treated with high dose cisplatin for stage III ovarian
carcinoma and followed for a minimum of 3 years had an actuarial survival
of 35% at 3 and 4 years (3).

The use of cisplatin is, however, severely compromised by its
toxicity. In early studies nephrotoxicity was apparent (4). Acute
clinical problems due to nephrotoxicity are now usually averted by the
selection of patients with good renal function, the use of hydration and
diuresis, and by restricting the number of treatment courses (usually to
about 6) (5). Nevertheless both renal and tubular function are affected
and convulsions may be induced by hypomagnesaemia (6).

Cisplatin also causes prolonged and intractable vomiting which is
poorly controlled by antiemetics, and may lead to patients refusing
treatment. Anaemia is common and high frequency hearing loss occurs in
about 50% of patients although it is not always symptomatic (7).

These toxic limitations of cisplatin have probably restricted its use
in other tumours such as head and neck cancer, where its activity is
undoubted but may not be sufficient to justify the side effects.

The analogue development programme, from which the compound JM8 (cis-diammine-1,1-cyclo butanedicarboxylate platinum II, CBDCA, carboplatin) emerged, was thus aimed at identifying a compound which maintained the therapeutic efficacy of cisplatin while lacking some or all of its toxicities. The programme was a collaborative venture between Johnson Matthey Research, Reading, England and The Institute of Cancer Research, London, England.

PRECLINICAL DEVELOPMENT OF JM8

Over 300 platinum containing compounds were made with variations both of the leaving groups and of the ammine ligands to span a wide range of reactivities and solubilities. These analogues were tested both for toxicity (LD50) and antitumour efficacy in mice. The animal tumours employed were the L1210 ascites tumour and the ADJ/PC6 plasmacytoma. From these data it became clear that the toxicity of a compound was usually related to the reactivity of the leaving groups. Compounds with labile leaving groups (eg sulphate) had a low LD50 while those with more stable leaving groups (eg malonate) had a high LD50. In contrast the antitumour activity was unrelated to the reactivity of the leaving groups, active compounds being found throughout the range(8).

A selection of 8 compounds with antitumour activity similar to that of cisplatin but having a range of physical and chemical properties was made. These compounds were studied in detail for their toxicity in rats. (9). Nephrotoxicity was assessed by serial measurement of blood urea, haematological toxicity by measurements of haemoglobin levels and differential white cell counts. In addition major organs were examined histologically. The majority of these compounds were less toxic than cisplatin. Both JM8 and CHIP seemed to be completely free from nephrotoxicity. All the eight compounds were tested for activity against the P246 human lung tumour xenograft. JM8 was distinctly more active than any of the others, achieving complete inhibition of tumour growth at a non-toxic dose. The results are summarised in table I.

Table 1. Summary of Toxicity and Activity of 8 platinum analogues

analogue	L1210/ PC6	P246 xenograft	toxicity renal	toxicity body wt.	renal histology
cisplatin	+	B	++	+++	necrosis PCT
1	+	C	0	++	CT
2	+	C	0	++	necrosis DCT
3	+	A	0	0	CT
4	+	C	0	++	0
5	+	B	0	+	0
6	+	B	0	++	0
7	+	C	+	++	necrosis DCT
8	+	B	0	++	0

Key:
1 Cis-dichlorobis(isobutylamine)platinum II (JM2)
2 Diammine(2-hydroxymalonato)platinum II (JM5)
3 Cis-diammine(1,1-cyclobutanediacrboxylato)platinum II (JM8, CBDCA)
4 Cis-dichloro-trans-dihydroxybis(ispropylamine)platinum IV (JM9, CHIP)
5 Cis-diammine(2-ethylmalonato)platinum II (JM10)
6 Cis-dichlorobis(cyclopropylamine)platinum II (JM11)
7 Cis-diisopropylaminebis(chloroacetato)platinum II (JM16)
8 1,2-diamminocyclohexane(sulphato)platinum II (JM20)

A - >90% inhibition at non toxic dose
B - substantial inhibition only at toxic dose
C - no activity at a toxic dose

JM8 CLINICAL STUDIES - PHASE I

A phase I study of JM8 was performed at The Royal Marsden Hospital in 1981 (10). The dose limiting toxicity was myelosuppression, with thrombocytopenia being the most prominent feature. This occurred over the range of doses from 200-520 mg/m2 given as a 1 hour infusion. However, when good risk patients were selected on the basis of renal function and previous treatment, a dose of 400 mg/m2 was found to be well tolerated, while 500 mg/m2 was not. When myelosuppression occurred, the platelet nadir occurred about 3 weeks after treatment. The recommended "phase II" dose was thus 400 mg/m2 given every 4 weeks. Evidence for nephrotoxicity was sought during this trial but was largely lacking. Serial measurements of glomerular filtration rate by the use of 51Cr EDTA (11) failed to reveal a consistent downward trend either with increasing doses or numbers of courses. Patients with severe pre-existing renal impairment were also treated without any further decline in renal function. Serial measurement of urinary N-acetylglucoseaminidase, leucine aminopeptidase and beta 2-microglobulin levels showed transient 2-5 fold elevations at therapeutic dose levels, and were thought to represent only slight and reversible tubular damage. Vomiting occurred but was reported to be less severe than that seen with cisplatin. Modest reductions in haemoglobin were noted. Evidence for peripheral neuropathy was found in a few patients, but no audiometric or symptomatic hearing loss was seen. However a substantial amount of antitumour activity was observed in patients with carcinoma of the ovary.

A number of other phase I studies of JM8 have now been performed and reported in abstract form (12-17), the results of which are summarised in table 2. The main additional information available from these studies is the documentation of WBC suppression in addition to thrombocytopenia. The nadir of the white count appears to be later than that of the platelets, particularly following a 5 day schedule where it was reported to occur between 34-38 days after treatment. Further, two of these studies reported nephrotoxicity occrring in patients with impaired renal function, a finding which disagrees with our own study.

In conclusion, 7 phase I studies of JM8 have all reported very similar findings. All found myelosuppression to be dose limiting and somewhat delayed. All found negligible evidence for nephrotoxicity and greatly reduced emesis compared to cisplatin. Three of these studies also reported evidence of antitumour efficacy derived from their phase I data.

Table 2. Phase I Studies of JM8

Schedule	Interval	MTD	RD	Tox	Other Toxicities Reported	Ref
IV 1 hr	4 wks	-	400	T	nausea/vomiting mild elevations of urinary enzymes	10
IV bolus	4 wks	520	400	T	mild nausea malaise	12
IV bolus	5-6 wks	550	-	M	nausea/vomiting nephrotoxicity in patients with impaired renal function	13
24 hrs	4 wks	320	-	T	nausea/vomiting nephrotoxicity in patients with impaired renal function	14
IV daily x 5	6 wks	125/day	100/day	M/T	nausea minimal nephrotoxicity	15
IV daily x 5	4-5 wks	99/day	77/day	M	mild nausea and vomiting	16
IV	1 wk	100	-	T	elevations in B_2-microglobulin	17

Key   T - thrombocytopeia   Tox - dose limiting toxicity
       M - myelosuppression   MTD - maximum tolerated dose
       RD - recommended dose

JM8 - PHASE II STUDIES

The promising results obtained in the phase I study at The Royal Marsden Hospital led to a number of phase II studies being initiated. Many of these are "on-going" but nevertheless it is possible to draw conclusions about the activity of the drug in certain tumour types. They have also permitted a more detailed documentation of the toxicities of JM8 in reasonably homogenous groups of patients.

Ovarian Cancer. A phase II study of the effects of JM8 in 33 patients previously treated with cisplatin or cisplatin containing combinations was conducted (18). These patients all had either recurrent disease following treatment with cisplatin or a cisplatin containing combination, or had been primarily resistant to such a combination. Many of these patients had received extensive myelosuppressive therapy and had impaired renal function as a result of therapy. Responses were documented according to WHO

criteria using clinical examination, ultrasonic, isotope or computer
assisted tomographic scanning and "second look" surgical procedures, as
appropriate. The results are shown in table 3, stratified according to the
reason for JM8 treatment. Although the overall response rate to JM8 was
low (21%), it is notable that responses occurred in patients who had been
primarily resistant to cisplatin therapy. Indeed, one patient who had had
progressive disease while receiving cisplatin at a dose of 100 mg/m2 4
weekly had a surgically confirmed complete response following subsequent
therapy with JM8.

Table 3. Response to JM8 of Patients With Ovarian Cancer Previously
Treated with Cisplatin

reason for stopping cisplatin	Response				total
	CR	PR	NR	NA	
end of course	0	1	3	1	5
NR to cisplatin	1	4	12	2	19
neuropathy	0	0	2	1	3
ototoxicity	0	0	1	0	1
renal toxicity	0	1	2	2	5
totals	1	6	20	6	33

Key   CR - complete response
      PR - partial response
      NR - minor response, stasis or progressive disease
      NA - not assessable for response

Patients not previously treated with cisplatin (19) these data are
presented in an abstract from elsewhere in this volume. thirty four
patients referred for treatment were included. Seven had received prior
therapy with bifunctional alkylating agents or other combination therapy;
eight had received previous abdominal or pelvic irradiation. The standard
dose of JM8 was 400 mg/m2 but this was reduced if myelosuppression was
encountered in 2 successive courses.   The results are summarised in table
4. The overall response rate was 56% with 24% of complete responses. Of
these complete responses, 4/8 were confirmed by a second look surgical
procedure.

Table 4. JM8 in Ovarian Cancer, Patients Not Previously Treated
with Cisplatin

---

complete response	- surgical 4	24%
	- clinical 4	
		56%
partial response	11	32

(two early patients may become complete, 2 were clinically complete)

MR,NC or PD   9

not assessable for response   6
- 2 received 1 course and were lost to follow up
- 2 stage III, but no second look procedure
- 2 carcinomatosis, patients died early

total   34

The only toxicities definitely attributable to JM8 which were observed in these studies were nausea, vomiting and myelosuppression. Peripheral neuropathy was also observed in 1 patient.

Small cell lung cancer (20). JM8 used in the treatment of small cell lung cancer primarily resistant to combination therapy (usually vincristine adriamycin and VP16) produced only a low response rate (1/12). However, in patients who had responded initially to combination therapy, but subsequently relapsed the results were considerably better (1 cr, 4 pr out of 8 patients). In new patients with extensive disease, or who were medically unfit to receive combination therapy the overall response rate was 50% (6/12). The response rate for all the small cell cases treated was 34% (12/35). In this study standard antiemetic therapy (Lorazepam 2 mg given 5 hours after JM8 and metoclopramide 10 mg given at the same time and repeated as necessary) was used. In 17 patients who remained as in-patients the incidence of nausea and vomiting was recorded and is summarised in table 5. It is notable that only 50% of the patients studied experienced nausea or vomiting.

Table 5.   JM8 for Small Cell Carcinoma of The Bronchus,
Nausea and Vomiting

days of symptom duration	nausea	vomiting
0	7	9
<1	2	4
2-3	4	3
>3	4	1

(all patients received metoclopramide and lorazepam)

Non small cell lung cancer. Only limited results are available in this disease.   There have been 2 partial responses in 11 patients treated.

Testicular teratoma. The known responsiveness of this tumour to a number of other chemotherapeutic agents means that all the patients treated have had advanced recurrent disease resistant to a variety of other drugs. No significant therapeutic responses have been seen although transient reductions in tumour markers has been observed in 1/5 patients. Four patients not previously treated with combination therapy who had extremely advanced disease received 1 course of JM8 as a single agent. Response was assessed by measurement of the tumour markers 4 weeks later prior to commencing combination therapy. All of these 4 patients responded to therapy although in one case the drop in HCG was only 33%.

Testicular seminoma. Complete responses have been seen in 2 of 3 patients treated.

Mesothelioma. Eight patients with mesothelioma were studied, with one peritoneal and nine pleural primaries. One clincally complete response and one partial response have been seen. One patient with extensive lung disease remained static for 14 months and a further patient had a minor response of parenchymal lung metastases but died of cardiac tamponade. The overall response rate stands at 25%, but the clinical observations are encouraging enough to warrant continuation of this study.

248

Thyroid carcinoma. Of five patients treated, one has had a partial response.

PHASE III STUDIES

Ovarian carcinoma. The encouraging single agent data for JM8 in ovarian cancer, the lack of universal cross-resistance with cisplatin and the good survival obtained previously in this disease by treatment with cisplatin led us to undertake a randomised crossover study of JM8 versus cisplatin for the treatment of new patients with FIGO stage III and IV ovarian cancer. New patients, diagnosed at laparotomy who were assessed medically and found to be fit enough to withstand high dose cisplatin therapy were then randomised to receive either cisplatin 100 mg/m2 4 weekly with hydration, or JM8 400 mg/m2 4 weekly. Patients were reassessed clinically after two courses. If the patient was apparently showing tumour regression treatment was continued until 5 courses, following which a laparotomy or laparoscopy was done. Patients having a complete or partial response confirmed surgically continued to receive 5 further treatments. while those without response changed to the other platinum complex. Therapy was also changed if toxicity precluded continuation of the initial derivative. This trial is on-going, but the preliminary analysis shows that the complete and partial response rates are identical in both arms, while all aspects of toxicity are reduced in the JM8 arm except for the possibility of a slightly increased incidence of mild myelosuppression. These data, published in preliminary form elsewhere (21) are summarised in table 6.

Table 6. JM8 in New Patients With Ovarian Cancer, Randomised
Study, JM8 Versus Cisplatin

	JM8	cisplatin
patients entered	22	26
stage III	18	19
stage IV	4	7
CR	3	3
PR	6	8
NA*	4	5
WBC <3,000 x10^9/1	8	8
platelets <100 x10^9/1	2	0
GFR fall >20%	2	18
audiometric hearing loss	0%	65%
sensory neuropathy	0	5

Key   WBC - total white total blood cell count
      GFR - glomerular filtration rate measured by the ^{51}Cr
            EDTA method
    * Patients awaiting second look procedure

CONCLUSIONS

JM8 is a well tolerated analogue of cisplatin with reduced non
haematological toxicities being reported by all of the 7 phase I studies.
Different schedules, and, presumably different patient populations were
used for these studies, but when the administration dose is divided by the
interval used there is a remarkable consistency of a recommended dose rate
of about 100 mg/m2/week. The reduced nephrotoxicity and emesis were well
predicted by preclinical studies. The myelosuppression (particularly
thrombocytopenia) was not predicted prospectively by the preclinical
studies, possibly because animal studies were not continued long enough to
reach the rather late nadir. When our phase I study was started,
preclinical data on ototoxicity and neurotoxicity were not available.

The facts that JM8 is well tolerated and may therefore be given to
patients in poorer medical condition than would be possible with cisplatin,
and that the dose tolerated by individual patients is relatively consistent
makes it an ideal candidate for phase II. So far, activity has been
obvserved in all the tumour types studied suggesting that JM8 may be a

broad spectrum antitumour agent with far wider indications than those of cisplatin.

The early data available from a randomised phase III study confirm the greatly reduced non-haematological toxicity of JM8 compared to that of cisplatin, while the antitumour activity appears to be maintained. Hopefully, the myelosuppression induced by JM8 will not preclude its incorporation into combination schemes containing other potentially myelosuppressive agents, since the day of the nadir is rather late.

AKNOWLEDGEMENT.

We should like to aknowledge the staff of The Royal Marsden Hospital for their collaboration and assistance with these trials. We should like to thank Johnson Matthey Ltd, Reading England, Bristol-Myers International Corp. and The National Cancer Institute, Bethesda, Maryland USA for the provision of JM8.

References
1   Newlands ES, Rustin GJS, Begent RHJ, Parker D, Bagshawe KD:
     Further advances in the management of malignant teratomas of the
     testis and other sites
     The Lancet Vol 1(1983) No 8331 984-951
2   Wiltshaw E and Kroner T: Phase II study of cis-dichlorodiammine
     platinum (II) (NSC 119875) in advanced adenocarcinoma of the ovary
     Cancer Treat. Rep. (60) 55-60, 1976
3   Wiltshaw E, Evans BD, et al: A randomised trial of high-dose cisplatin
     versus low low dose cisplatin and chlorambucil in carcinoma of the
     ovary
     proc. 14th Int. Congress of Chemotherapy, Vienna 1983 (in press)
4   Prestayko AW, D'Aoust JC, Issel IF, Crooke ST: Cisplatin (cis-diammine
     dichloro platinum (II))
     Cancer Treat. Rev. (6) 17-39, 1979
5   Krakoff IH: Nephrotoxicity of cis-dichlorodiammineplatinum (II)
     Cancer Treat. Rep. (63) 1527-1532, 1979

6   Macauley VM, Begent RHJ, Phillips ME, Newlands ES: Prophylaxis against hypomagnesemia induced by cis-platinum combination chemotherapy
Cancer Chemother. Pharmacol (in press)

7   Reddel RR, Kefford RF, Grant JM, Coates AS Fox RM Tattersall MHN: Ototoxicity in patients receiving cisplatin: Importance of dose and method of drug administration
Cancer Treat. Rep. (66) 19, 1982

8   Harrap KR: Platinum Analogues:Criteria for selection In: Cancer Chemotherapy Muggia FM (ed) Martinus Nijhoff, Massachusets (in press)

9   Harrap KR, Jones M, Wilkinson CR, Clink H McD, Sparrow S, Mitchley BCV, Clarke S, Veasey A: Antitumour, toxic and biochemical properties of cisplatin and eight other platinum complexes. In: Cisplatin Current status and New developments, Prestayko AW, Crooke ST, and Carter SK (eds)
New York Academic Press 1980 ppp 193-212

10   Calvert AH, Harland SJ, Newell DR, Siddik ZH, Jones AC, McElwain TJ, Raju S, Wiltshaw E, Smith IE, Baker JW, Peckham MJ and Harrap KR: Early clinical studies with cis-diammine-1,1-cyclobutane dicarboxylate platinum II
Cancer Chemother. Pharmacol (9) 140-147, 1982

11   Chantler C, Garnett ES, Parsons V: Glomerular filtration rate measurement in man by the single injection methods using Cr^{51} EDTA
Clin. Sci. Mol. Med. (37) 169, 1969

12   Koeller JM, Earhart RH, Davis TE, Trump DL, Tormey DC: Phase I trial of carboplatin (NSC 241240) by bolus intravenous injection
Proc. 74th Meeting of The Am. Assoc. for Cancer Res. (24) 162, 1983

13   Kaplan S, Joss R, Sessa C, Goldhirsch A, Cattaneo M, Cavalli F: Phase I trials of cis-diammine-1,1-cyclobutane dicarboxylate platinum II (CBDCA) in solid tumours.
Proc 74th Meeting of The Am. Assoc. for Cancer Res. (24) 132, 1983

14   Curt CA, Grygiel JJ, Weiss R, Corden B, Ozols R, Tell D Collins J,, Myers CE: A phase I and pharmacokinetic study of CBDCA (NSC 241240)
Proc. of the 19th Meeting of The Am. Soc. of Clin. Oncology (2) 21, 1983

15   Nicaise C, Rozencweig M, Beer M, Piccart M, Crespeigne N, Anton Aparicio L, Van Rijmenant M Lenaz L, Kenis Y: Phase I clinical trial of carboplatin (CBDCA) administered at a five-day schedule
Proc 74th Meeting of The Am. Assoc. for Cancer Res. (24) 164, 1983

16   Egorin MJ, Van Echo DA, Whitacre MY, Olman EA, Aisner J: Phase I study and clinical pharmacokinetics of carboplatin (CBDCA) (NSC 241240)
Proc. 19th Meeting of The Am. Soc. of Clin. Oncology (2) 28, 1983

17   Priego V, Luc V, Bonnem E, Rabman A, Smith F, Schein P, Woolley P: A phase I study and pharmacology of diammine (1,1) cyclobutane dicarboxylato (2-1-0) platinum (CBDCA) administered on a weekly schedule
Proc. 19th Meeting of The Am. Soc. of Clin. Oncology (2) 30, 1983

18   Evans BD, Raju S, Calvert AH, Harland SJ, Wiltshaw E: A phase II study of JM8, a new platinum analogue in advanced ovarian carcinoma
Cancer Treat. Rep. (in press) 1983

19   Calvert AH, Baker JW, Dalley VM, Harland SJ, Jones AC, Staffurth J:
     Phase II trial of cis-diammine-1,1-cyclobutane dicarboxylate platinum
     II (CBDCA, JM8) in patients with carcinoma of the ovary not previously
     treated with cisplatin
     Proc. 4th Int. Symp. on Platinum Coordination Complexes In Cancer
     Chemotherapy, Vermont 1983
20   Harland SJ, Smith IE, Smith N, Alison DL, Calvert AH: Phase II study
     of cis-diammine-1,1-cyclobutane dicarboxylate platinum II (JM(, CBDCA)
     in carcinoma of the bronchus
     Proc. 4th Int. Symp. on Platinum Coordination Complexes in Cancer
     Chemotherapy, Vermont, USA 1983
21   Wiltshaw E, Evans BD, Jones AC, Baker JW, Calvert AH: JM8, successor
     to cisplatin in advanced ovarian cancer?
     Lancet 1(1983) (No 8324) p 587

POSTER PRESENTATIONS

IV-1   ANTITUMOR DIAMINEPLATINUM (II) PHOSPHATE COMPLEXES.
A.R. Amundsen, J.D. Hoeschele and E.W. Stern.

IV-2   PRE-CLINICAL AND PHASE I CLINICAL TRIAL WITH bis(PYRUVATO) 1,2-DIAMINOCYCLOHEXANE PLATINUM (II).
A. Khan, R.J. Speer, H. Ridgway, R. Young, J. Tseng, D. Stewart, N.O. Hill, A. Pardue, C. Aleman, R. Hilario, M. Lakho, K. Osther and J.M. Hill.

IV-3   SYNTHESIS AND ANTITUMOUR ASSAYS OF NEW Pt(II) AND Pt(IV) COMPLEXES.
D. Craciunescu, R. Maral, G. Mathe and A. Doadrio.

IV-4   ANALOGS OF SULFATO 1,2-DIAMINOCYCLOHEXANE PLATINUM (II).
D. Craciunescu, G. Atassi, A. Doadrio and C. Ghirvu.

IV-5   PHASE II TRIAL OF 1,1-DIAMINO-METHYLCYCLOHEXANE-SULFATE PLATINUM II NSC 311056 (TN06).
C.R. Franks, G. Nys, E. Materman, R. Canetta, L. Lenaz and S.K. Carter.

IV-6   MOLECULAR ORBITAL STUDIES ON SOME cis-PLATINUM AND PALLADIUM AMINE ANTI-TUMOR COMPLEXES.
E.A. Boudreaux and B.K. Park.

IV-7   STRUCTURE-ACTIVITY RELATIONSHIPS FOR INDUCTION OF BACTERIOPHAGE LAMBDA BY PLATINUM (II) AND PLATINUM (IV) COMPLEXES.
R.K. Elespuru, S.K. Daley and B. Das Sarma.

IV-8   SYNTHESIS AND BIOLOGICAL EFFECTS OF A NEW FLUORESCENT PLATINUM COMPOUND.
B.L. Bergquist and J.C. Chang.

IV-9   NEW ANALOGS OF 4-CARBOXYPHTHALATO (1,2-DIAMINOCYCLOHEXANE)-PLATINUM(DACH-Pt).
P.J. Andrulis, Jr., P. Schwartz and G.R. Gale.

IV-10   IN VITRO PHASE II EVALUATION OF CISPLATIN AND THREE ANALOGS AGAINST VARIOUS HUMAN CARCINOMAS.
A.H. Rossof, P.A. Johnson, B.D. Kimmell, G.D. Wilbanks, E.L. Yordan, Jr., J.E. Graham, C.F. Kittle and S.G. Economou.

IV-11   BIOPHYSICAL AND BIOCHEMICAL STUDIES OF A NEW SPIN-LABELED Pt (II) COMPLEX IN MAMMALIAN CELLS.
H.G. Claycamp, A. Mathew, R. Morgan, E.I. Shaw and J.D. Zimbrick.

IV-12   NEW PLATINUM COMPLEXES AS RADIOSENSITIZERS.
K.A. Skov, N.P. Farrell, T.G. de Carneiro, F.W.B. Einstein and T. Jones.

IV-13   PLATINUM-METAL COMPLEXES AS DUAL FUNCTION AGENTS IN CHEMOTHERAPY.
N.P. Farrell, J. Williamson and D.J. McLaren.

IV-14   PREPARATION OF A NEW ANTITUMOR OXALATO (1R,2R-CYCLOHEXANE-DIAMINE PLATINUM (II)) COMPLEX.
Y. Kidani, M. Noji, K. Inagaki, T. Tashiro and M. Miyazaki.

IV-1 ANTITUMOR DIAMINEPLATINUM(II) PHOSPHATE COMPLEXES. Alan R. Amundsen*, James D. Hoeschele, and Eric W. Stern. *Research and Development Dept., Engelhard Industries Division of Engelhard Corp., Menlo Park, Edison, NJ 08818.

A series of platinum phosphate compounds are formed by the interaction of cis-$[PtA_2(H_2O)_2](NO_3)_2$ with $H_nPO_4^{(3-n)-}$, and various organophosphate ions. When A=NH_3, at least two different orthophosphate compounds (light yellow and gray) are formed. The nature of the product depends chiefly on the initial pH of the reaction solution. When A_2=ethylenediamine and 1,2-diaminocyclohexane, pyrophosphate complexes of the type $[\{PtA_2\}_2P_2O_7]$ may be prepared. When A=NH_3, soluble blue phosphate ester compounds are formed with α-D,L-glycerophosphate, α-D-glucose-1-phosphate, β-glycerophosphate, and D-glucose-6-phosphate. Insoluble blue phosphate ester compounds are formed with D-fructose-6-phosphate, D-galactose-6-phosphate, D-ribose-5-phosphate, and D-fructose-1,6-diphosphate. All of the above exhibit antitumor activity against Sarcoma 180 ascites in Swiss mice, featuring in most cases high %ILS values, broad active dose ranges and high therapeutic ratios. Activity is also shown by some of these materials against L1210 and P388 leukemias, B16 melanoma, epindymoblastoma, Lewis lung carcinoma, CD8F1 mammary tumor and colon 26 tumor in mice.

IV-2 PRE-CLINICAL AND PHASE I CLINICAL TRIAL WITH bis(PYRUVATO) 1,2-DIAMINOCYCLOHEXANE PLATINUM(II). Amanullah Khan, Robert J. Speer, Helen Ridgway, Robert Young, Julia Tseng, David Stewart, N. O. Hill, Ayten Pardue, Cesar Aleman, Rufina Hilario, Mazhar Lakho, Kurt Osther, and J. M. Hill. The Cancer Center at Wadley Institutes of Molecular Medicine, 9000 Harry Hines, Dallas, Texas 75235.

bis(Pyruvato) 1,2-diaminocyclohexane platinum(II) (PYP) was found to have 25 X higher therapeutic index than cisplatin in leukemia L1210. It is soluble (>10 mg/ml) and stable for several hours in 5% dextrose solution. PYP achieved 66% cure rate in L1210 bearing BDF1 mice at doses of 25-80 mg/kg and had an LD50 of 90 mg/kg. In mice, 75-120 mg/kg caused thrombocytopenia, leukopenia and toxicity to spleen, kidney and intestine. PYP inhibited antibody formation at 70 mg/kg and delayed hypersensitivity at 100 mg/kg in mice (P 0.05). PHA and PWM induced transformation of human lymphocytes was inhibited (P<0.05) by 4.5 µg/ml PYP in vitro. Phase I clinical trial was initiated in November, 1982 at 2 mg/kg dose which was escalated to 4, 6.6,10,14,18 and 22 mg/kg. Sixteen patients were included in the trial. Their Karnofsky score varied from 20-40. At doses below 10 mg/kg the only side effect was mild nausea. At 10 and 14 mg/kg, nausea, vomiting and mild diarrhea were observed. At 14 mg/kg hypomagnesemia was noted in one patient. Six patients received 18 mg/kg dose on 9 occasions (3 patients received 2 doses each). Nausea and vomiting occurred on 8 and diarrhea on 2 of 9 occasions. Elevated SGOT was seen once. Seven patients received 22 mg/kg dose. All of them had nausea and vomiting. Five patients had diarrhea, 4 patients developed neutropenia and thrombocytopenia, 4 patients showed temporary elevation of SGOT and 2 patients had hypomagnesemia. Nephrotoxicity was seen in 2 patients. Both had low creatinine clearance (52 and 41 ml/min prior to treatment). Analyses of sera revealed that after 18 mg/kg dose, platinum peaked at ~210 µg/g during the last 30 minutes of infusion and cleared with T½ of ~20 hours. Analyses of urine revealed platinum excretion of ~30% of dose during the first 24 hours after infusion and little thereafter. Platinum content of autopsy tissues (14 days after 18 mg/kg) showed tumor (breast) with 12 µg/g dry weight; spleen and lung, 5; kidney, liver, small intestine, bone marrow and pancreas, ~5; adrenal, <4; and brain and skeletal muscle, 0. Partial response in one patient with AGL and one patient with CGL in blastic crisis was seen at 22 mg/kg. A drop in CEA was noted in one patient with Ca of the breast who received escalating doses of PYP. The maximum tolerated single dose was in the range of 18 mg/kg. Partial responses in phase I trial in 2 patients with leukemia suggest that this compound deserves further investigation.

IV-3 SYNTHESIS AND ANTITUMOUR ASSAYS OF NEW Pt(II) AND Pt(IV) COMPLEXES.

D. Craciunescu, R. Maral, G. Mathé, A. Doadrio. Dptº. of Inorganic and Analytical Chemistry, Faculty of Pharmacy, Madrid (3), Spain.
** "Institut de Cancerologie et d'Immuno-genetique", Villejuif, France.

Thirty five new Pt(II) and Pt(IV) complexes, belonging to the structural formulation cis-Pt(L)(X)$_n$ and Pt(L)(X)$_n$(OH)$_2$ (Where L = 1, 2 Diamino-cyclohexane and X$^-$ or of the classical antitumour drugs "MELPHALAN", "LEUKERAN", n = 1 or 2) were synthesized and assayed against mice bearing the established L$_{1210}$ tumours, in an attempt to found more active compounds (comparing with the cis-Pt(NH$_3$)$_2$Cl$_2$) and/or compounds with an increased water solubility. Some of those complexes were retained for detailed and expanded antitumour assays, namely those in which X^{2-} = = fumarate (T/C = 194% for a dose of 16 mg/Kg); X^{2-}=tetramethyleneglutarate (T/C = 211% for a dose of 211%); X$^-$ = = hexahydroxyheptanoate (T/C = 188 for a dose of 20 mg/Kg); X^{2-} = sulphosalycilate (T/C = 188 % for a dose of 40 mg/Kg); X^{2-} = 2-oxoglutarate (T/C = 200% for a dose range of 75-100 mg/Kg), X$^-$ = the anion of the polygalacturonic acid (T/C = 222% for a dose of 8 mg/Kg). As a general matter, Pt(II) complexes were more active compared with the Pt(IV) complexes (only Pt(L)(OH)$_2$(X)$_2$ where X$^-$= hexahydroxy heptanoate produced T/C = 194% for a dose of 100 mg/Kg). Complexes in which the leaving ligand was chosen between.the dicarboxylates were more active comparing with those in which the leaving ligand was a monodentate anion. The use of the classical antitumour agents "MELPHALAN" and "LEUKERAN" as monodentate leaving ligand was not effective. Complexes were administered i.p. days 1, 5, 9, as suspensions in oil and/or dissolved in "saline".

No clear structure-activity relationship has yet emerged, between the T/C % values and, on the other hand, the strength of the Pt-O bonding, as appreciated from the detailed study of the I.R. spectra (4000-250 cm^{-1}).

IV-4 ANALOGS OF SULFATO 1, 2 DIAMINOCYCLOHEXANE PLATINUM (II). *D.Craciunescu;**G.Atassi; *A.Doadrio; ***C.Ghirvu. *Department of Inorganic and Analytical Chemistry, Faculty of Pharmacy, Madrid-3. **"Institut des tumeurs Jules Bordet", 1000 Brussels, Belgium. ***Chair of Physical Chemistry, "Institutul Politehnic Iasi", Iasi Romania.

Efforts to improve the therapeutic index of the somewhat toxic and unstable sulfato (1, 2 Diaminocyclohexane) Platinum (II) have led to the synthesis of 4-carboxyphtalato (1, 2 Diaminocyclohexane) Platinum (II) by Gale and co-workers. In this paper we report the synthesis and antitumour data (against mice bearing the established L$_{1210}$ tumour) of the following analogues: a) cis-Pt(L)(X); b) cis-Pt(L)(X)$_2$; c) Pt(L)(X)(OH)$_2$; d) Pt(L)(X)$_2$(OH)$_2$, where L = 1, 2 Diaminocyclohexane and X$^-$ or X^{2-} = the anions of the organic acids (derivatives of the phthalic, isophthalic, and homophthalic acids). They presented a good solubility (4-30 mg/ml) in 1% NaHCO$_3$. Among them, the neutral Pt(II) complexes of the 1, 2, 3, Benzenetricarboxylic acid; 1, 3, 5, Benzenetricarboxylic acid; 5-Sulphoisophthalic acid; Isophthalic acid; Homphthalic acid; Pyromellitic acid; Hemimellitic acid induced T/C% values higher than 350% (for an average dose range 50-100 mg/Kg, administered i.p. days 1, 5, 9, in 1% NaHCO$_3$ or in "saline"). This represented and interesting degree of activity. Others complexes, in which X$^-$= the monoanion of an organic indicator("Methyl-orange"), or even of an N-acethylated aminoacid (N-acethyl valine) or the anion of the galacturonic, gluco-heptonic acids presented in addition excellent water solubilities (~10-20 mg/ml) good stabilities and T/C% values between 195-250%. We were impressed with the good water solubility (~10 mg/ml), low toxicity (LD$_5$ ~ 320 mg/Kg) of the Pt(L)(X)$_2$ complex (Where X$^-$= the anion of the 2, 5 Dihydroxy Benzenesulphonic acid), which induced T/C ~ 375% for the dose range 50-100 mg/Kg. Structure-activity relationship data were drawn, thus thaking into consideration the results of the EHMO calculations performed on the leaving ligands molecules (X$^-$ or X^{2-}), as well as the results of the I.R. spectroscopic studies performed in the 4000-250 cm^{-1} range.

IV-5 PHASE II TRIAL OF 1,1-DIAMINO-METHYLCYCLOHEXANE-SULPHATE
PLATINUM II NSC 311056 (TNO6). C.R. Franks, G. Nys,
E. Materman, R. Canetta, L. Lenaz and S.K. Carter.
Bristol Myers International Corporation, Pharmaceutical Research &
Development Division, 185 Chaussee de la Hulpe, B-1170 BRUSSELS,
Belgium.

Representing: Drs. ADENIS, Lille, ARNOLD, Freiburg, BLACKLEDGE,
Birmingham, CALABRESI, Latina, CALMAN, Glasgow, DE LENA, Bari,
MARANGOLO, Ravenna, METZ, Vandoeuvre-les-Nancy, MOURIDSEN,
Copenhagen, NEWTON, London, ROSSO, Genova, SCHULTZ, Aarhus, SLEVIN,
London, TIMOTHY, London, VILLANI, Rome, WAGENER, Nijmegen.

A new platinum analogue TNO6 (1,1-diamino-methylcyclohexane-
sulphate platinum II, NSC 311056) is currently under study on a
multicenter basis. Two protocols are activated both using an intermittent dose schedule. The first compares cisplatinum with TNO6 in
tumours known to be responsive to platinum, such as ovary, cervix,
bladder and head and neck tumours. Patients are randomised to receive either cisplatinum or TNO6; on progression of disease, cis-
platinum treated patients receive TNO6, and TNO6 treated patients
cisplatinum. This protocol is designed to: 1) define the activity
of TNO6 in tumours known to be responsive to cisplatinum 2) define
whether cross resistance occurs between cisplatinum and TNO6
3) define and compare the toxicity of cisplatinum with that of TNO6.

The second protocol is a broad phase II protocol and accrues
patients with a wide variety of tumour types, including tumours
which have demonstrated some response to platinum, such as melanomas
and small cell lung tumours. The objectives of this protocol are to:
1) define the activity of TNO6 in tumours not known to be overtly
responsive to cisplatinum 2) define further the toxicity of TNO6.

One hundred and fifty seven patients have now been accrued to the
studies, 50 to the randomised trial and 107 to the broad phase II
trial. Since it is too early to evaluate the data from the randomised
trial, only data from the broad phase II trial are presented. The
preliminary analysis does not allow firm conclusions with reference
to antitumour activity. However it is interesting to note the wide
spectrum of biological activity. The predicted myelosuppression did
not occur at the dose level used, which suggests that the starting
dose may be increased. However, since there is an increasing trend
in BUN and proteinuria, the question relating to dose escalation
is still under debate. A further analysis on 60 evaluable patients
will be carried out shortly.

IV-6 MOLECULAR ORBITAL STUDIES ON SOME CIS-PLATINUM AND
PALLADIUM AMINE ANTI-TUMOR COMPLEXES
Edward A. Boudreaux* and Byung K. Park. *Department of Chemistry,
University of New Orleans, New Orleans, Louisiana 70148, U.S.A.
and Department of Chemistry, Yeungnam University, Gyongsan 632,
KOREA.

A variety of complexes having the general formula cis-$[MA_2Cl_2]$,
where A=ammonia, primary or secondary methyl amine, saturated
straight chain, heterocyclic or alicyclic amine containing from
two to five carbons and M=Pt(II) and Pd(II), are currently being
investigated theoretically via a non-empirical, non-parameterized
molecular orbital method previously developed by the primary
author. The computational details may be found in Chem. Biol.
Interactions, 30 (1980) 189-201, and references cited therein.

The results obtained thus far include: $Pd(NH_3)_2Cl_2$, $Pt(NH_3)_2Cl_2$,
$Pt(en)Cl_2$, $Pt(PR)_2Cl_2$, $Pt(NH_2CH_3)_2$ and $Pt[NH(CH_2)_2]Cl_2$ for which
net atomic charges, interatomic populations and orbital characteristics of the highest occupied MO's (HOMO) are compared. While
several unanticipated electronic structural features have been
noted, a most significant correlation is that those complexes
whose HOMO's have a high percent chlorine character show the
greatest anti-tumor activity. This no doubt relates directly to
the ease of solvolysis in situ, a requirement necessary to render
the drug active.

These and other aspects of this investigation will be discussed
in terms of rationalizing whether or not the electronic structure
and chemical bonding per se play a pertinent role in dictating the
anti-tumor behavior of these complexes.

258

IV-7 STRUCTURE-ACTIVITY RELATIONSHIPS FOR INDUCTION OF BACTERIO-
PHAGE LAMBDA BY PLATINUM (II) AND PLATINUM (IV) COMPLEXES.
R.K. Elespuru, S.K. Daley and B. Das Sarma*, NCI-Frederick Cancer
Research Facility, Frederick, MD 21701 and *West Virginia State
College, Department of Chemistry, Institute, West Virginia 25112.

Several structure-activity studies with neutral coordination
compounds of platinum have been carried out utilizing animals with
transplanted tumors. While these experiments may offer a good
chance of finding metal complexes with therapeutic utility, they are
impractical on a routine basis. Moreover, consistent differences in
activity resulting from variations in structure have not been found.
A simpler assay was sought that could be used as a prescreen for
evaluation of structurally diverse platinum coordination complexes.
While small numbers of Pt compounds have been tested in several short
term assays (e.g. Salmonella mutagenesis and E. coli prophage induction), an extensive study with a substantial number of compounds
appears not to have been made.
    A colorimetric assay of lambda prophage induction was used to
compare the activity of approximately 60 Pt complexes (B. Das Sarma,
S.K. Daley and R.K. Elespuru, Chem.-Biol. Interact., in press). Induction of a lambda-lacZ fusion phage was monitored quantitatively
by the synthesis of β-galactosidase, product of the lacZ gene, five
hrs after addition of test substance. In general, assays were run
50 at a time (10 compounds at 5 doses). The inducing capacity of
the compounds tested varied over a 25-fold range, as measured by the
quantity of β-galactosidase induced. Optimum doses for induction
were generally in the range of 100 to 300 μg/ml.
    We have analyzed the data by noting trends in induced β-gal.
enzyme levels, as a result of variations in structure. Dose-
response curves for compounds grouped by structure will be shown.
Consistent changes in activity were seen as a result of several
structural variations. Activity declined with increasing chain
length of alkyl groups substituted on amines, while the addition of
hydroxyl to alkyl groups increased activity. Trans-hydroxy Pt (IV)
compounds were more active than their Pt (II) equivalents. Among
ethylenediamine Pt (IV) complexes, the order of activity was Cl > Br
for halogens in equatorial positions, but the reverse for halogens
in axial positions. Seven Pt complexes were shown to have greater
inducing activity than cisplatin, while others were less toxic.
These data may be useful in the determination of some of the structural requirements for effective DNA interaction of a diverse set of
platinum complexes. Results will be compared with in vivo data on
antitumor activity.

IV-8 SYNTHESIS AND BIOLOGICAL EFFECTS OF A NEW FLUORESCENT
PLATINUM COMPOUND. Barton L. Bergquist and James C.
Chang, Depts. of Biology and Chemistry, University of Northern
Iowa, Cedar Falls, Iowa 50614, U.S.A.

A new analog of cisplatin, having interesting physical and
biological properties, has been synthesized. The molecule is
highly fluorescent and can therefore be monitored by fluorescence
techniques.

The compound, bis(5-aminofluorescein) dichloroplatinum (II) (abbreviated CFP) was synthesized from
K₂[PtCl₄] and 5-aminofluorescein.

Replicate preparations, elemental analysis plus UV, visible,
and IR spectra confirm the existence of the desired
compound. The molecule consists of a central Pt attached to two
chlorines and two 5-aminofluorescein groups bonded through their
nitrogens. It is soluble in water, methanol, DMSO plus other
organic solvents.

The molecule has been demonstrated to undergo complexation
with nucleotides in vitro. Biological studies with the bacteria
S. typhimurium and protozoan Tetrahymena thermophila indicate a
relatively low toxicity as compared to cisplatin.

CFP serves well as a fluorescent cell label in vitro.
The compound readily labels cellular inclusions (e.g. vacuoles)
in living cells and the membranes of dead (fixed) cells. It
also exhibits shifts in visible, UV and fluorescent spectra
relative to pH.

CFP has also shown potential as a radiosensitizer. Work
on isomeric differences is continuing.

259

IV-9 NEW ANALOGS OF 4-CARBOXYPHTHALATO(1,2-DIAMINOCYCLOHEXANE)-
PLATINUM(DACH-PT). Peter J. Andrulis, Jr.*, Paul Schwartz*
and Glen R. Gale. *Andrulis Research Corporation, 7315 Wisconsin
Avenue, Suite 650N, Bethesda, Maryland 20814, U.S.A. and USVA
Medical Center, Charleston, South Carolina 29403, U.S.A.

In studying structure-activity relationships of platinum
compounds, it was found that complexes having the chelating ligand
1,2-diaminocyclohexane were the most active in the L1210 murine
leukemia screen. In addition, complexes with this ligand were active
in cisplatin-resistant L1210 and P388. In clinical trials, such a
complex with the 4-carboxyphthalate ligand has exhibited substantially
reduced renal toxicity and quantitatively less nausea and vomiting
than cisplatin. Positive responses were observed in patients with
cisplatin-resistant tumors, including gastric cancer and lung
adenocarcinoma.

We have now prepared and screened new analogs of this complex and
have related aromatic substitution effects to antitumor activity. In
addition, novel complexes with unusual dimeric structures have been
synthesized and found to be active in several screening systems.

IV-10 IN VITRO PHASE II EVALUATION OF CISPLATIN AND THREE
ANALOGS AGAINST VARIOUS HUMAN CARCINOMAS.
A.H. Rossof, P.A. Johnson, B.D. Kimmell, G.D. Wilbanks, E.L. Yordan, Jr.,
J.E. Graham, C.F. Kittle, S.G. Economou. Rush-Presbyterian-St. Luke's
Medical Center, 1753 West Congress Parkway, Chicago, IL 60612, U.S.A.

Using the Hamburger-Salmon human tumor stem cell assay, the respective activities of cisplatin and 3 new platinum coordination compounds, cis-
diisopropylamine transhydroxydichloroplatinum IV (JM9; NSC 256927), 2-
ethylmalonato-cisdiammine platinum II (JM10; NSC 241240), and diaminocyclohexane platinum II (JM74; NSC 224964) were evaluated and compared.
Drugs were tested at the following concentrations: cisplatin, 0.2 mcg/ml;
JM9, 0.6 mcg/ml; JM10, 3.6 mcg/ml; and JM74, 3.2 mcg/ml. This represents
one-tenth the peak plasma concentration of cisplatin and equitoxic concentrations of the 3 analogs using published animal toxicity data. Single cell
suspensions of 500,000 tumor cells were incubated with the above concentrations of drug for 1 hour at 37°C, washed free of drug, and then plated in
triplicate in 0.3% agar in enriched CMRL 1066 on previously prepared semi-
solid underlayers consisting of 0.5% agar in enriched McCoy's 5A medium.
After incubation for 14 days at 37°C in a 7% CO_2 atmosphere and 100%
humidity, colonies consisting of 30 or more cells were counted and the mean
colony counts on the drug-treated and control plates were compared. Only
experiments in which control plate mean colony counts were $\geq$ 30 are
considered for this report. Percentage inhibition by an analog $\pm$ 20% (an
arbitrary figure) compared to the parent compound cisplatin was seen in the
following tumor types: Ovary, 5 of 8 experiments; endometrium, 1 of 1;
bladder, 1 of 2; kidney, 0 of 1; lung, 2 of 4; and colon, 1 of 3. Analog
inhibition $\pm$ 30% compared to cisplatin was seen in the following experiments:
Ovary, 4 of 8; endometrium, 1 of 1; bladder, 0 of 2; lung 1 of 4; and colon 0 of
3. No single analog was consistantly more active although in ovarian
carcinoma JM9 was better in 3 of 9 and worse in 1 of 9 experiments while
JM10 was better in 3 of 7 experiments. There seem to be sufficient numbers
of experiments in which these 3 cisplatin analogs demonstrate deviations $\pm$
20% and $\pm$ 30% inhibition compared with cisplatin that we conclude that each
compound should be evaluated separately and thoroughly for activity in
human cancer.

IV-11 BIOPHYSICAL AND BIOCHEMICAL STUDIES ON A NEW SPIN-LABELED Pt (II) COMPLEX IN MAMMALIAN CELLS. H. Gregg Claycamp, Abraham Mathew, Robert Morgan, Edward I. Shaw and John D. Zimbrick, University of Kansas, Radiation Biophysics, Nuclear Reactor Center, Lawrence, Kansas 66045, U.S.A.

We have synthesized several new spin-labeled cis-Pt analogs for use as intracellular probes of cis-Pt interactions, and for investigation as potential dose-modifying agents for combined radiation-drug cancer therapy. Electron Paramagnetic Resonance (EPR) studies on one of these Complexes, cis-Pt (2,2,6,6-tetramethyl-4-amino-piperidine-N-oxyl)$_2$dichloride (PDN-1) shows that it converts rapidly from cis to trans configuration in pure DMSO ($T_{1/2} \approx 3$ minutes) but is relatively stable in pure dimethylformamide (DMF). If the complex (1 X 10^{-4}M) is added to Hams F-12 cell culture medium and incubated at 37°C, the conversion of cis to trans configuration occurs in a temperature and time dependent manner. The uptake and removal of cis-PDN-1 in CHO fibroblasts was studied by use of EPR techniques wherein the signal from extracellular drug was effectively removed from the spectrum by the broadening agent potassium trioxalatochromate. Intracellular drug could be detected as early as 4 minutes after its addition to cell suspensions. The effective removal constant for the spin-labeled complex from CHO cells is approximately 0.3/hr. This constant is composed of two components: the actual removal of the drug and the reduction of the nitroxyl radicals by intracellular sulphydryls. The toxicity of PDN-1 and its ability to act as a radiation dose-modifying agent was studied in hypoxic and euoxic CHO cells. A drug dose (concentration X time) of 0.24 millimole-hours results in 50% survival. (Supported by Grant #CA 28339 from NIH/NCI, DHHS).

IV-12 NEW PLATINUM COMPLEXES AS RADIOSENSITIZERS Kirsten A. Skov⁑, Nicholas P. Farrell+, Tania Gomes de Carneiro+, Frederick W.B. Einstein++ and Terry Jones++.

⁑Medical Biophysics Unit, B.C. Cancer Research Centre, 601 West 10th Avenue, Vancouver, B.C. V5Z 1L3, Canada, +Departamento de Quimica - ICEx, Universidade Federal de Minas Gerais, Cidade Universitaria, 30.000 Belo Horizonte, Brazil, and ++Department of Chemistry, Simon Fraser University, Burnaby, B.C. V5A 1S6, Canada.

Control of some tumors by radiotherapy may fail due to the presence of hypoxic cells which are relatively radioresistant. Certain nitroimidazoles, such as misonidazole and metronidazole, have potential as adjuncts to treatment by ionizing radiation in that they radiosensitize the hypoxic cells. We are investigating the possibility that the attachment of such compounds to a DNA-binding metal such as platinum will result in a drug with improved properties. The radiosensitizing molecule would be located near the DNA, which is the target of radiosensitization. In addition, the toxic properties which limit the use of the nitroimidazoles might be affected in a favourable way. The fact that many platinum complexes are known to interact with radiation damage is also an advantage.

Using mammalian cells, several series of such complexes are being investigated for their toxicity and radiosensitizing abilities. Both cell inactivation and DNA damage are being studied. The cis-[PtCl$_2$ (misonidazole)$_2$] complex is a better sensitizer than the trans isomer; both complexes are far less toxic than cis-[Pt Cl$_2$ (NH$_3$)$_2$]. Complexes with other ligands as well as other metals (palladium, ruthenium) are being investigated. The E_1 values of misonidazole and metronidazole are altered by 0.14 and 0.22 respectively upon platination. Nitroimidazoles are more labile than amines, and the decomposition products involving loss of non-Cl ligand are being investigated.

Supported by the B.C. Cancer Foundation and the Conselho Nacional de Desenvolvimento Cientifico e Technologico.

IV-13 PLATINUM-METAL COMPLEXES AS DUAL FUNCTION AGENTS IN CHEMOTHERAPY. Nicholas P. Farrell*, Depto de Quimica, Univ. Federal de Minas Gerais, Belo Horizonte, Brazil, and James Williamson, National Institute for Medical Research, Mill Hill, London NW7, England.

Accepting that the primary mode of attack of platinum-metal complexes in their antineoplastic activity is in DNA template inactivation, a pertinent question is how to increase the selectivity toward the designated target molecule. In this context, a dual-function nature can be ascribed to cis-PtCl$_2$(NH$_3$)$_2$ whereby the amine moiety reacts initially with DNA by electrostatic interaction with phosphate groups and the PtCl$_2$ unit (or some hydrolysed version thereof) subsequently forms inactivating Pt-base linkages. It is therefore of some considerable interest to study metal complexes of DNA-binding ligands (but not amines per se) and evidence for the utility of this approach has been accumulated in in vivo studies in both trypanosomiasis and cancer. The known activity of cis-PtCl$_2$ (NH$_3$)$_2$ vs. Trypanosoma rhodesiense allows this comparison and, apart from the inherent interest, confirms the advantage of trypanosomiasis as a cancer "model". Initially, complexes of Berenil were studied and later these were extended to Ethidium and Samorin, all known trypanocides. Representative results are:

	LD$_{50}$ (mg/kg)	CD$_{50}$ (mg/kg)	LD$_{50}$/ CD$_{50}$	Maximal % T/C (mastocytoma P815)
PtCl$_2$ (dac)	28	-	-	128, 179
Berenil	140	1.90	74	87
PtCl$_2$-Berenil	221	1.60	138	
Rh$_2$(acetate)$_4$Berenil$_2$	118	0.97	122	103
Ethidium Bromide	38	3.8	10	109
(Ethidium)$_2$ PtCl$_4$	125	2.3	54	104, 105, 156
Samorin	44	0.42	105	110
(Samorin) PtCl$_4$	38	0.48	288	114

Structure-activity relationships on these and a number of other species amplifying this picture will be presented.

IV-14 PREPARATION OF A NEW ANTITUMOR OXALATO(1R,2R-CYCLOHEXANE-DIAMINE PLATINUM(II) COMPLEX. Yoshinori Kidani, Masahide Noji, Kenji Inagaki*, Tazuko Tashiro** and Motoichi Miyazaki***. *Faculty of Pharmaceutical Sciences, Nagoya City University,Tanabe-dori, Mizuho-ku, Nagoya 467 Japan, **Cancer Chemotherapy Center, Kamiikebukuro, Toshima-ku, Tokyo 170 Japan, ***Faculty of Pharmaceutical Sciences, Kanazawa University, Takaramachi,Kanazawa 920 Japan.

1,2-Cyclohexanediamine(=dach) has been developed as one of the most antitumor active carrier ligands and the leaving groups of 1R, 2R-dach Pt(II) complex have been varied to prepare highly antitumor active and least toxic Pt complexes. The authors prepared antitumor active Pt(oxalato)(1R,2R-dach) (ℓ-OHP) with the least toxicity. ℓ-OHP is soluble in water, 7.9 mg/ml, and very stable more than a week in water, determined by means of HPLC, using TSK G1000PW column. The stability, a half life in 0.9% NaCl solution was found to be 11.2 hr and the acute toxicity for mice was found to be about 15-20 mg/kg. Antitumor activity of ℓ-OHP showed that, at a dose of 6.25 mg/kg, T/C was 380% and 5 mice out of 6 survived, tested according to the NCI Pt Analog Study Protocol, using L1210 bearing CDF$_1$ mouse, by ip-ip administration on days 1, 5 & 9. In order to develop this complex to clinical trials, we studied the extensive basic and preclinical examination. At a dose of 12.5 mg/kg, 3 mice survived, being administered on days 5, 9 & 13 by ip-ip. On ip-iv administration, optimum dose was 6.25 mg/kg and T/C was more than 200%, in both systems of administrating on days 1, 5 & 9 and 5, 9 & 13. It was also effective against Lewis lung carcinoma, B 16 melanoma, Colons 26 and 38, and MX-1. ℓ-OHP did not show any cross-resistance to the DDP-resistant L1210 leukemia. At the dose of 3.12 and 6.25 mg/kg, all of 6 mice of one group survived without showing any cross-resistance against DDP-resistant L1210 leukemia. It was rather much efficacious against DDP-resistant L1210 leukemia. Combination therapy of ℓ-OHP with the other antitumor agents was also performed and they showed to be very effective. As to the most severe toxicity of Pt complexes, ℓ-OHP did not show any nephrotoxicity. The BUN value in serum was found to be 14 mg/dl, control being 17 mg/dl, the creatinine value was 0.6 mg/dl, control being 0.6 mg/dl, and any kidney toxicity using Wistar rats had not been observed. The distribution of ℓ-OHP, when 2.0 mg Pt/kg were injected by iv to rabbits, after 24 hr examination, showed that 3.3 ppm in kidney, that of DDP being 12.4 ppm and 0.7 ppm in liver, that of DDP being 4.3 ppm were observed. These findings suggested us to proceed further advanced studies aiming clinical use. The authors recommend ℓ-OHP as one of the most promising cancer chemotherapeutic agents to be exploited.

262

IV-15 ONE APPROACH TO TARGETED PLATINUM DRUG ACTIVITY --- DESIGN
OF A SYNTHETIC ANTIESTROGEN-Pt(II) COMPLEX
Robert C. Richmond. Norris Cotton Cancer Center,
Dartmouth-Hitchcock Medical Center, Hanover, NH 03755,U.S.A.
Thomas J. Curphey. Dartmouth Medical School, Hanover, NH 03755,U.S.A.
John A. Katzenellenbogen. School of Chemical Sciences, University
of Illinois at Urbana-Champaign, Urbana, IL 61801,U.S.A.

Continuing advancement in cancer therapy with cis-dichlorodiammine Pt(II) (cis-DDP) seems to suffer a plight common to established antitumor drugs. This is, improved tumor response is slow in
greatly advancing from presently realized levels. Although continued improvement in cancer cure is sure to follow from continued research on current treatment protocols, much of this improvement will
be due to optimizing existing variables within these protocols, i.e.,
a situation at some point of diminishing returns. It is likely that
dramatic improvement in cancer therapy will require the use of new
classes of antitumor agents. Targeted drugs are one such class.
We have added Pt(II) to a malonic acid-containing ligand synthesized as a methylethylstilbene analog, i.e., (E)-2-carboxy-4,5-
diphenyl-4-heptenoic acid. The Pt(II) complex formed is identical
to JM-10, i.e., cis-(2-ethylmalonato)(diammine) Pt(II), but with the
ethyl group replaced by linkage to the methyl group of methylethylstilbene. The final complex (abbr. TDP) was synthesized in expectation of achieving activity similar to the non-steroidal antiestrogen
and antitumor drug, tamoxifen.
Tamoxifen binds to the cytoplasmic estrogen receptor. This complex translocates to the nucleus of the cell, removing it from cycle.
Metastatic breast carcinoma often responds to tamoxifen drug treatment. Tamoxifen does not kill cells per se, and a tamoxifen resistance eventually develops. Addition of a killing factor to this
targeted tamoxifen system is therefore desirable. Substitution of
tamoxifen with TDP was planned ideally to: 1) maintain tamoxifen
antiestrogen activity; 2) incorporate relatively specific antitumor
toxicity; 3) provide relatively specific tumor cell Pt(II)-induced
radiation sensitization and/or potentiation.
Exposure of the estrogen receptor positive, human breast tumor
cell line MCF-7 to 4 micromolar TDP in tissue culture causes 90%
inactivation in 31 hr by CFU assay. In comparison, exposure of MCF-7
to 4 micromolar JM-10 causes 90% inactivation in 40 hr. This toxic
activity of TDP is not likely related to specific delivery via the
estrogen receptor system, however, as TDP does not bind to rat
uterine estrogen receptor in a competetive binding assay. Redesign
of the antiestrogen ligand in TDP is needed for targeted action.

IV-16 ANTITUMOR ACTIVITY OF SULFADIAZINE COMPLEXES
OF PLATINUM(II). Alessandro Pasini* and
Franco Zunino** *Dipartimento di Chimica Inorganica e
Metallorganica, the University,via Venezian 21,
20133-Milano, Italy, and ** Oncologia Sperimentale B,
Istituto Nazionale per lo Studio e la Cura dei Tumori,
via Venezian 1, 20133-Milano, Italy.

In the attempt to find cis-platin analogues with
lower toxicity, we are studying complexes of platinum
with low molecular weight carriers. Platinum complexes
of 2-sulfanilamidopyrimidine (sulfadiazine) of formula
cis-$[PtCl_2(sdH)_2]$ and cis-K$[PtCl_2sd]$ (sdH=sulfa-
diazine; sd=its anion) have been synthesized and
characterized. They are cytotoxic in vitro to HeLa
cells, and cis-K$[PtCl_2sd]$ shows significant activity
(% T/C > 170) against P388 leukemia in mice. Both
compounds showed lower toxicity, but also lower
potency than cis-platin when administered i.p.
The difficulty of i.v. administration of high doses,
however, precluded further in vivo tests.
Some discrepancies between cytotoxicity and
farmacological properties of these compounds suggest
that the changes in the chemical structure of the
carrier molecule influence both transport characteristics
and drug uptake by the target cells.

IV-17 SYNTHESIS AND CHARACTERIZATION OF TNO-PLATINUM CHEMOTHERA-
PEUTIC AGENTS. Harry A. Meinema, Frans Verbeek, Jan W.
Marsman and Eric J. Bulten. Institute of Applied Chemistry TNO,
Croesestraat 79, P.O. Box 5009, 3502 JA Utrecht, The Netherlands.

Investigations into platinum antitumor agents of the types L_2PtX_2
and $L_2PtX_2Y_2$ have demonstrated that ligands of the type $L_2=2,2$-di-
substituted-1,3-propanediamines are of particular advantage in that
they may give rise to complexes having
- exclusively the active cis-structure
- high antitumor activity
- little (if any) renal toxicity
- little (if any) cross-resistance.
The synthesis of a series of novel platinum (II) and -(IV) antitumor agents of the types (A) and (B) will be presented.

n = 0,1; R',R" = Alkyl; R'-R" = $(CH_2)_n$, n = 3,4,5
X = halogen, NO_3; X_2 = SO_4^{2-}, Oxalate, (substituted)malonate,
a.o. dicarboxylates
Y = halogen, OH^-

One specific representative of such a platinum complex cis-1,1-
bis(aminomethyl)cyclohexane platinum (II) sulphate - (TNO-6) is
currently undergoing Phase (I) and Phase (II) clinical trials.

TNO-6

Investigations into the analysis, characterization, detection and
stability of TNO-6 both in the solid state and in aqueous solution
will be presented.

SECTION V

NON-PLATINUM METAL COMPLEXES AS ANTITUMOR AGENTS

Chaired by B. Rosenberg

Structure Activity Relationship of Antitumor Palladium Complexes
D.S. Gill

INTRODUCTION

The discovery of cisplatin[1] as an antineoplastic agent has sparked a tremendous interest in the development of new platinum complexes and complexes of other metals as anticancer drugs. Recently, a number of platinum(II) complexes have been shown to be highly active as broad-spectrum antitumor agents. However, there are several drawbacks associated with the use of platinum complexes to treat tumors. Generally, the platinum complexes are highly nephrotoxic, sparingly soluble in water and are relatively inactive against gastro-intestinal tumors.[2] It was, therefore, of interest to explore the possibility of developing antitumor palladium complexes as the coordination chemistry of palladium(II) and platinum(II) is usually similar. In all instances reported in the literature the palladium complexes tested had either little or marginal antitumor activity. The low activity of the palladium complexes has been attributed to the rapid formation of aquated complexes in vivo[3]. By suitable choice of the ligands, a variety of palladium complexes have been synthesized whose antitumor activities are comparable to, and in some instances greater than, the platinum complexes currently in widespread use in cancer chemotherapy.

In order to design and develop potent anticancer drugs involving different metal complexes, it is important to have some understanding of the relationship between structural parameters and antitumor activity. Based upon the antitumor properties of a number of platinum and palladium complexes, the following empirical rules were formulated relating the antitumor activity of metal complexes to physiochemical properties.

1. Complexes that have antibacterial activity do not necessarily have antitumor activity.
2. Complexes should contain a pair of inert ligands (e.g., amines).
3. Complexes should contain a pair of leaving groups of intermediate lability.
4. Complexes should be neutral.
5. Other heavy metals (e.g., palladium) give complexes inactive or less active than the platinum analog.

In this paper, exceptions to the last three rules will be presented and discussed. Also, an attempt will be made to define structure-activity relationship of antitumor palladium complexes.

EXPERIMENTAL SECTION

Syntheses.

Preparation of Dichloro(cis-1,2-diaminocyclohexane)palladium.

1,2-Diaminocyclohexane (dach) as an isomeric mixture of trans- and cis-dach, respectively, was separated into trans-dach dihydrochloride, and cis-dach sulphate by the method of Saito et al.[4]

To a solution containing 5.0 g (0.017 mole) of sodium tetrachloropalladate(II) in 200 ml of water containing sodium hydroxide was added cis-dach sulphate (0.017 mole). The mixture was stirred at room temperature. Within 10 minutes, a yellow precipitate was obtained. The mixture was stirred for another 12 hours. The yellow precipitate was collected by filtration, washed with 0.01 N HCl, cold water, hot water, alcohol and ether to give a quantitative yield of the product. This was further purified by treatment with silver nitrate in water and precipitation of the dichloro complex with 1N HCl. Elemental analysis gave: H, 4.84; C, 24.63; N, 9.60; Cl, 24.67; Pd, 36.43. Calculated for $H_{14}C_6N_2Cl_2Pd$: H, 4.81; C, 24.70; N, 9.61; Cl, 24.40; Pd, 36.51.

Other Pd(bidentate amine)Cl$_2$ complexes such as dichloro(trans-1,2-diaminocyclohexane)palladium, dichloro

(1,2-diaminoethane)palladium, dichloro(1,2-diaminopropane)
palladium and dichloro(1,3-diaminopropane)palladium were
prepared in a similar manner from the respective amine salt and
sodium tetrachloropalladate(II).

Preparation of Dinitrato(trans-1,2-dimanocyclohexane)palladium.

A mixture of Pd(trans-dach)Cl_2 (5.828 g, 0.02 mole and
silver nitrate (6.664 g, 0.0196 mole) in 100 ml of water,
acidified with HNO_3, was stirred for 24 hours in a low actinic
glass flask. Silver chloride was removed by filtration and
the pale yellow solution was concentrated on a flash evaporator
and allowed to crystallize. It was recrystallized from dilute
nitric acid/saturated sodium nitrate solution. Elemental
analysis gave: H, 4.13; C, 20.87; N, 16.13; Pd, 30.67.
Calculated for $H_{14}C_6N_4O_6Pd$: H, 4.06; C, 20.90; N, 16.26; Pd,
30.89.

The dinitratopalladium complexes of other amines reported
in this paper were prepared by similar methods.

Preparation of [Hydroxo-Bridged Oligomeric (1,2-diaminocyclo-
hexane)palladium] Nitrate.

Pd(dach)$(NO_3)_2$ (5.0 g) was dissolved in 70 ml water.
The pH of the solution was raised to 6.45 by dropwise addition
of 1.5 N NaOH. The flask was stoppered and allowed to stand at
room temperature for 30 minutes. The volume of the solution
was reduced to 30 ml on a flash evaporator at 30°C and the
solution was allowed to stand at 5°C for a week. During this
time, the oligome   crystallized out of the solution as a yellow
colored complex. The pH of the filtrate was raised to 6.45
again and the above procedure was repeated to get more of the
complex. The overall yield of the complex was 60%. The complex
analyzed as: H, 5.08; C, 23.95; O, 21.42; N, 13.98; Pd,
35.35. Calculated for $[H_{15}C_6N_3O_4Pd]_n$: H, 5.01; C, 24.05;
O, 21.38; N, 14.03; Pd, 35.54.

Preparation of Tartronato(1,2-diaminocyclohexane)palladium.

To a solution containing 1.0332 g (0.003 mole) of
dinitrato(dach)palladium was added tartronic acid (1.52 g,
0.0096 mole), neutralized with 2N NaOH. A yellow crystalline
precipitate was obtained. This was filtered, washed with
ethanol and acetone, then dried at room temperature and reduced
pressure. The yield was 90%. The complex analyzed as H, 4.79;
C, 31.95; N, 8.23; O, 23.54, Pd, 31.28. Calculated for
[$C_9H_{16}N_2O_5Pd$: H, 4.73; C, 31.91, N, 8.27; O, 23.64; Pd, 31.44.

The dicarboxylatepalladium complexes of other bidentate
amines were prepared similarly.

Measurement of Antitumor Activity of Palladium Complexes.

Animal tests for evaluating antitumor activities of
palladium complexes were performed on ICR random-bred, white,
female, 4-5 week old (18-20 g) mice. Ascites sarcoma-180J
cells (4 x 10^6) were injected intraperitoneally into animals
on day 1 and the compounds (6 animals/dose level) were injected
as solutions or slurries on day 1. Evaluations were made on
2x the average day of death of the negative control. 7 mg/kg
of cisplatin is injected as a positive control of the testing
situation. The % Increase Life Span (ILS) is computed as
follows: The average day of death of test animals minus the
average day of death of the negative control , divided by the
average day of death of control x 100. Cisplatin gave a
% ILS of 60-75.

RESULTS AND DISCUSSION

Syntheses

There are few published details on the syntheses of
dichloropalladium complexes of bidentate amines. The syntheses
of dichloro(ethanylenediamine)palladium(II) and dichloro
(2.2'-bipyridine)palladium complexes as described in the
literature[5] are tedious, and give a mixture of products whose
separation is cumbersome. The syntheses described herein are
simple and give pure products in improved yields. The
dinitrato and dicarboxylato complexes were synthesized by slight
modifications of the literature methods for analogous platinum

271

complexes. The similarities between the absorption and
vibrational spectra of the hydroxo-bridged oligomeric complex
and the cyclo-tris(μ-hydroxo)tris(1,2-diaminocyclohexane
platinum] Nitrate indicate that the palladium complex is also
a trimer. The crystal structure of the complex is under
investigation. The purity of the complexes was checked by
elemental analysis and by spectroscopic methods. Of the various
techniques, ^{13}C NMR has proved to be quite useful since it gives
widely separated resonances. Figure 1, gives the ^{13}C chemical
shifts for dinitrato(1,2-diaminocyclohexane)palladium
complexes.

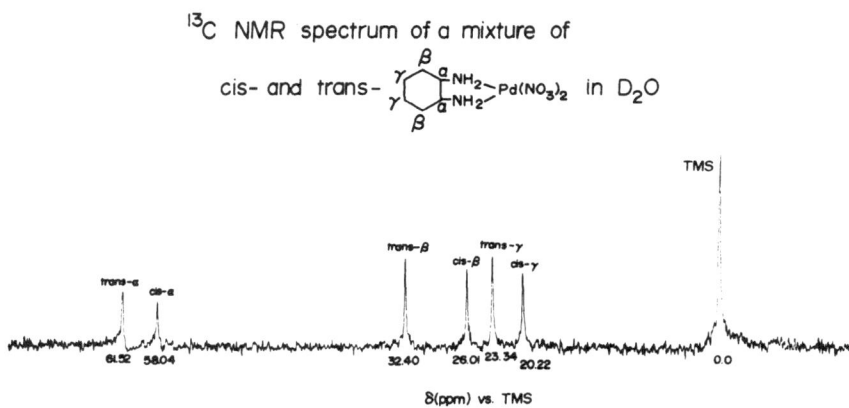

Figure 1. ^{13}C NMR of a mixture of <u>cis</u>- and <u>trans</u>-dinitrato
(1,2-diaminocyclohexane)palladium.

Antitumor Activity and Kinetic Considerations.

The coordination chemistries of platinum and palladium
are similar in terms of their oxidation state, coordination
number, geometry associated with each oxidation state and
affinity for similar ligands. The palladium(II) complexes,
however, are somewhat less stable in both the thermodynamic
and the kinetic sense and the chemistry of palladium(IV) is
relatively limited. The marginal activity or the

lack of antitumor activities of Pd(II) complexes tested
heretofore, was explained on the basis of fast reactivity
of the leaving groups. The order of reactivities for
isoelectronic complexes of nickel, palladium, gold, and
platinum is given below[3d]:

Ni (II)	Pd (II)	Au(III)	Pt (II)
5×10^6	10^5	10^4	1

Thus, in order to develop active antitumor palladium
complexes, it is imperative to moderate the lability of the
leaving groups. Three different approaches were adopted in
the design and development of new active antitumor palladium
complexes. The first approach was realized from the studies
with dinitrato(trans-1,2-diaminocyclohexane)platinum(II)
complex.[6] During the investigation of the hydrolytic behavior
of the complex by ^{195}Pt NMR at different pH's, the presence of
oligomeric species was detected. (Figure 2). These complexes

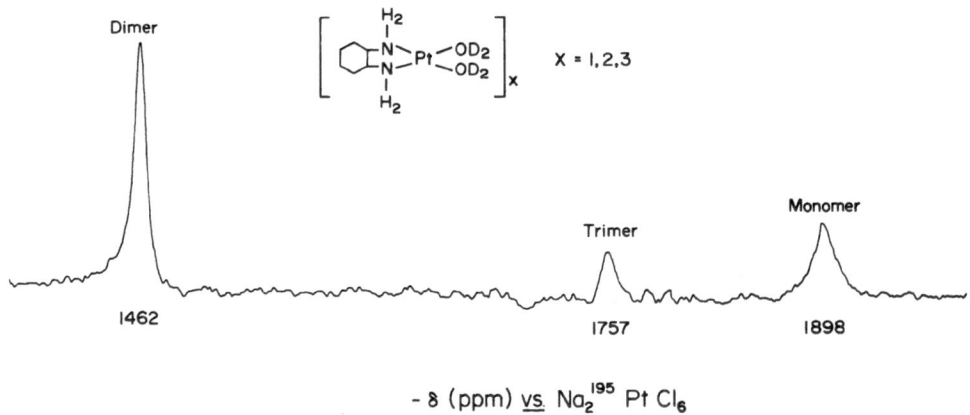

$$- \delta \text{ (ppm) } \underline{vs} \text{ Na}_2{}^{195}\text{Pt Cl}_6$$

Figure 2. The ^{195}Pt Spectrum Pt (trans-dach) (NO3)2 and
Oligomeric Complexes.

were then obtained on a preparative scale and were tested for
their antitumor activity. The structures and pH equilibria of
their formation is given in Scheme 1. It was observed that the
dimer and the trimer were more active and less toxic than the

scheme I

momomer. An interesting feature of these complexes was their reactions with physiological concentrations of sodium chloride. The monomer gave the corresponding dichloro complex instantaneously, but the dimer and the trimer required about two weeks for complete conversion to the dichloro complex. The hydroxo-bridged complexes have also been shown to be substitutionally inert by Lim and Martin.[7] The reactivity of the hydroxo-bridged oligomer of palladium towards sodium chloride was examined and it was qualitatively similar to its platinum analog. The complex was, therefore, tested for anticancer activity.

The second approach was based on the in vivo modification of the labile groups to relatively inert ligands. The determination of the acidity constant of ionization of Pd (trans-dach)(H_2O)$_2^{2+}$ clearly indicated the very fast oligomerization of the monohydroxo species.[9] A similar dimerization process was observed for diaquo(ethylenediamine palladium.[7] The dimerization was accelerated at pH-values close to physiological pH. Thus formation of the hydroxo-bridged complexes from the dinitratopalladium complexes is expected to occur in vivo.

The third approach towards moderating the reactivity of the

leaving groups comprised the use of chelate groups such as dicarboxylates.

The antitumor activities of these three classes of compounds are given in Table 1. As illustrated all three types of complexes

Table 1.   Antitumor Effects of 1,2-Diaminocyclohexanepalladium Complexes Against Sarcoma 180-J.

Complex	Dose (mg/kg)	Maximum % ILS
$[Pd(dach)(OH)]_n(NO_3)_n$	80	75
$Pd(dach)(NO_3)_2$	80	65
$Pd(dach)malonate$	150	76

show antitumor activity comparable to cisplatin.

The dinitrato complexes of other bidentate amines also showed anticancer activity comparable to or greater than cisplatin (Table 2).

Table 2.   Antitumor Activities of Dinitratopalladium Complexes Against Sarcoma 180-J.

Complex	Dose (mg/kg)	Maximum % ILS
$Pd(NH_3)_2(NO_3)_2$	10-80	Inactive
$Pd(1,2\text{-diaminopropane})(NO_3)_2$	100-200	70
$Pd(1,3\text{-diaminopropane})(NO_3)_2$	60	81
$Pd(1,2\text{-diaminoethane})(NO_3)_2$	80	94
$Pd(\underline{trans}\text{-dach})(NO_3)_2$	60	81
$Pd(2,2'\text{-bipyridine})(NO_3)_2$	80	70

The fact that the oligomeric species are considered to be active and are formed in vivo from monomeric complexes is evident from the dose response data of dachPd complexes (Table 3).

Table 3.   Antitumor Activities of Palladium Complexes at Different Dosage Levels.

Complex	Dose (mg/kg)	Percent ILS
$Pd(dach)(NO_3)_2$	40	27
	60	35
	80	65

Complex	Dose (mg/kg)	Percent ILS
$[Pd(dach)(OH)]_n(NO_3)_n$	20	23
	30	53
	50	48
	80	75

The oligomer showed a wider dose response whereas the monomer was active only at higher doses.

Comparison of Activities of Trans-dach and Cis-dach Complexes.

It has been shown by Kidani and coworkers that for platinum, trans-dach complexes have higher antitumor activities than the cis-dach complexes.[8] Similar behavior was observed in the case of palladium complexes (Table 4). This may be explained on the basis of the instability of cis-dach complexes as compared with the trans-dach complexes.[9]

Table 4. Antitumor Effects of Cis-dach and Trans-dach Palladium Complexes.

Complex	Dose (mg/kg)	Maximum % ILS Trans-	Cis-
Pd(dach)(NO_3)_2	60	81	50
Pd(dach)oxalate	30	46	31
Pd(dach)cyclobutanedicarboxylate	100	55	35
Pd(dach)malonate	150	76	46

Antitumor Activities of Diamminepalladium Complexes

The maximum antitumor activities of diamminepalladium complexes are given in Table 5. It is clear from the Table that the complexes having monodentate leaving groups were inactive. This may be due to the rapid isomerization of cis- complexes to the inactive trans- complexes.[10] However, the diammine complexes having bidentate leaving groups were active because chelation prevents isomerization to the inactive trans- form.

Table 5. Antitumor Activities of Diamminepalladium Complexes.

Complex	Dose (mg/kg)	Maximum % ILS
Pd(NH_3)_2Cl_2	50	4
Pd(NH_3)_2(NO_3)_2	20	14
Pd(NH_3)_2 oxalate	50	37

Complex	Dose (mg/kg)	Maximum % ILS
$Pd(NH_3)_2$ glutarate	100	80
$Pd(NH_3)_2$ malonate	100	50

Comparison of Antitumor Activities of Palladium Complexes with their Platinum Analogs.

A comparison of antitumor activities of the two series of complexes is given in Table 6. It is evident from the antitumor data that there is no strict correlation between the activities of palladium complexes and their platinum analogs.

Table 6. Comparison of Antitumor Activities of Dinitratopalladium Complexes and their Platinum Analogs.

Complex	M = Pd	M = Pt
$M(1,2$-diaminoethane$)(NO_3)_2$	Active	Marginally Active
$M(1,2$-diaminopropane$)(NO_3)_2$	Active	Marginally Active
$M(trans$-dach$)(NO_3)_2$	Active	Active
$M[dach(OH)]_n(NO_3)_n$	Active	Active
$M(2,2'$-bipyridine$)(NO_3)_2$	Active	Inactive
$M(NH_3)_2(NO_3)_2$	Inactive	Marginally Active

Biological Activity of Palladium Complexes and their Relevance to the Treatment of Gastric Tumors.

Biologically, the formation of polynuclear complexes and their antitumor properties are interesting. The formation of these complexes is favored in the pH range close to the physiological pH. Cleare and Hoeschele have correlated the antitumor activity of platinum complexes to charge neutrality and ligands of moderate stability. The charged complexes or complexes having ligands with fast leaving rates were shown to be inactive and toxic.[3d] Later reports by Schwartz[11], and confirmed in our laboratory, have shown that dinitrato(dach) platinum, I, and the oligomers II and III were very active. The activity of I was attributed to the formation in vivo of oligomeric complexes.[6] The hydroxo-bridged complexes have been shown to be substitutionally inert and thus may not be easily converted to an ineffective and possibly toxic form by extracellular reactions. However, in intracellular reactions, the polynuclear complexes may undergo a slow equilibrium to the monomeric form. This may be promoted by the facile reaction with DNA bases. This may provide the basis for a slow conversion of the polynuclear complexes to a monomeric aquated form that is responsible for the activity in intracellular reactions.[6] The dinitratopalladium complexes are capable of forming hydroxo-bridged complexes relatively easily and a similar mechanism is proposed for the antitumor activities of monomeric as well as polymeric palladium complexes.

It is also hypothesized that the palladium complexes may have a particular relevance for the treatment of tumors of gastro-intestinal region where cisplatin fails. It is widely believed that cisplatin retains its integrity in the extracellular fluid where chloride concentration is high ($\sim$ 100 meq, but inside the cell ($[Cl^-]\sim4$ meq), it undergoes the following aquation reactions and it is the aquated products which react with DNA causing the anticancer effect. However, in the gastro-

$$Pt(NH_3)_2Cl_2 \; \underset{\longleftarrow}{\longrightarrow} \; \begin{array}{c} Pt(NH_3)_2Cl(H_2O) \\ Pt(NH_3)_2Cl(OH) \end{array} \; \underset{\longleftarrow}{\longrightarrow} \; \begin{array}{c} Pt(NH_3)_2(OH)_2 \\ Pt(NH_3)_2(OH_2)_2 \\ Pt(NN_3)_2OH(H_2O) \end{array} \; \rightleftharpoons \; oligomers$$

intestinal region the chloride concentration is quite close to the extracellular fluid. Therefore, it is unable to undergo aquation reactions which accounts for its inactivity against gastric cancers. On the other hand, the palladium complexes are capable of undergoing aquation reactions in this environment[9] and should be investigated for the treatment of gastro-intestinal tumors.

CONCLUSIONS

From these results of antitumor activities of a variety of palladium complexes against sarcoma-180J in swiss white female mice, the following conclusions may be drawn for the antitumor activities of palladium complexes: (1) The dinitrate complexes and the hydroxo-bridged oligomers of bidentate amines show anticancer activities comparable to or greater than cisplatin. (2) Complexes having monodentate amines and monodentate leaving groups are inactive. (3) Complexes having monodentate amines or bidentate amines as inert ligands and bidentate group as the leaving group are generally active. (4) In case of dachpalladium complexes, the trans-dach complexes are more effective than the cis-dach complexes. (5) There does not seem to be a strict correlation between the activities of palladium complexes and their platinum analogs. (6) The criteria of charge neutrality and moderate lability of leaving groups for anticancer activity are not strictly observed.

ACKNOWLEDGEMENT

The author would like to thank Professor Barnett Rosenberg for the encouragement, valuable discussions, and support of this work.

REFERENCES

1. B. Rosenberg, L. van Camp, J.E. Trosko, and V.H. Mansour, Nature (London), 222, 385 (1969).
2. "Cisplatin--Current Status and New Developments," A.W. Prestayko, S.T. Crooke, and S.K. Carter, Eds., Academic Press, New York, 1980.
3. (a) S. Kirschner, Y-K. Wei, D. Francis, and J.G. Bergman. J. Med. Chem., 9, 369 (1966). (b) R.D. Graham and D.R. Williams, J. Inorg. Nucl. Chem. 41, 1245 (1979). (c) T.A. Connors, M.J. Cleare, and K.R. Harap, Cancer Treat. Rep. 63, 1499 (1979). (d) M.J. Cleare and J.D. Hoeschele, Bioinorg. Chem. 2, 187 (1973).
4. R. Saito and Y. Kidani, Chem. Lett. 2, 123 (1976).
5. J. McCormick, E.N. Janyes, Jr., R.L. Kaplan; Inorg. Synth., 13, 216 (1972).
6. D.S. Gill and B. Rosenberg, J. Amer. Chem. Soc. 104, 4598 (1982).
7. M.C. Lim and R.B. Martin, J. Inorg. Nucl. Chem. 38, 1911 (1976).
8. Y. Kidani, K. Inagaki, and R. Saito, J. Clin. Hemat. and Onc., 197 (1976).
9. D.S. Gill, Unpublished results.
10. (a) R.A. Walton, Spectrochim. Acta 21, 1795 (1965). (b) Y.N. Kukushkin, G.N. Sedova, L.Y. Pyzhova, Russ. J. Inorg. Chem. 24, 1257 (1979). (c) L. Cattalini and M. Martelli, J. Amer. Chem. Soc. 91, 312 (1969). (d) P-C. Kong and F.D. Rochon, Can. J. Chem. 59, 3293 (1981).
11. P. Schwartz, S.J. Michen, G.R. Gale, L.M. Atkins, A.B. Smith and E.M. Walker, Jr., Cancer Treat. Rep. 61, 1519 (1977).

The Metallocene Dihalides — A Class of Organometallic Early Transition Metal Complexes as Antitumor Agents
P. Köpf-Maier and H. Köpf

1. INTRODUCTION

The metallocene dihalides $(C_5H_5)_2MX_2$ represent a group of organometallic compounds which are known as chemical compounds since about thirty years. They were firstly prepared by Wilkinson and Birmingham in 1954 (1), whereas their antitumor activity was detected only in 1979 (2-4).

2. CHEMICAL CHARACTERISTICS

From a chemical point of view, the metallocene dihalides $(C_5H_5)_2MX_2$ are characterized by the following features:

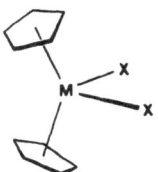

- The molecular geometry of the complexes is that of a distorted tetrahedron.
- As central metal atom M, they contain early transition metals, e.g., Ti, V, Nb, or Mo.
- The ligands X represent acido ligands, e.g., halide or pseudo-halide ligands, which are arranged in adjacent positions.
- The sites of the other two ligands are occupied by two cyclopentadienyl rings which are bonded to the central atom by carbon-to-metal bonds.

3. STRUCTURE-ACTIVITY RELATION

To gain information on the structure-activity relation, the influence of chemical modification on the antitumor properties of the metallocene dihalides was studied using the Ehrlich ascites tumor in mice. The investigations revealed the following main results (5,6):

There is a pronounced dependence of the tumor-inhibiting potency upon the central atom M involved. Whereas the metallocene dichlorides with M = Ti, V, Nb, and Mo exhibit strong tumor-inhibiting potencies, the cytostatic properties are markedly reduced in the case of the analogous complexes with M = Ta, W, Zr, or Hf (2-4,7,8).

Considering the dependence of the antitumor activity upon the acido ligands X within the titanocene system, equally strong tumor inhibition could be demonstrated for the halide ligands X = F, Cl, Br, I as well as for the pseudohalide ligands X = NCS or N_3 (9).

The third possibility of modification offered by the titanocene dichloride model system is to formally substitute hydrogen atoms of the cyclopentadienyl rings by other residues R. When monosubstituted complexes, symmetrically 1,1'-disubstituted complexes, or 1,1'-bridged complexes (e.g., R = CH_3 or $Si(CH_3)_3$; Z = CH_2 or $Si(CH_3)_2$)

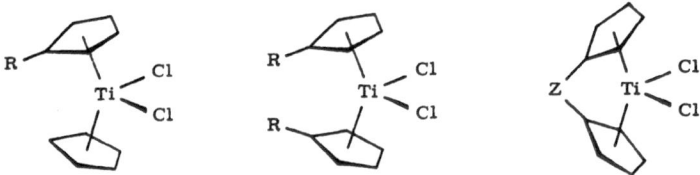

were tested against the Ehrlich ascites tumor, a reduction of tumor-inhibiting potency was the general finding (10). Because, however, there exist some contradictory results with substituted titanocene derivatives against other tumor systems (11), the effect of modification at the cyclopentadienyl ring ligands upon the cytostatic activity is not yet clear.

4. SPECTRUM OF BIOLOGICAL ACTIVITY

Up to now, several biological activities of the metallocene dichlorides have been discovered.

The compounds inhibit the growth of the intraperitoneally growing Ehrlich ascites tumor (2-4,7-9,12) as well as the growth of the solid, subcutaneously growing form of the same tumor (12). Moreover, the metallocene dichlorides are active against Lewis lung tumor (13) and, marginally, against the leukemias L 1210 and P 388 (12).

In vitro, the metallocene dihalides affect the growth of animal and human tumor cells, e.g., Ehrlich ascites tumor cells (14), HeLa cells, or KB cells (11). The representative most effective in vitro is $(C_5H_5)_2VCl_2$.

Against various DNA and RNA viruses in the extracellular phase, titanocene dichloride has been found to exhibit significant antiviral activity (15).

5. CELLULAR MODE OF ACTION

To elucidate the cellular mode of action of the metallocene dihalides, diverse cytobiological experiments were performed.

Incorporation studies using ^{3}H-labeled specific precursors of the DNA, RNA, or protein syntheses indicated the DNA synthesis to be that metabolic way which is most sensitive to treatment with metallocene dichlorides (M = Ti, V) (16,17).

Electron energy loss-spectroscopic studies demonstrated the accumulation of metal-containing species in those cellular areas which are rich in nucleic acids, mainly in the nuclear heterochromatin which is rich in DNA (18,19).

The cytokinetic studies revealed the appearance of a G_2 block as a common result after in vivo or in vitro application of metallocene dichlorides (Fig. 1) (20,21). During in vitro exposure, additionally, accumulations of cells at the G_1/S boundary occurred; following short exposure periods, these cells escaped the arrest at G_1/S and continued their transit through the cell cycle as synchronized populations (Fig. 2).

From the morphologic point of view, two main developments could be pursued by light and electron microscopy (22):
(i) Within 24 to 48 h after application of metallocene dichlorides, numerous giant cells were formed; most of them were mononucleated, some of them multinucleated; the giant cells mostly exhibited degenerative features in the cytoplasm, such as the appearance of large vacuoles or the accumulation of lipid

282

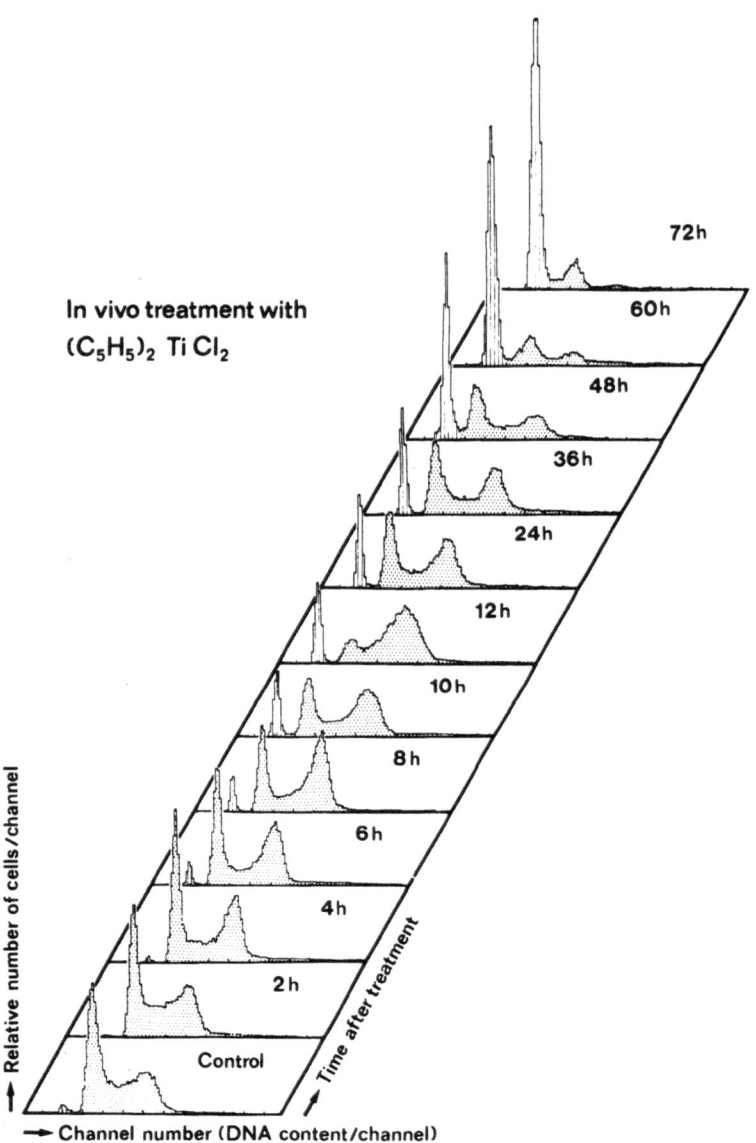

In vivo treatment with
$(C_5H_5)_2$ Ti Cl_2

72h
60h
48h
36h
24h
12h
10h
8h
6h
4h
2h
Control

Relative number of cells/channel

Time after treatment

Channel number (DNA content/channel)

FIGURE 1. Pulse-cytophotometric distribution curves of the DNA content of ascitic cells (▒▒▒ Ehrlich ascites tumor cells; ▥▥▥ immigrated macrophages, leukocytes, and lymphocytes) at various intervals after a single application of titanocene dichloride (80 mg/kg) in vivo.

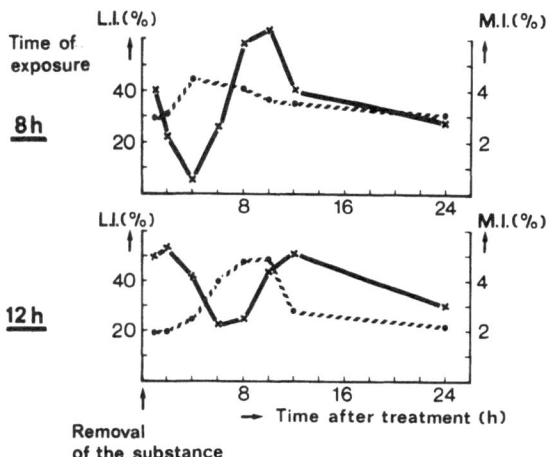

FIGURE 2. Mitosis index (M.I.) and ^{3}H-thymidine labeling index
(L.I.) of Ehrlich ascites tumor cells cultured in vitro, at the
end of increasing intervals (abscissa) of restitution following
an 8 h (above) or a 12 h (below) exposure to titanocene dichloride
(10^{-4} mol/l).

droplets. (ii) Within the same period, numerous cells became

necrotic; the first signs of this development consisted in nuclear

segmentation and chromatin condensation at 8 to 12 h after sub-

stance application. In vivo, the giant cells as well as the

necrotic ones were eliminated by phagocytosis performed by

macrophages, whereas in vitro the cells disintegrated and de-

composed.

In addition to these events, the morphogenesis of endogenous,

previously unexpressed viruses could be observed in the ultra-

structural picture of diverse tumor cells, e.g., of Ehrlich

ascites tumor cells or KB cells, after treatment with titanocene

FIGURES 3, 4, and 5. Parts of Ehrlich ascites tumor cells after
application of titanocene dichloride (80 mg/kg) in vivo.
Fig. 3: Numerous condensed, worm-shaped figures within a nucleo-
lus. Fig. 4: Accumulated condensed figures within a cytoplasmic
invagination; note the close proximity to the nucleoli (Nu).
Fig. 5: Numerous intracytoplasmic spherical particles (→)
representing type A viruses.

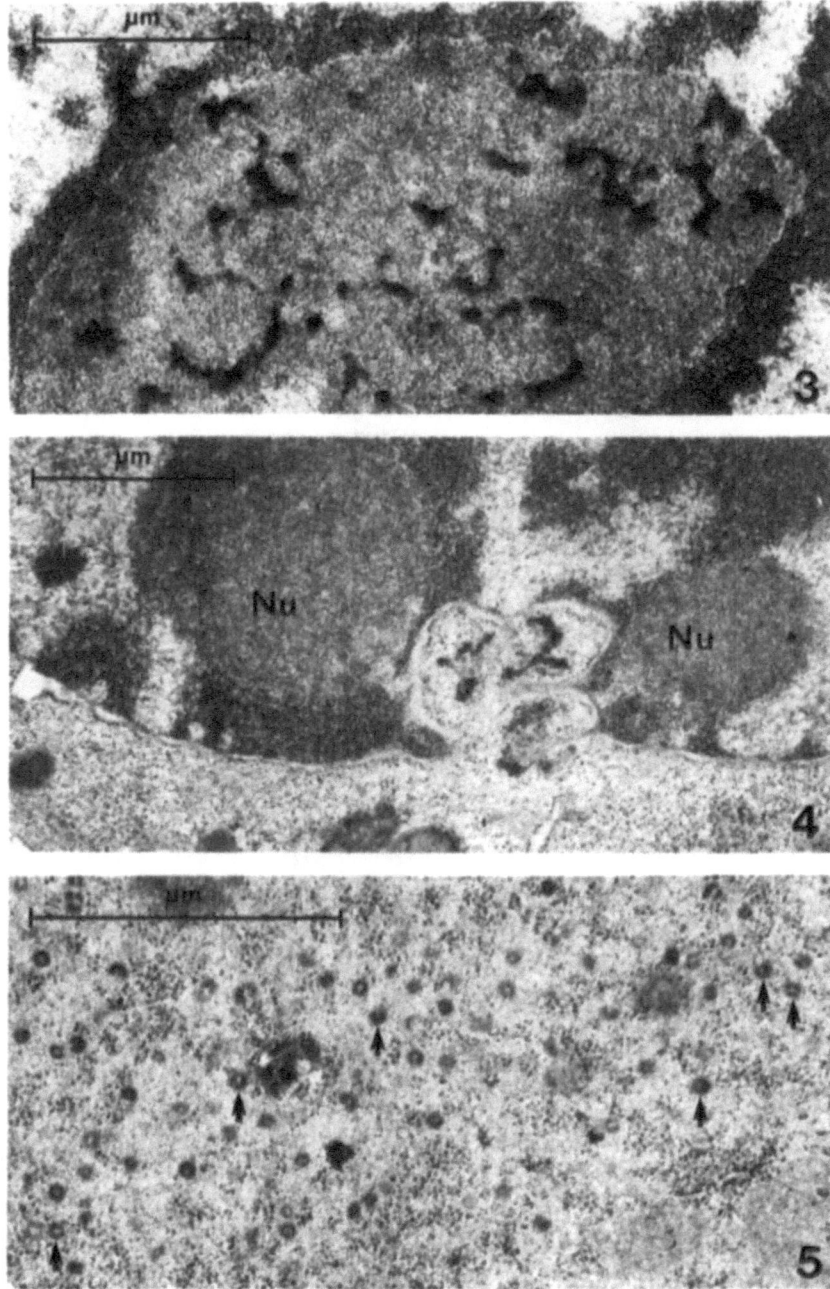

285

dichloride in vivo or in vitro (22): This development started with the appearance of oblong, worm-shaped condensed figures within the nucleoli (Fig. 3); it can be assumed that these figures represent early stages of viruses. Some hours later, the condensed figures occurred outside of the nucleus within cytoplasmic invaginations into the nucleus (Fig. 4). Again some hours later, i.e., about 24 to 48 h after substance application, numerous uniformly shaped, spherical particles, which probably represent structurally completed stages of activated endogenous viruses, were detectable in the cytoplasm of the tumor cells (Fig. 5). It seems to be possible that this event of virus activation, which has been observed up to now only after application of few substances, e.g., of 5-bromodeoxyuridine and 5-iododeoxyuridine (23,24) or of cis-platinum (31,32), might induce unspecific or specific immunologic processes in vivo and thus enhance the tumor defense in vivo.

The postulated stimulation of immunologic events may be confirmed by the observation that animals which had borne Ehrlich ascites tumor and had been treated with titanocene dichloride, rejected reimplanted tumor cells during at least several months after treatment, whereas this phenomenon was not observable to the same extent after treatment with cis-diamminedichloroplatinum(II) or after previous inoculation of inactivated Ehrlich ascites tumor cells (11).

Summarizing the results of the cytobiological experiments, it can be stated that there is high probability for DNA to be the target for the primary attack of the metallocene species.

6. TOXICOLOGIC STUDIES

The antitumor drug cis-diamminedichloroplatinum(II) is burdened by severe nephrotoxic effects which are probably heavy metal-promoted and which are manifested morphologically by structural lesions of the epithelial cells of the proximal as well as of the distal convoluted tubules (25-28) (Figs. 6,7). In contrast to these results after treatment with cis-diamminedichloroplatinum(II), no apparent pathologic alterations were detectable after application of titanocene or vanadocene dichlorides in equitoxic, effective doses: The glomeruli as well as the epithelial cells of the proximal and distal tubules and of the collecting ducts showed light-microscopically and ultrastructurally normal structural features (Figs. 8,9) from 24 h up to 16 d after substance application (11). It must be supposed that this lack of effect on the kidneys by the metallocene dichlorides investigated is due to the toxicologic metal character of titanium and vanadium.

Another toxicologic feature, the problem of teratogenicity of the metallocene dichlorides, has also been studied. For this purpose, the morphologic appearance of proliferating embryonal and fetal tissues was studied after maternal application of titanocene dichloride on day 10, 11, 12, or at later stages of murine pregnancy. It was surprising that neither on day 10, 11, or 12, i.e., during the murine organogenesis, nor later, any histologic alterations became manifest within proliferating tissues (11). Considering the probable intracellular attack of the metallocene dichlorides upon the DNA, these results are highly unexpected and, moreover, very uncommon for a cytostatic agent. Analogously, we could demonstrate an inability of the inorganic cytostatic drug cis-diamminedichloroplatinum(II) to pass the placental barrier during organogenesis (29,30). Thus, it seems to be plausible that the metallocene dichlorides which exhibit certain chemical similarities to cis-diamminedichloroplatinum(II) (2) are apparently incapable of traversing the placenta during long phases of pregnancy and that this effect might be responsible for the lack of effect on proliferating embryonal or fetal tissues by the metallocene dichlorides.

ACKNOWLEDGMENT

This work was supported by financial grants of the Deutsche Forschungsgemeinschaft and the Fonds der Chemischen Industrie.

FIGURES 6 and 7. Epithelial cells of a proximal (Fig. 6) and of a distal (Fig. 7) convoluted tubule of the kidney 4 days after application of cis-diamminedichloroplatinum(II) (10 mg/kg) in vivo. Note the severe structural disintegration phenomena within the tubular cells.

FIGURES 8 and 9. Parts of a proximal (Fig. 8) and of a distal (Fig. 9) convoluted tubule of the kidney 4 days after application of 40 mg titanocene dichloride / kg (Fig. 8) or 70 mg vanadocene dichloride / kg (Fig. 9). The ultrastructural features of the renal cells shown do not differ from those of untreated control cells.

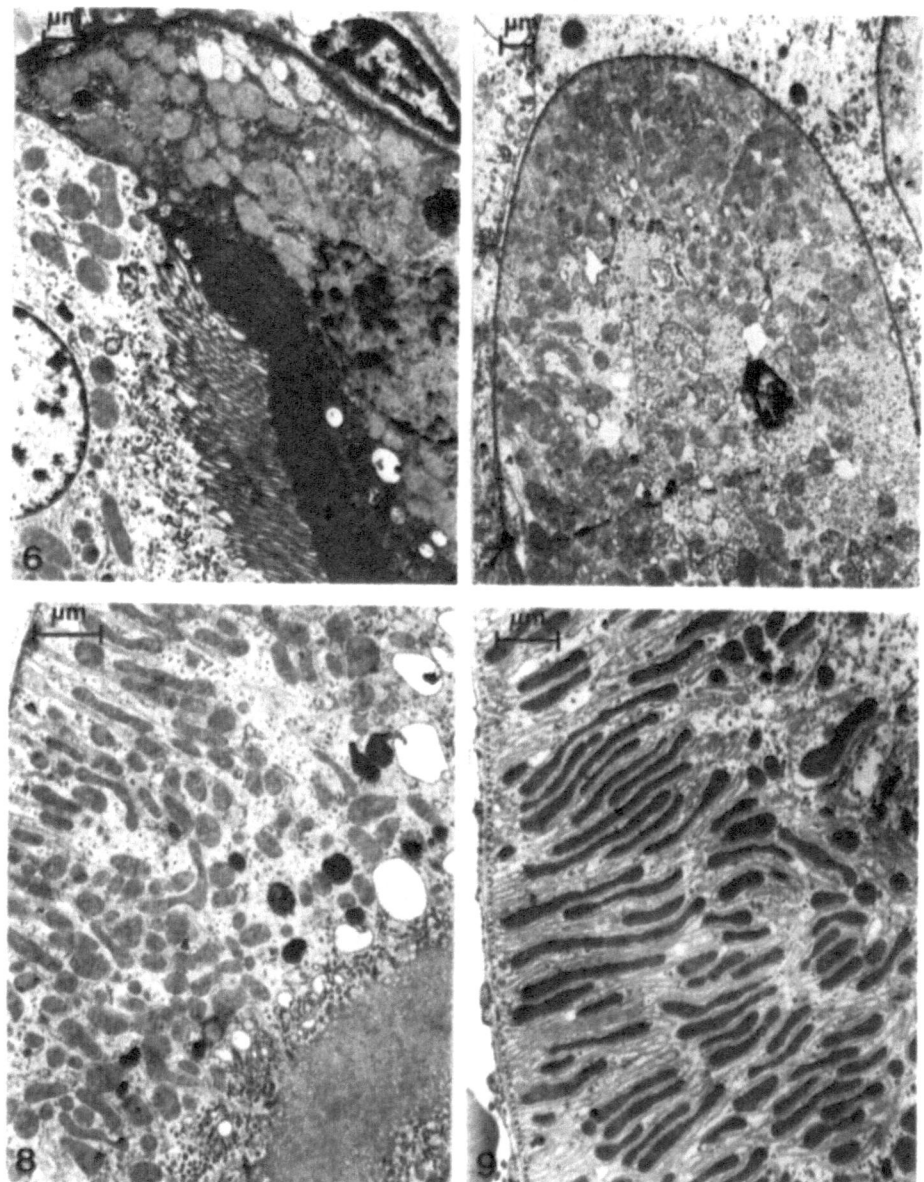

REFERENCES

1. Wilkinson G, Birmingham JM. 1954. Bis-cyclopentadienyl compounds of Ti, Zr, V, Nb and Ta. J. Am. Chem. Soc. 76, 4281-4.
2. Köpf H, Köpf-Maier P. 1979. Titanocen-dichlorid - das erste Metallocen mit cancerostatischer Wirksamkeit. Angew. Chem. 91, 509; Angew. Chem. Int. Ed. Engl. 18, 477-8.
3. Köpf-Maier P, Köpf H. 1979. Vanadocen-dichlorid - ein weiteres Antitumor-Agens aus der Metallocenreihe. Z. Naturforsch. 34b, 805-7.
4. Köpf-Maier P, Leitner M, Voigtländer R, Köpf H. 1979. Molybdocen-dichlorid als Antitumor-Agens. Z. Naturforsch. 34c, 1174-6.
5. Köpf H, Köpf-Maier P. 1981. Metallocendihalogenide als potentielle Cytostatika. Nachr. Chem. Tech. Lab. 29, 154-6.
6. Köpf H, Köpf-Maier P. 1983. Tumor inhibition by metallocene dihalides of early transition metals: Chemical and biological aspects. ACS Symp. Ser. 209, 315-33.
7. Köpf-Maier P, Hesse B, Köpf H. 1980. Tumorhemmung durch Metallocene: Wirkung von Titanocen-, Zirconocen- und Hafnocen-dichlorid gegenüber Ehrlich-Aszites-Tumor der Maus. J. Cancer Res. Clin. Oncol. 96, 43-51.
8. Köpf-Maier P, Leitner M, Köpf H. 1980. Tumor inhibition by metallocenes: Antitumor activity of niobocene and tungstocene dichlorides. J. Inorg. Nucl. Chem. 42, 1789-91.
9. Köpf-Maier P, Hesse B, Voigtländer R, Köpf H. 1980. Tumor inhibition by metallocenes: Antitumor activity of titanocene dihalides $(C_5H_5)_2TiX_2$ (X = F, Cl, Br, I, NCS) and their application in buffered solutions as a method for suppressing drug-induced side effects. J. Cancer Res. Clin. Oncol. 97, 31-9.
10. Köpf-Maier P, Kahl W, Klouras N, Hermann G, Köpf H. 1981. Tumorhemmung durch Metallocene: Ringsubstituierte und ring-überbrückte Titanocen-dichloride. Eur. J. Med. Chem. 16, 275-81.
11. Unpublished results.
12. Köpf-Maier P, Wagner W, Hesse B, Köpf H. 1981. Tumor inhibition by metallocenes: Activity against leukemias and detection of the systemic effect. Eur. J. Cancer 17, 665-9.
13. Chang SI et al. 1981. Die Synthese von Metallverbindungen und experimentelle Untersuchungen über die tumorhemmende Wirkung von Substanzen aus der IV. Nebengruppe. Yao Hsueh T'ung Pao 16, 57.
14. Köpf-Maier P, Wagner W, Köpf H. 1981. In vitro cell growth inhibition by metallocene dichlorides. Cancer Chemother. Pharmacol. 5, 237-41.
15. Tonew E, Tonew M, Heyn B, Schröer HP. 1981. Über biologische Wirkungen von Koordinationsverbindungen der Übergangsmetalle. 4. Zur antiviralen Wirkung der Metallocendihalogenide des Titans und Molybdäns. Zbl. Bakt. Hyg., I. Abt. Orig. A 250, 425-30.
16. Köpf-Maier P, Köpf H. 1980. Tumor inhibition by titanocene dichloride: First clues to the mechanism of action. Naturwiss. 67, 415-6.

17. Köpf-Maier P, Wagner W, Köpf H. 1981. Different inhibition pattern of the nucleic acid metabolism after in vivo treatment with titanocene and vanadocene dichlorides. Naturwiss. 68, 272-3.
18. Köpf-Maier P, Krahl D. 1981. Intracellular distribution of titanium after treatment with the antitumor agent titanocene dichloride: An electron energy loss spectroscopic study. Naturwiss. 68, 273-4.
19. Köpf-Maier P, Krahl D. 1983. Tumor inhibition by metallocenes: Ultrastructural localisation of titanium and vanadium in treated tumor cells by electron energy loss spectroscopy. Chem.-Biol. Interact., in press.
20. Köpf-Maier P, Wagner W, Liss E. 1981. Cytokinetic behavior of Ehrlich ascites tumor after in vivo treatment with cis-diamminedichloroplatinum(II) and metallocene dichlorides. J. Cancer Res. Clin. Oncol. 102, 21-30.
21. Köpf-Maier P, Wagner W, Liss E. 1983. Induction of cell arrest at G_1/S and in G_2 after treatment of Ehrlich ascites tumor cells with metallocene dichlorides and cis-platinum in vitro. J. Cancer Res. Clin. Oncol., in press.
22. Köpf-Maier P. 1982. Development of necroses, virus activation and giant cell formation after treatment of Ehrlich ascites tumor with metallocene dichlorides. J. Cancer Res. Clin. Oncol. 103, 145-64.
23. Aaronson SA. 1971. Chemical induction of focus-forming virus from nonproducer cells transformed by murine sarcoma virus. Proc. Nat. Acad. Sci. USA 68, 3069-72.
24. Lowy DR, Rowe WP, Teich N, Hartley JW. 1971. Murine leukemia virus: High-frequency activation in vitro by 5-iododeoxyuridine and 5-bromodeoxyuridine. Science 174, 155-6.
25. Gonzalez-Vitale JC, Hayes DM, Cvitkovic E, Sternberg SS. 1977. The renal pathology in clinical trials of cis-platinum(II)diamminedichloride. Cancer 39, 1362-71.
26. Dentino M, Luft FC, Yum MN, Williams SD, Einhorn LH. 1978. Long term effect of cis-diamminedichloride platinum (CDDP) on renal function and structure in man. Cancer 41, 1274-81.
27. Dobyan DC, Levi J, Jacobs C, Kosek J, Weiner MW. 1980. Mechanism of cis-platinum nephrotoxicity: II. Morphologic observations. J. Pharm. Exp. Ther. 213, 551-6.
28. Chopra S, Kaufman JS, Jones TW, Hong WK, Gehr MK, Hamburger RJ, Flamenbaum W, Trump BF, Chase DH. 1982. Cis-diamminedichloroplatinum-induced acute renal failure in the rat. Kidney Internat. 21, 54-64.
29. Köpf-Maier P. 1983. Stage of pregnancy-dependent transplacental passage of ^{195m}Pt after cis-platinum treatment. Eur. J. Cancer Clin. Oncol. 19, 533-6.
30. Köpf-Maier P, Merker HJ. 1983. Effects of the cytostatic drug cis-platinum on the developing neocortex of the mouse. Teratol., in press.
31. Sodhi A, Aggarwal SK. 1974. Effects of cis-dichlorodiammine platinum (II) in the regression of sarcoma 180: A fine structural study. J. Nat. Cancer Inst. 53, 85-9.
32. Sodhi A. 1976. Ultrastructural changes of sarcoma-180 cells after treatment with cis-dichlorodiammine platinum (II), in vivo and in vitro. Ind. J. Exp. Biol. 14, 383-90.

The Design of Metal Complexes as Anticancer Drugs
P.J. Sadler, M. Nasr and V.L. Narayanan

1. INTRODUCTION

In the past, the focus of the National Cancer Institute's (NCI) efforts has been principally directed towards the acquisition and screening of diverse ranges of organic compounds to identify new leads. The discovery of the excellent anti-tumour activity of cisplatin (1) has drawn attention to the potential for activity exploration amongst other inorganic compounds (2-6).

An important step in this process is the establishment of structure-activity relationships. In general, platinum compounds have shown excellent activity in L1210 leukaemia, in addition, the 13 (non-discreet) compounds currently known to have the highest activity (DN2 activity, a reproducible T/C > 150 against B16 melanoma) fall into three related classes. Their structures are shown in Figure 1. All have two cis N ligands which are primary amines, except NSC-312605, and either two cis chlorides or oxy-acids as the remaining ligands. One is a Pt(IV) complex (NSC-256927). These features suggest that, with the appropriate choice of metal oxidation state and the types and numbers of coordinated ligands, it may be possible to design anti-cancer complexes of a variety of metals.

In this paper we survey compounds of the three Group 1B elements copper, silver and gold which have been evaluated for anticancer activity at the NCI. Copper is one of some 25 elements which are thought to be essential for normal animal metabolism, whereas Ag aud Au, like Pt, are non-essential. Our choice of this Group was for two reasons. Firstly, they can share with Pt(II) a d^8 electronic configuration and in the cases of Au(III) (strictly) and Cu(II) (loosely) square-planar coordination geometries.

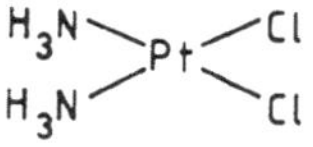

Figure 1. Highly-active platinum anticancer complexes

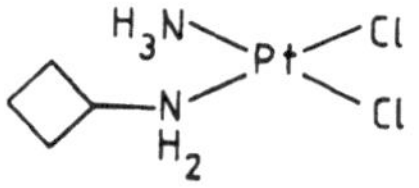

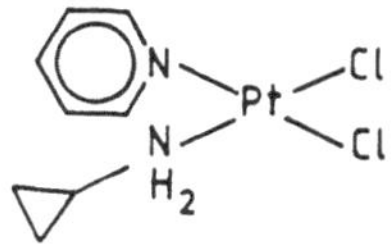

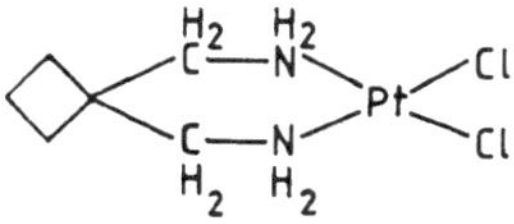

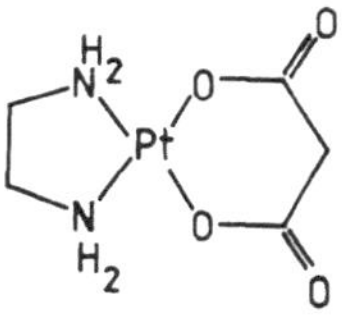

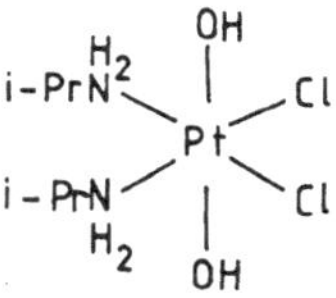

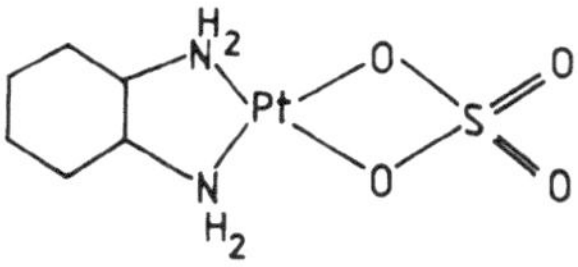

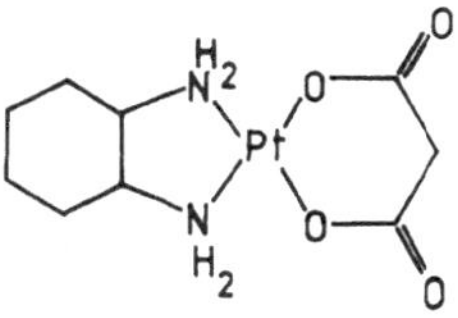

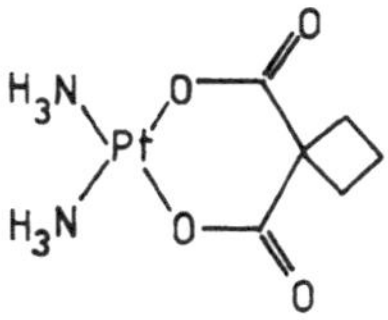

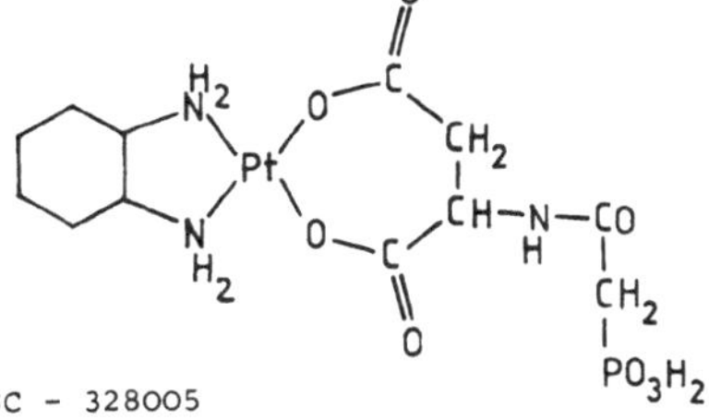

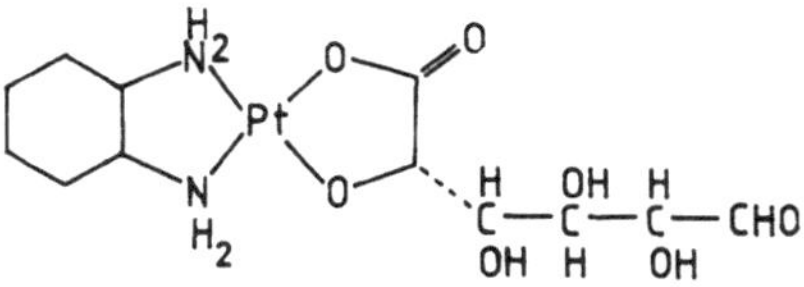

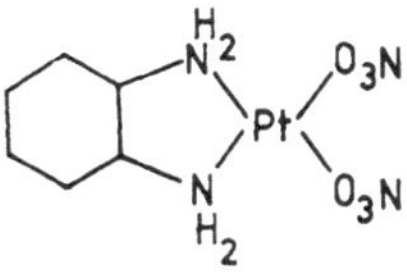

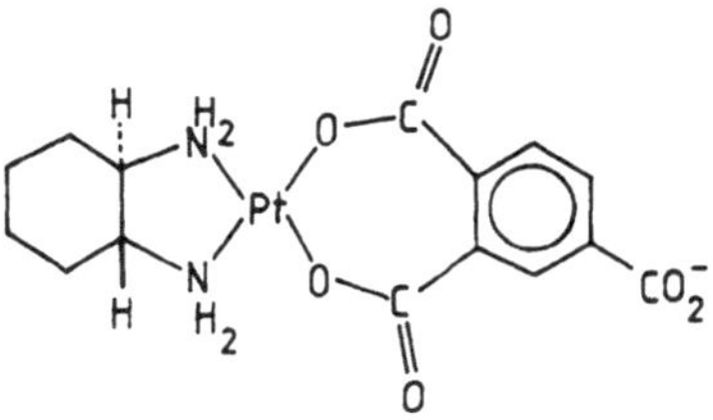

Table 1. A comparison of Group IB Ions with Pt(II).

Metal ion[a]	Preferred geometry	$pK_a(H_2O)$[b]
d^8:Pt(II)		7.0^c
Cu(III)	?	?
Ag(III)	?	?
Au(III)		0.7
d^9:Cu(II)		5.6^c
Ag(II)	?	0.5
Au(II)	?	?
d^{10}:Cu(I)		?
Ag(I)		10.0
Au(I)		?

(a) Common oxidation states underlined   (b) ref (7)
(c) $MCl_3(H_2O)$, others refer to aquo ions.

However, the common oxidation states, Table 1, do not include Cu(III), Ag(III), Ag(II) or Au(II) and we shall say little more about them, although this does not imply any lack of anti-cancer potential. The high polarising power of Pt(II) toward e.g. coordinated water may play a role in the intracellular biochemistry of Pt drugs through the formation of reactive hydroxy complexes. This property is also shared by Cu(II) and, even more so, Au(III), Table 1. Even amines coordinated to Au(III) would be expected to undergo ready proton dissociation at physiological pH (7.4), Table 2. A complex such as $[Au(en)Cl_2]^+$ may therefore be uncharged and readily enter cells.

Ligand exchange rates on Pt(II) tend to be slower than those of Au(III), see (9), but those of Cu(II) can be very rapid (8) (H_2O exchange rate on aquated Cu(II) is ca. 10^9 sec^{-1}). Therefore we have to choose ligands (polydentate and/or lipophilic) which undergo slow exchange reactions with Cu(II) so that the complex reaches the desired attack site.

Our second reason for considering Group 1B was the knowledge that both Cu and Au are known modulators of immunological reactions. We now discuss this further.

Table 2. pK_a Values for amines coordinated to Pt(II),
Pt(IV) and Au(III)[a].

	pK_1		pK_1
$Pt(NH_3)_3(DMSO)^{2+}$	9.1	$Au(NH_3)_4^{3+}$	7.5
$Pt(NH_3)_6^{4+}$	8.0	$Au(en)_2^{3+}$	6.5
$\underline{cis}Pt(NH_3)_4Cl_2^{2+}$	9.6	$[Au(dien)Cl]Cl_2$	4.0

(a) For refs. see (7) and (9)

1.1. Immunoregulation

Immunological reactions may play a role in the mechanism of action of Pt drugs (1). Fairlie and Whitehouse have recently summarized the evidence for both immunosuppressant and immuno-stimulating effects (10) and have suggested that the profound lymphotoxic effects of Pt drugs, which resemble those of nitrogen mustards, may be of value in suppressing cell-mediated immuno-pathies. Rheumatoid arthritis is thought to involve an autoimmune response and some Pt amines show antiarthritic activity in animal models (10). Interest has arisen in comparisons between the molecular pharmacology of platinum and gold (11).

Gold(I) thiolates, such as Myocrisin given by intramuscular injection, and gold(I) phosphines such as auranofin (on clinical trial), given orally, are in use for the treatment of rheumatoid arthritis (12), Fig. 2. They are capable of suppressing or enhanc-ing immune responses dependent on the circumstances (12).

Interest in the possibility of the involvement of copper in immunoregulation has been greatly stimulated by Lipsky and Ziff's observations (13) that Cu(II) salts in the presence of a large excess of thiols, especially D-penicillamine, markedly inhibit mitogen-triggered DNA synthesis in human peripheral blood lympho-cytes. Since thiols reduce Cu(II) to Cu(I), it is possible that Cu(I) plays a natural role in the regulation of lymphocyte function.

2. ANTICANCER ACTIVITY

Table 3 lists the numbers of copper, silver and gold compounds evaluated by the NCI. The copper compound (NSC-175462) shows a

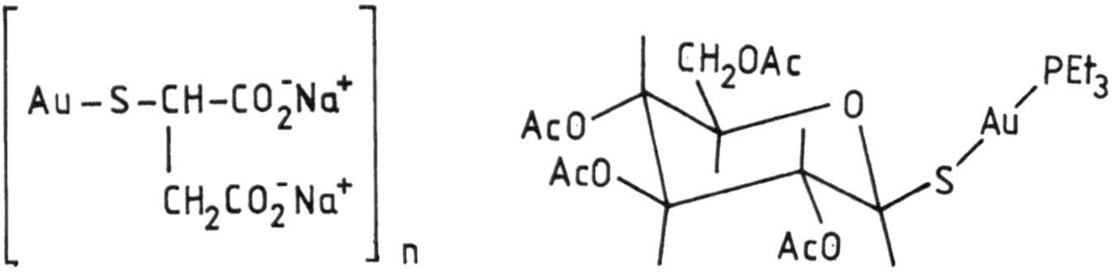

Figure 2.   Antiarthritic gold drugs : aurothiomalate ('Myocrisin') and auranofin ('Ridaura')

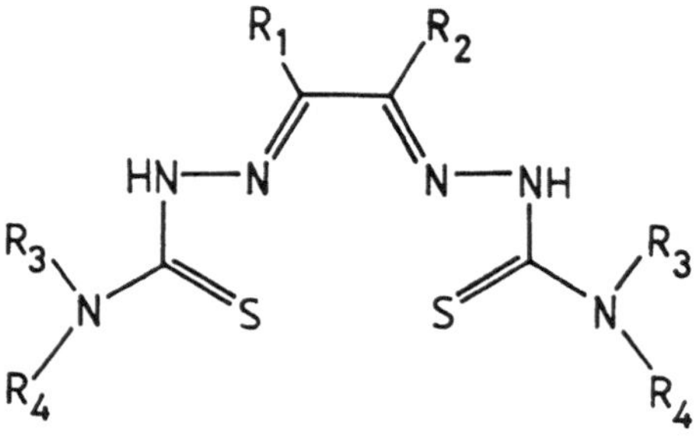

H₂KTS : R_1 = $-CH(CH_3)OC_2H_5$
         R_2 - R_4 = H

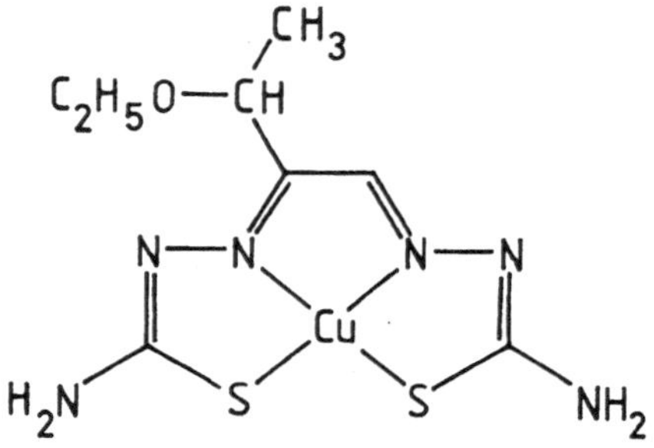

Cu KTS

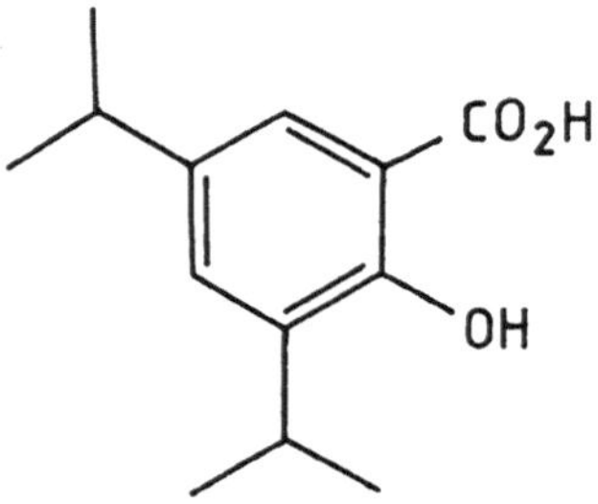

DIPS - H

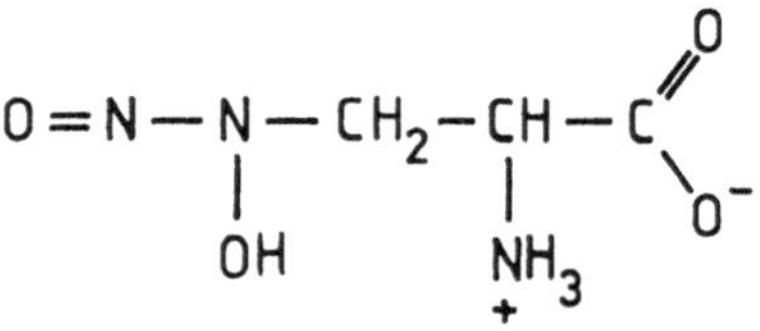

L - Alanosine

Figure 3. The structure of bisthiosemicarbazone and other ligands for copper, and CuKTS. In crystals of the latter there are two longer Cu...S bonds above and below Cu (21).

Table 3.   Copper, silver and gold compounds evaluated by the
          NCI (up to 1982).

| Metal | Evaluated | Active | | High Activity[a] |
		in vitro	in vivo	
Copper	1109	14	27	1
Silver	134	2	5	0
Gold	106	-	22	0

(a) a reproducible T/C > 150% against B16 melanoma.

DN2 level of activity in B16 melanoma (reproduced T/C > 150%) and
is the only other metal compound apart from the 13 Pt compounds
described above, on the NCI panel which showed such activity.   In
our discussions of Cu, Ag and Au, we also include other literature
reports of activity.

2.1. Copper

In 1947 Co(II), Ni(II) and Cu(II) phthalate complexes were
reported to cause favourable regression of human leukaemia (11)
but when Co(II), Ni(II), Cu(II) and Zn(II) butylphthates were
tested against the ADJ/PC6A tumour in 1974 they were inactive (4).
In 1959 Takamiya reported the anti-tumour activity of bis(dimethyl-
glyoximato) Cu(II) : 200-300% increase in lifespan with Ehrlich
ascites and S180 tumours (15,16).   The ligand alone was inactive,
as were some other copper oximes.   It should be noted that not
all Cu(II) oximes will have the same solid-state structures.
$Cu(DMG)_2$ itself has a dimeric structure whereas the salicylald-
oximes form infinite chains (17).   There are many examples of
Cu(II) compounds with four short bonds in an approximate square-
planar configuration and two additional longer axial bonds (tetragonal coordination, so-called Jahn-Teller distortion).   The
intermolecular interactions which exist in many solid Cu(II)
complexes could play a role in their pharmacological activity.

The idea that strong chelating agents may interfere with the
transport of metals into cells or their subcellular distribution
lead French and Freelander to screen bisthiosemicarbazones (18).
Subsequently H.G. Petering and coworkers reported that 3-ethoxy-
2-oxobutyraldehyde (H_2KTS) given i.p. or orally lead to complete

regression of Walker 256 (and nitrogen mustard resistant) carcinoma, a solid sarcoma 180, and had a wide range of activity against transplantable solid tumours but not leukaemias (19). The cytotoxicity of H_2KTS was shown to depend on the presence of Cu(II) either in culture media or animals' diet (20). CuKTS has a tetragonal structure, Fig. 3 (21).

Copper(II) has a high affinity for KTS^{2-}, log K = 18.4, and CuKTS (E_o = -120 mV at pH 6.6) is readily reduced by thiols (22). The RSH/RSSR reduction potential for intracellular thiols being ca. -200 mV. The substituents R_1 -R_4, Figure 3, have a marked effect on cytotoxicity which correlates with the rates of ligand substitution with ethylenediamine and reduction by dithiotheitol. D.H. Petering has summarised the evidence for intracellular reduction of CuKTS giving a Cu(I)-thiolate complex followed by release of H_2KTS into the extracellular medium (22). DNA synthesis within Ehrlich cells is inhibited within 5 minutes.

In Table 4 are listed some of the active Cu compounds evaluated by the NCI. It is notable that the Cu(I) complex NSC-55475 and the Cu(II) complex NSC-76505 are active in several systems. These have 6-mercapto-purine (NSC-755) and thioguanine (NSC-752) as ligands, respectively, which are themselves active compounds. Similarly, several complexes with alkylating groups on the ligand have shown activity e.g. NSC-68292.

The most active complex is NSC-175462, a Cu(II) dichloride complex of the closed macrocyclic ligand, tetrabenzo[b,f,j,n] [1,5,9,13] tetraazacyclohexadecine (TAAB). Fig. 4. The diperchlorate salt NSC-175464, is also active. The complexes can be prepared by a template synthesis reaction by self condensation of o-aminobenzaldehyde in the presence of Cu(II), or Ni(II) (23). The ligand provides a distorted square-planar geometry for Cu(II) and, with complete electron conjugation, also shows a strong resemblance to a porphyrin. Cu(II)(TAAB) is easily reduced to the Cu(I) complex, E½-10mV vs normal hydrogen electrode in dimethylformamide (24). The unusually high stability of Cu(I)(TAAB) is attributable to the extensive delocalisation of the added electron onto the ligand, which can probably distort toward the tetrahedral geometry preferred by Cu(I). Cu(TAAB) is inactive, however, in

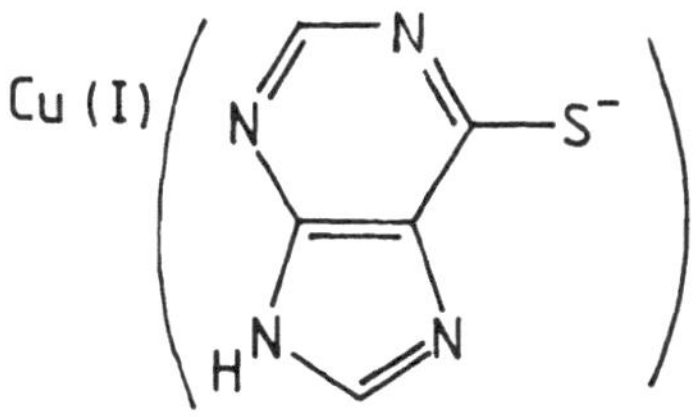

NSC - 55475

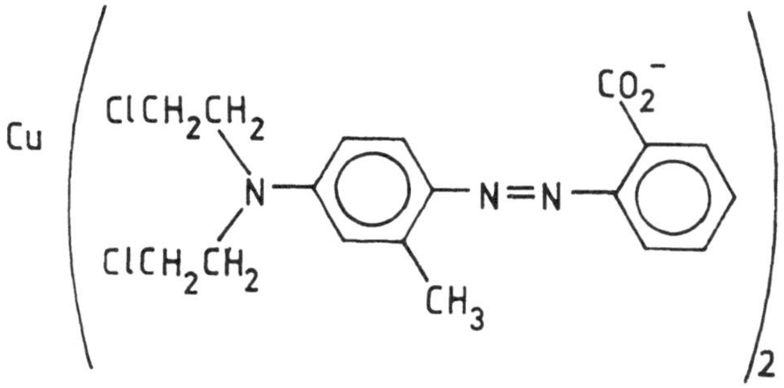

NSC - 68292

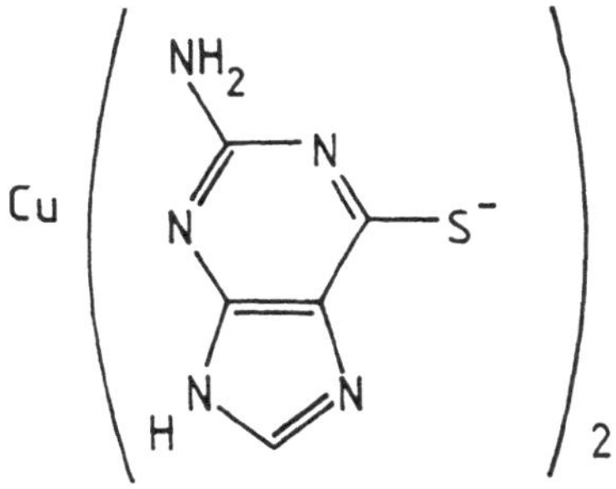

NSC - 76505

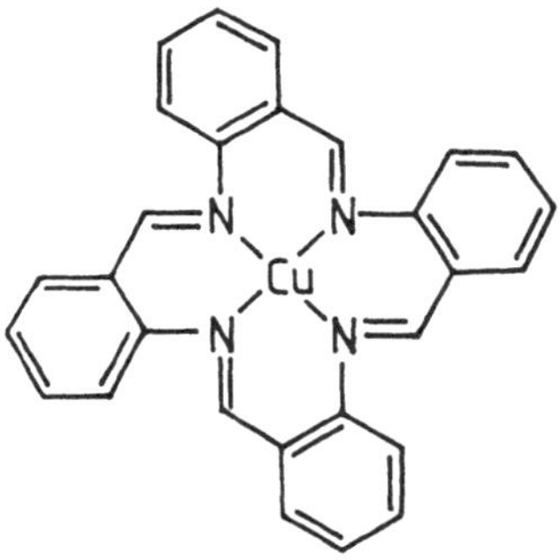

NSC - 175462 (2Cl⁻)
NSC - 175464 (2ClO₄⁻)

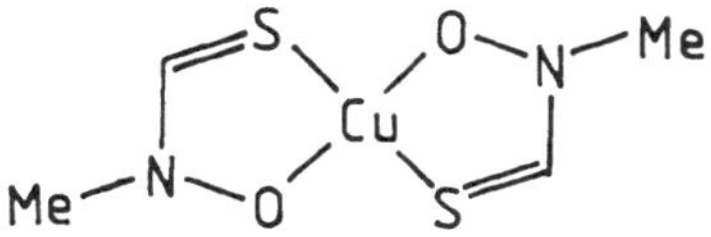

NSC - 178262

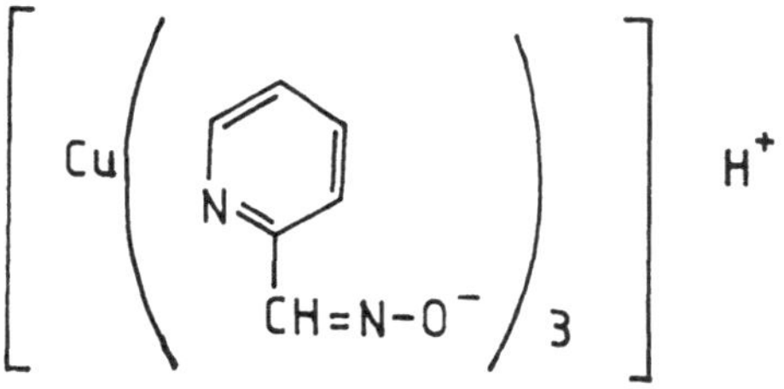

NSC - 284613

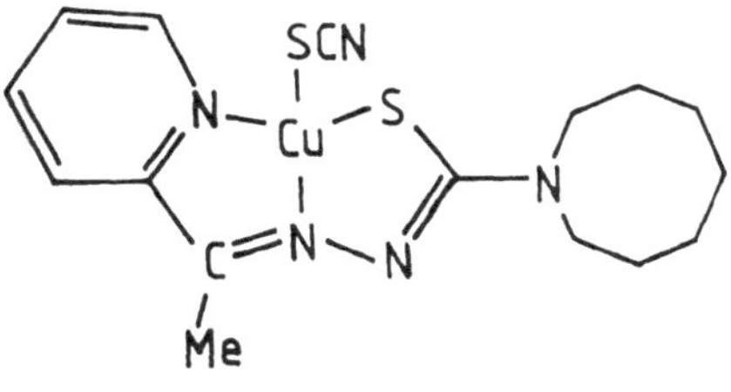

NSC - 338305

Figure 4. Some copper compounds exhibiting anticancer activity.
In several cases the structures are not known with certainty.

Table 4. Copper compounds exhibiting anti-cancer activity.

Compound[a]	Tumour[b]	Schedule	Dose[c]	T/C%[d]
NSC-55475	A755	ip,d 1-11	3.7-50	(0)
	L1210	ip,d 1-14	18.8	147
	P388	ip,d 1-9	20-50	150
	S180	ip,d 1-7	70-254	(19)
NSC-68292	P388	ip,d 1-9	12.5	209
	W256	ip,d 1-5	0.4-28	(5)
NSC-76505	A755	ip,d 1-11	5.0	(5)
	L1210	ip,3dx	0.8-10	142
NSC-175462	B16	ip,d 1-9	6.25-12.5	170
	P388	ip,d 1-9	3.12-6.25	144
NSC-175464	B16	ip,d 1-9	12.5	164
	P388	ip,d 1-9	6.25-12.5	150
NSC-178262	CD8F$_1$	ip,d 7,14,35	0.75-3.0	(21)
	Lewis L	ip,d 1-9	0.12-0.5	143
NSC-284613	L1210	ip,3hx8	3.0-6.0	335
NSC-338305	CX-1	sc,d4x4	300	(39)
	LX-1	sc,d4x3	150	(40)
	P388	ip,d 1-5	6.25	164

(a) for structures see Fig.4 (b) mouse, A755 adrenocarcinoma, L1210 lymphoid leukaemia, P388 lymocytic leukaemia, S180 sarcoma 180, W256 Walker carcinoma 256, B16 melanocarcinoma, CD8F, mammary tumour, CX-1 human colon xenograph, LX-1 human lung xenograph (c) mg/kg (d) mean tumour weight changes (in brackets), and median survival times for treated (T)/ control (C).

the remaining 7 tumour panel systems of the NCI.

Sorenson and coworkers have shown that a copper aspirin complex and several Cu(II) salicylates are effective in a solid Ehrlich tumour model produced by injecting Ehrlich cells intramuscularly in the hind limbs of female mice (25,26). One of the most effective is bis(diisopropylsalicylato)Cu(II), Cu(DIPS)$_2$, a lipophilic complex which is probably polymeric in the solid state via bridging carboxylates. They reasoned that since many tumour cells contain lowered levels of (Cu, Zn) and Mn superoxide dismutases (27,28) compared to their mature, normal cell counterparts, then a copper complex with superoxide dismutase activity may lead to the appearance of the normal cell phenotype. The Cu salicylates (im injection) decreased tumour growth, increased survival and decreased metastasis. The latter was attributed to a possible increase in a copper-dependent immune response. There was little

Table 5. Some active, silver anti-tumour compounds.

Compound[a]	Tumour	Schedule	Dose	T/C%
$Ag(CF_3(CF_2)_6CO_2H)$	A755	ip,d 1-11	3.5-14	(38)
$Ag(SCH_2CH_2CO_2H)$	S180	ip,2xd 1-14	125-281	(38)
$Ag(MP)$	L1210	ip,d 1-9	25-800	154
$Ag(CP)$	P388	ip,d 1-9	3.1	153

(a) MP is 6-mercaptopurine, CP is cyclopropane carboxylic acid.

evidence that tumour cell killing accounted for the effectiveness of the complexes since the LD_{50} for $Cu(DIPS)_2$ is 240 mg/kg in rats and > 320 mg/kg in mice (sc), whereas an effective dose is 25 mg/kg.

Several organic drugs bind Cu(II) tightly. Bleomycin (NSC 125066) is isolated as a Cu(II) complex and could act as a Cu transport agent (29). L-Alanosine, NSC-153353 (Fig. 3) has anti-viral, immunosuppressive and antitumour activity (including P388, mammary CD8F) but the strong Cu(II) complex (log K, 22.7 at pH 7.2) is reported to be inactive (30,31).

Finally, Cramp and coworkers (32) have observed that mammalian cells treated with Cu(I) become more sensitive to radiation.

2.1.2. Role of metallothionein ? Recently metallothionein has been implicated in the absorption, transport and detoxification of Cu (33,34), in the regulation of Zn, Cu and SH levels in cells and the insertion of metals into apoenzymes. The role of metallo-thioneins in cancer cells is not known. It is possible to assume that the concentration and distribution of these metallothioneins may be different in cancer cells versus normal cells. It may be possible to exploit these differences in the design of novel Cu complexes as anticancer agents.

2.2. Silver

Silver compounds are potent antibacterials and silver sulpha-diazine (2-sulphanilamidopyrimidine) has been used for the treat-ment of infections in burn wounds (35). Ligand exchange reactions of linear or tetrahedral Ag(I) complexes are likely to be very rapid but little attempt appears to have been made to design complexes in which these are slowed down. A few complexes

Table 6. Effect of gold compounds on P388 leukaemia in mice
(doses usually ip from 4-200 mg/kg in saline-Tween 80).

Class	Active[a]	Inactive[b]
Au(III)	$[AuMe_2Cl_2]AsPh_4$	$AuCl_2(Ph)(py), AuCl_2(Ph)(SBu_2)$
	$Me_2Au(SCN)_2AuMe_2$	$[Au(en)_2]Cl_3, [Au(DACH)_2]Cl_3$
		$AuCl_3(pyridine), [AuCl_4]X^c$
Au(I)	$K[Au(CN)_2]$, auranofin[f]	Au(thiomalate)
	$BrAuS(CH_2Ph)_2$	
Ph$_3$PAu-Y	Y = thymidine[d]	2-thiouracil[d]
	5-fluorouracil[d], 6-mercapto-	
	purine[d]	N_3^-, $CH_3CO_2^-$
	5-fluorodeoxyuridine[d]	
	Cl^-, $TACP^{-[e]}$	

(a) T/C 120-174% the highest value is for Ph$_3$PAuCl (b) T/C < 120%
(c) X includes a wide range of N bases, except those which are
alkylating agents   (d) ref (36) (e) various N-bound substituted
tetraazacyclopentanes   (f) ref (37), see fig. 2 for auranofin
structure

evaluated by the NCI have shown marginal anticancer activity but
most are probably polymeric, and of uncertain structure, Table 5.

2.3. Gold

Both Au(III) and Au(I) complexes exhibit antineoplastic
activity against P388 leukaemia in mice, Table 6. However, in
some compounds of structure Ph$_3$PAuY gold is complexed with known
anticancer agents. Ligand exchange reactions of Au(I) are usually
very rapid, and Au(I) unlike Pt(II) would not be expected to form
kinetically-inert bonds with N or O ligands of DNA. A mechanism
of action which contrasts with Pt(II) may therefore be involved.

The Au(III) derivatives $AuCl_4^-$ and $AuCl_3(py)$ are strong oxidizing agents. They may undergo rapid hydrolysis and reduction to
Au(I) in vivo, bind to plasma proteins and not enter cells. The
antiarthritic drug aurothiomalate (Myocrisin) which is polymeric in aqueous solution does not promote the entry of gold into
cells. On the other hand the orally-active antiarthritic drug
auranofin, Fig. 2, is highly lipophilic. We have shown (38) by
^{1}H and ^{31}P nmr, that, once inside red cells, some of the tetra-

301

Table 7. Mouse survival after auranofin treatment of lymphocytic
leukaemia P388 (ref. 32).

Dose[a]	Cures	T/C%
3 daily	0/8	155
3 (2 x daily)	4/8	185
6 (2 x daily)	7/8	220

(a) mg/kg ip, in 50% EtOH/0.9% NaCl

acetylthioglucose is displaced by glutathione and that PEt_3 is
displaced only slowly. Lorber and coworkers (39,40) found that
auranofin inhibited DNA synthesis irreversibly in HeLa cells, as
does cisplatin, and to a lesser extent RNA and protein synthesis.
Auranofin also interferes with membrane tranport.

Subsequently it was shown that auranofin increased the survival
of mice with P388 leukaemia, Table 7, and caused regression of
Sarcoma 180 tumours (37) without evidence of nephrotoxicity.
However, Sutton has reported (41) that auranofin exhibited only
minimal activity in the P388 system at maximum non-toxic doses.
Patients receiving auranofin show marked suppressive effects in
response to mitogens and to skin-test antigens, but do not seem
to experience increased susceptibility to opportunistic infections
(39,40).

The preferred ligands for R_3PAu^+ would be (approx.):
PR_3, CN^-, $RS^- \gg -C=S > I^- > Br^- >$
$R_2S > R_1R_2N^- > Cl^- > -C=N- \gg RCO_2^- > H_2O$
However this order applies to aqueous media and may be quite
different in hydrophobic environments. For example, we find (42)
that Et_3PAuCl causes dramatic spin-state changes of haemoglobin
irrespective of whether its free SH groups are blocked. Little
is known about aquated complexes of Au(I), although $Au(H_2O)_x^+$
does not exist. Clearly these areas need further chemical investigation.

Perhaps the most curious behaviour is shown by $K[Au(CN)_2]$
which exhibits significant activity against several tumours,
Table 8, including a 50% cure rate for Lewis Lung carcinoma. This
complex was originally used for the treatment of tuberculosis
over 70 years ago (9), but was abandoned because of its toxicity.

Table 8. Comparison of the activity of KAu(CN)$_2$ (in saline)
against different mouse tumours.

Tumour	Schedule	Dose	Eval.	T/C%	Cures
Intra-renal CX-1 colon xenograph	sc, d 1,5,9,13	20.0	d 15	7[a]	0/6
Lewis lung carcinoma	ip, d 1-9	2.5	d 60	200[b]	5/10
P388	ip, d 1-9	6.25	d 30	150[b]	0/6

(a) mean tumour weight change   (b) median survival time

The transport pathways for Au(I) cyanide complexes into cells
require investigation. It is possible that gold merely acts as a
transport agent for CN^-, a potent inhibitor of many metalloenzymes.
Au(I) itself is an effective inhibitor of many enzymes including
collagenase, an enzyme which may provide an invasive mechanism
when tumours spread (12).

In strict contrast to Pt(II), the available data for Au(I) and
Au(III) compounds appears to indicate that active compounds have
tightly bound ligands with high trans influences (R_3P, CH_3^-, RS^-).
They are probably responsible for lowering the reactivity of gold
toward extracellular proteins and its transport into cells where
metabolism may occur. Au(III) alkyls readily form hydroxy-bridged
complexes in aqueous media (43).

There is an opportunity for the design of Au(III) compounds.
We have shown (44) that their oxidizing power can be considerably
reduced by the appropriate choice of ligands. Au(III) is likely
to form more stable bonds to N bases of DNA than Au(I). Imidazole,
for example, undergoes slow exchange reactions with Au(III), on
the nmr timescale, but for Au(I) they are rapid (45). Au(III)
complexes of nucleotides are known (46).

3. CONCLUSION.

It is clear that a systematic search should now begin for anticancer activity amongst a wide range of elements. The compounds
designed should be well-characterised and should possess reasonable water solubility and stability. Our survey of data on copper,
silver and gold suggests that it may be possible to design new

303

complexes of these metals which would exert anti-tumour activity. Copper is attractive because it is a natural metal ion, and gold because of widespread clinical familiarity through its use in rheumatoid arthritis treatment.

Copper complexes in which the ligand exchange rates are slow and/or in which Cu(I) is stabilized appear to be particularly suitable for exploration. Cu(II) compounds are often cross-linked in the solid state and care must be taken to achieve reproducibility if they are administered as suspensions or when dissolution is a-chieved. The same comment will apply to many other metal complexes.

Au(I) and Au(III) complexes with strong π-acceptor ligands e.g. phosphines, alkyls, thiolates, cyanide are worthy of further investigation, including new Au(III) complexes with lowered redox potentials. There is a need to test a wide range of well-characterised Ag complexes.

Addendum. Elsewhere in this volume the anticancer activity of TNO-6 is described. This should be added to the other 13 compounds shown in Figure 1. Although only tested once against B16 melanoma by the NCI, it did show a DN2 level of activity.

Acknowledgements. PJS thanks Dr. T. Sadler for assistance with collation of data, and H. Robbins for drawing the Figures.

REFERENCES

1. Rosenberg B. (1980) Metal Ions in Biol. Syst. 11, 168.
2. Narayanan VL. (1983) In "Development in Pharmacology" (Reinhoudt DN, Connors TA, Pinedo HM, Van De Pall KW. eds.) Vol. 3, p5. Martinus Nijhoff, The Hague/Boston/London.
3. Wolpert-DeFillippes MK. (1980) In "CisPlatin: Current Status and New Developments" (Prestayko AW, Crooke ST, Carter SK. eds) pp 183-191 Academic Press, New York.
4. Cleare MJ, Hydes PC. (1980) Metal Ions in Biol. Syst. 11, 1.
5. Sadler PJ. (1983) Chem. Brit. 18, 12.
6. Platinum, Gold and Other Chemotherapeutic Agents, ACS Symposium Series (1983), 209.
7. Burgess J. (1978) Metal Ions in Solution, Ellis Horwood, Chichester, U.K.
8. Martell AE. ed. (1978) Coordination Chemistry, ACS Monograph 174, ACS Washington, D.C.
9. Sadler PJ. (1976) Structure and Bonding (Berlin) 29, 171.
10. Fairlie DP, Whitehouse MW. (1980) Agents and Actions Suppl. 8, 399.
11. Crooke ST. (1982) J. Rheumatol. 9 (suppl. 8), 61.
12. Lewis AJ, Walz DT. (1982) Progress in Med. Chem 19, 2.
13. Lipsky PE, Ziff M. (1978) J. Immunol. 120, 1006.
14. Geschickte CF, Reid EE. (1947) in Approaches to Tumor Chemotherapy, Moulton, ed. AAAS Washington, D.C. p.431.

15. Takamiya K. (1960) Nature $\underline{185}$, 190.
16. Takamiya K. (1959) Gann. $\underline{50}$, 265.
17. Wells AF. (1975) Structural Inorganic Chemistry 4th Ed. Clarendon Press, Oxford.
18. French FA, Freelander BL. (1960) Cancer Res. $\underline{21}$, 505 and (1958), $\underline{18}$, 1298.
19. Petering HG, Birskirk HH, Underwood GE. (1964) Cancer Res. $\underline{24}$, 267.
20. Petering HG, Birskirk HH, Crim JA. (1967) Cancer Chem. $\underline{27}$,
21. Taylor MR, Glusker JP, Gabe EJ, Minkin JA. (1974), Bioinorg. Chem. (1974), $\underline{3}$, 189.
22. Petering DH. (1980) Metal Ions in Biol. Syst. $\underline{11}$, 197.
23. Melson GA, Busch DH. (1964), J. Amer. Chem. Soc. $\underline{86}$, 4834.
24. Gagné RR, Allison JL, Ingle DM. (1979) Inorg. Chem. $\underline{18}$, 2767.
25. Sorenson JRJ, Oberley LW, Oberley TD, Leuthauser SWC, Ramakrishna K, Vernino L, Kishore V. (1982) Proc. Conf. Trace Sub. Envir. Health XVI, Hemphill DD, ed., Univ. Missouri Press, Columbia, Mo.
26. Sorenson JRJ, Oberley LW, Crouch RK, Kensler TW, Kishore V, Lenthauser SWC, Oberley TD, Pezeshk A. (1982) Proc. 3rd Inst. Conf. Inorg. and Nut. Asp. Cancer and Other Diseases, La Jolla, 11-13 Nov. 1982.
27. Oberley LW, Buettner GR. (1979) Cancer Res. $\underline{39}$, 1141.
28. Fee AJ. (1982) Metal Ions in Biol. Syst. $\underline{13}$, 259.
29. Umezawa H, Takita T. (1979) Structure and Bonding (Berlin) $\underline{40}$, 73.
30. Murthy YKS, Thiemann JE, Coronelli C, Semsi P. (1966) Nature $\underline{211}$, 1198.
31. Purvis G, Kovach JS. (1981) Biochem. Pharmacol. $\underline{30}$, 771.
32. Hesslewood IP, Cramp WA, McBrien DCH, Williamson P, Lott KAK. (1978) Br. J. Cancer $\underline{37}$, 95.
33. Kägi JHR, Nordberg M. eds. (1979) Metallothionein, Birkhauser Verlag, Basel.
34. Lerch K. (1982) Metal Ions in Biol. Syst. $\underline{13}$, 299.
35. Fox CL. (1968) Arch. Surg. $\underline{96}$, 184.
36. Agrawal KC, Bears KB, Marcus D, Jonassen HB. (1978) Proc. Am. Assoc. Cancer Res. $\underline{19}$, 28.
37. Simon TM, Kunishima DH, Vibert GJ, Lorber A. (1981) Cancer Res. $\underline{41}$, 94.
38. Razi MT, Otiko G, Sadler PJ. (1983) ACS Symposium Ser. $\underline{209}$, 371.
39. Simon TM, Kunishima DH, Vibert GJ, Lorber A. (1979), Cancer $\underline{44}$, 1965.
40. Simon TM, Kunishima DH, Vibert GJ, Lorber A. (1979) J. Rheum. $\underline{6}$ (Suppl. 5) 91.
41. Sutton BM. (1983) ACS Symposium Ser. $\underline{209}$, 305.
42. Otiko G, Sadler PJ. Unpublished, and Otiko G. PhD thesis (1982) Univ. of London.
43. Glass GE, Vonnent JH, Britton D, Tobias RS (1968) J. Amer. Chem. Soc. $\underline{90}$, 1131.
44. Calis GHM, Trooster JM, Razi MT, Sadler PJ. (1982) J. Inorg. Biochem. $\underline{17}$, 139.
45. Malik NA (1980) PhD thesis Univ. of London, and Malik NA, Sadler PJ. unpublished.
46. Gibson DW, Beer M, Barrett RJ. (1971) Biochemistry $\underline{10}$, 3669.

SECTION VI

UNIQUE THERAPEUTIC APPROACHES USING PLATINUM COORDINATION COMPLEXES

Chaired by J. Burchenal

Overview
J. Burchenal

In this session on unique techniques of platinum administration two general areas were covered: (1) new clinically studied analogues which might cut down the undesirable side effects of a broad spectrum of anti-tumor activity and, (2) new techniques of administration which, again, might avoid some of the undesirable side effects of the present derivatives and at the same time increase the anti-tumor activity.

It was mentioned in the introduction that the formal papers in this session would deal with the clinical trials of two of the new derivatives, the 1,2-diaminocyclohexane, 4-carboxyphthalato platinum (JM-82), DACCP, and the 1,1-diaminomethylcyclohexane (sulfato) platinum II (TNO-6), and that the much more thoroughly studied analogue cis-diammine 1,1 cyclobutanediboxylate platinum II (CBDCA or JM-8) would only be presented as a poster in this session but would be discussed in detail in the next session. Similarly, the use of hypertonic saline administered with the cis-platinum to prevent the renal toxicity and allow the administration of much higher and more effective doses of cis-platinum was covered by a paper in this session, whereas such other methods of administration of cis-platinum as the intraarterial and intraperitoneal administration were covered only in the posters and in the discussion.

The inferences to be drawn from this session were that of the new analogues clinically evaluated to date, CBDCA, or JM-8, appears the most promising. It has produced both complete and partial remissions in patients with ovarian carcinoma; in 34 patients not previously treated with cis-platinum, 8 complete remissions and 11 partial responses occurred. No renal toxicity or ototoxicity were noted in these patients, and peripheral neuropathy was observed in only 1 patient. The limiting toxicity was myelosuppression, with nausea and vomiting being rather regular but generally considered as less than with cis-platinum. Even in the group of 33 patients previously treated with cis-platinum, 21% remissions were seen in small cell lung cancer, and overall response rate was 34%. In testicular tumors, with known resistance to other therapy, only 1 out of 5 patients had a minor regression, but in 4 patients previously untreated but with advanced disease, all responded to therapy.

In contrast, JM-82, the carboxyphthalato analogue DACCP, which had shown interesting effects in patients with nasopharyngeal, cervical, lung and gastic cancer previously treated, has not as yet had adequate Phase II trial in the signal tumors due to synthetic difficulties which limited the supply available. As with CBDCA the limiting toxicity was thrombocytopenia, and nephrotoxicity was uncommon in the Phase I trial except in 1 patient who was thought to be septic and was given an aminoglycoside antibiotic. Peripheral neuropathy was seen in patients treated with multiple courses of the agent.

Similarly with TNO-6, adequate Phase II trials have not as yet been done. In Phase I studies, one partial response was achieved in carcinoma of the lung, ovarian carcinoma, small cell lung cancer, and testicular cancer. Except for the patients with breast cancer, all patients had been shown to be resistant to cis-platinum. As with the other new analogues, thrombocytopenia was the limiting toxicity, although in addition there was also a significant occurrence of proteinuria which could be partially averted by giving TNO-6 in prolonged infusions over a four-hour period. Similar increase in creatinine was seen in patients receiving maximum tolerated doses of 35 mg/m^2 regardless of whether it was given rapidly or by prolonged infusion. Thus, of the three analogues discussed, JM-8 appears to be the most thoroughly tested and appears to demonstrate superiority over cis-platinum in that it is equally effective and produces no nephro- or ototoxicity. The other two, as well as the bis(isopropylamine)-dihydroxydichloroplatinum IV derivative (CHIP) will require further studies before their place in the therapeutic armamentarium can be evaluated.

Another approach to increasing the effectiveness of cis-platinum was the study by Ozols and the group at the National Cancer Institute who gave cis-platinum at 40 mg/m^2 daily x 5 dissolved in 250 ml of 3% sodium chloride and gave a total of 6 liters of saline daily x 5 days by continuous intravenous drip. In this way, they achieved a total platinum dosage of 200 mg/m^2 every four weeks and reported effects in far-advanced germ cell tumors much superior to those to be expected with conventional administration of cis-platinum, with no sign of nephrotoxicity.

Two other approaches which succeeded in increasing the concentrations of cis-platinum, at least in the localized tumor area while still allowing reasonably high concentrations in the systemic circulation, were the intra-peritoneal injections of cis-platinum in ovarian carcinoma with ascites and the intraarterial use of cis-platinum in localized but far-advanced osteo-genic sarcoma. Preliminary studies with both of these techniques suggested the value of this approach. Indeed, both the clinical trial of the newer analogues and clinical and pharmacologic evaluations of the unique approaches to the administration bode well for future progress in this areas.

Phase I and Early Phase II Trials of 4'Carboxyphthalato (1,2 Diaminocyclohexane) Platinum (II)

D.P. Kelsen, H. Scher and J. Burchenal

INTRODUCTION

Cisplatin (DDP) was the first heavy-metal antineoplastic
agent to enter clinical trial. During its initial studies,
nephrotoxicity limited use of the drug, and its clinical
utility was questioned.[1] By use of a variety of techniques,
which included prehydration and a mannitol-induced diuresis,
DDP's therapeutic index was increased, and broad Phase II
trials performed.[2] DDP has demonstrated substantial activity
in the treatment of a variety of solid tumors and is now part
of the first-line of therapy for patients with disseminated
testicular, ovarian, or bladder cancer.[3-5] However, nephrotoxicity remains the dose-limiting factor, and the drug causes
severe emesis in many patients. If higher dosages ($90-120mg/m^2$)
are used, hospitalization is usually required. There is, thus,
intense interest in the development of new, second generation
platinum analogues which may (1) have a broader therapeutic
index, (2) lack cross resistance with the parent compound,
(3) have activity in tumors resistant to DDP and (4) be at
least as active as Cisplatin in tumors responsive to that drug.

4'Carboxyphthalato (1,2 diaminocyclohexane) platinum (II)
(DACCP) is one of 4 cisplatin analogues which have recently
begun their initial trials. All were chosen because, in preclinical screening, they had less toxicity than did the parent
compound. In addition, the diaminocyclohexane (DAC) analogues
were of interest because of their activity in L-1210 cell lines
resistant to cisplatin.[6] Besides its in vitro lack of cross
resistance, DACCP has the advantage, over other DAC compounds,
of high solubility in alkaline solutions. The major disadvan-
tage of DACCP was a formulation problem. This question had

been addressed to the point that adequate supplies of clinically acceptable material were available for a Phase I and pilot Phase II trial, therefore, DACCP was chosen for study at the Memorial Sloan-Kettering Cancer Center.

MATERIALS AND METHODS

The Phase I clinical trial of DACCP was performed in 45 patients with advanced cancer. In all cases, patients had malignant tumors that were refractory to conventional therapy or for which no effective conventional treatment exists. In the disease-oriented Phase II trials, patients with diseases known to be responsive to conventional therapy (e.g. testicular cancer) had all received prior chemotherapy, but had relapsed. Patients with other malignancies, such as non-small cell lung cancer, gastric, or esophageal cancer, for which conventional therapy is unsatisfactory, could receive the Phase II agent as first-line chemotherapy. All patients had histologic proof of malignancy confirmed by the department of pathology, MSKCC.

Prior to entrance into the study, all patients underwent a complete blood count and differential, platelet count, 12-channel screening profile, chest roentgenogram, urine analysis, electrocardiogram, prothrombin and partial thromboplastin time and creatinine clearance. Radionuclide scans, computerized tomograms and audiograms were obtained when clinically indicated.

During the Phase I trial, complete blood counts and platelet counts and screening profiles were repeated twice weekly; during the Phase II studies, they were obtained every 2-3 weeks; prior to retreatment, [and a 24 hour creatinine clearance], they were repeated, as were studies needed to assess response.

DACCP was supplied as a lyophilized powder (synthesized by Johnson Matthey, Inc., Malvern, Penna and supplied by Bristol Laboratories, Syracuse, New York).

The drug was prepared, immediately prior to administration, by adding DACCP 10mg/m^2 to a solution of 8.4% sodium bicarbonate (U.S.P.): 5% dextrose in water at a ratio of 1:9. The DACCP solution was stirred vigorously for 2 minutes, and then filtered through a 0.20 micron Nalgene filter (Nalge Co., Rochester, N.Y.). The solution was then added to 50ml of 5% Dextrose in water, and administered as a rapid i.v. infusion over 15-20 minutes.

During the initial portion of the Phase I trial, 1000ml of 5% dextrose and 0.45% sodium chloride were given prior to DACCP; a second liter of the same solution was given after drug administration. Later in the study, it was found that at doses up to 640mg/m^2 only one liter of fluid was needed. At the 720mg/m^2 level, we continue to use 2 liters of hydration. The Phase I trial followed a modified Fibonnacci schema, and dose levels from 40-800mg/m^2 were studied. During the Phase II trials, 640-720mg/m^2 were given. For both trials, the interval between doses was 28 days.

For patients with measurable disease, the criteria of response used were similar to that of Miller et.al., with the addition of a minor response category (>25% but <50% decrease in tumor measurements).[7] For patients with esophageal cancer in whom the primary lesion was part of (or the only) evaluable lesion, criteria of response were identical to those previously reported.[8] Prior to the initiation of therapy, informed consent was obtained from all patients.

Pharmacokinetic analysis of platinum concentrations were performed during the Phase I trial, using flameless atomic absorption spectrophotometry. The techniques used were identical to those used to measure platinum concentrations after cisplatin administration; they have been previously reported.[9]

RESULTS

Therapeutic Activity - Phase I Trial

This portion of the study has already been reported in detail.[10] As one would expect for a Phase I trial, the vast majority of patients (80%) had received prior chemotherapy; two-thirds had received prior radiation therapy. Approximately 50% of patients had measurable disease. Fifteen patients had lung cancer, and 11 had sarcomas. Characteristics of the patient population are shown in Table I.

TABLE I

Patient Characteristics

	No. of Patients
Patients entered	45
Adults	34
Pediatric	11
Median age	42 (3-73)
Median performance status	70 (40-90)
Sex	
Male	31
Female	14
Prior therapy	
None	3
Chemotherapy	11
Radiation	5
Chemotherapy/radiation therapy	26

The major toxicities seen were myelosuppression and nephrotoxicity, and are discussed in detail below. The conclusion of the study was that the recommended starting dosage for Phase II trials was 640mg/m^2 with escalation to 720mg/m^2 level if toxicity was acceptable; during the Phase I trial, therapeutic activity was seen in patients with nasopharyngeal and cervical cancer (PR) with MR seen in lung and gastric cancer. The patients with lung, nasopharyngeal and gastric cancer had been previously treated.

Therapeutic Activity - Phase II Trial

On the basis of the Phase I study, pilot Phase II trials were initiated in non-small cell lung cancer, esophageal, gastric, ovarian, testicular, bladder and colon cancers. Only the lung cancer study has been completed.

Non-Small Cell Lung Cancer: Thirty-three patients were entered into this trial. Characteristics of the patient population are shown in Table II.

TABLE II

Non-Small Cell Lung Cancer

Entered	33
Evaluable	28
Median Age (Range)	55 (34-74)
M:F	28:5
Median P.S. (Range)	70 (50-90)
Prior Therapy	
None	12
Chemotherapy	10
Chemotherapy/Radiation	11
Prior Cisplatin	18

Although most had been heavily pretreated, 12 patients had not received prior chemotherapy. Only 1 partial response (PR) was seen among the 28 evaluable cases. This patient had previously been treated with cisplatin and vindesine, and had developed progressive disease after an initial partial response. His remission on DACCP lasted for 3 months. One additional patient had stabilization of disease. The 95% confidence limits for this trial are 0-17%.

Colon Cancer: To date, 11 patients with advanced cancer have received an adequate trial with DACCP. Eight had not received prior chemotherapy. No responses have been seen.

Ovarian Cancer: Eight patients with ovarian cancer, all of whom had received extensive prior chemotherapy with cisplatin containing combinations, have been treated with DACCP. One partial response, of 5 months duration, was noted.

Gastric Cancer: Nine patients with advanced adenocarcinomas of the upper gastrointestinal tract have had adequate trials with DACCP. Six of these patients had not received prior systemic therapy. One partial response, of 5 months duration, was seen. None of the 3 previously treated patients responded.

Epidermoid Carcinomas of the Esophagus: Nine patients with esophageal cancer have also had adequate trials. Four had received prior therapy with a cisplatin-containing regimen. One minor response was seen.

Testicular Cancer: Eight patients with advanced testicular cancer have been treated to date. All had received extensive prior chemotherapy with cisplatin containing combinations. None of these patients have responded.

Bladder Cancer: Five patients have received adequate trials. All but one were previously treated. One partial response was seen.

Toxicities: During the Phase I study, hematologic toxicity was first noted at the $280mg/m^2$ dose level and subsequently single patients at each level had moderate leukopenia. However, no decrease in the median white blood count nadir below 3,000 cells was observed even at the maximally tolerated dose. At $800mg/m^2$ the dose-limiting toxicity of thrombocytopenia was reached. The median platelet count nadir at 640mg/m^2 was 104,000 occurring on day 11. At 800mg/m^2, the median again occurred on day 11 but was 26,000, with three of the seven patients requiring at least one platelet transfusion. The recommended starting dose for Phase II trials was, therefore, 640mg/m^2 with dose escalation to 720mg/m^2 if no thrombocytopenia, granulocytopenia or nephrotoxicity were observed. In the Phase II trial, although many patients had prior therapy, hematologic toxicity was moderate. In patients with non-small cell lung cancer treated at 640 and 720mg/m^2, 3/29 or 11% had platelet nadirs below 125,000, and 2/29 or 7% had white blood count nadirs below 3,000 cells/mm^3. In the other Phase II trial the degree of prior therapy appears to have played a major influence as only patients with ovarian carcinoma and germ cell carcinoma have demonstrated significant thrombocytopenia. 5/9 adequately treated patients with ovarian and 2/7 adequately treated patients with germ cell malignancies have shown various platelet nadirs below 75,000.

Nephrotoxicity was uncommon in the Phase I trial. Using the hydration schedule outlined above, no elevations in serum creatinine above 1.6mg/m^2 were observed until the 360mg/m^2 dose level. At the 640mg/m^2 level, 3 patients had peak creatinines greater than 1.5 which returned to normal. At 80mg/m^2, 3 of 7 patients had peak creatinines greater than 1.5. There was one patient who developed irreversible, fatal, renal failure in the Phase I trial. She was noted to be febrile the night following treatment, and was felt to be septic. An aminoglycoside antibiotic was given. At post mortem, severe renal tubular necrosis was observed; she was considered to have a drug related death, although since an aminoglycoside was used, toxicity could not wholly be ascribed to DACCP. Since nephrotoxicity was minimal at the 640 level, a lesser degree of hydration (1 liter total) was used in 10 additional patients. When no toxicity was seen, this regimen was given thereafter. In the Phase II trials, minimal increases in the creatinine were noted even in a heavily pretreated population, such as ovarian and germ cell neoplasms, who had received a median of four courses of prior cisplatin.

Nausea and vomiting were observed at all dose levels throughout this Phase I trial although this was described as quantitatively less and of shorter duration than with cisplatin. It would usually occur approximately four hours after the dose and last anywhere from 4 to 8 hours. In general, patients were eating the next morning. In the Phase II trial, metaclopramide was used in selected cases. It did ameloriate the symptoms in most cases although this was not systematically studied. Diarrhea was observed in approximately 30% of patients above $640mg/m^2$. Fever was seen in seven patients during the Phase I study. Serial cultures and pyrogen testing were performed and were negative. Alopecia was not seen and in several cases hair growth resumed. A decrease in auditory function was observed in one patient who had received six courses of cisplatin and 6,000 Rads to the head and neck area for a nasopharyngeal carcinoma. He developed moderate ototoxicity following his eighth dose of DACCP and an audiogram showed high tone losses above 4000 hertz. In the Phase II trials a decrease in auditory acuity was observed in two patients both of whom had received prior cisplatin.

Allergic reactions were observed in both the Phase I and II trials. Two patients who had received prior cisplatin developed hives and urticaria on dose one. One patient developed anaphylaxis on the fourth dose of treatment, despite premedication with benadryl; she recovered uneventfully. Although allergic reactions were observed in the Phase II trials, patients who developed hives and urticaria were premedicated with benedryl and steroids for subsequent doses. No additional cases of anaphylaxis were observed.

More disturbing was the development of a peripheral neuropathy in patients treated with multiple courses of the agent. In the Phase I trial this was seen in four patients who had received four or more doses of the drug. However, two of these patients had received prior cisplatin and vinca alkaloids. Nerve conduction studies performed on these patients revealed a marked sensory loss. In the Phase II trial three patients

who received three courses of the agent developed a peripheral
neuropathy. Once again, these patients had been treated with
prior vinca alkaloids and cisplatin. One patient was removed
from the study because of significant toxicity. The symptoms
lasted approximately four to six months.

Hypomagnesemia was not seen in the Phase I trial except
in two patients who had decreased magnesium levels at the start
of thereapy.

Pharmacokinetics

During the Phase I trial, the pharmacokinetics of DACCP
were investigated in 9 patients at 3 dosage levels: 40, 200,
640Mg/m^2. The result of these studies, performed using flameless atomic absorption spectrophotometry, are summarized in
Table III. The T$\frac{1}{2}$ first was similar to that of cisplatin,
the T$\frac{1}{2}$ second phase was substantially shorter than that seen
with cisplatin.

Pharmacokinetic Behavior of DACCP

Drug Dosage (mg/sq m)	Mean Peak Plasma [platinum] (Mg/ml)		Mean T$\frac{1}{2}$ First (min)		Second (hr)	
	Total	Filterable	Total	Filterable	Total	Filterable
40	6.4	0.9	22	12	18.2	15.8
200	20.5	4.5	33	18	20.7	19.9
640	81.7	15.1	65	18	14.9	16

DISCUSSION

DACCP is one of the first cisplatin analogues to enter
clinical trial. It attracted interest because it was found
to be non-cross resistant with cisplatin in Ll210 leukemia.
In studies by Burchenal et.al., Ll210 cell lines that were
resistant to 2.5Mg/ml of cisplatin (Ll210/DDP) responded to
DACCP in concentrations of 0.23Mg/ml (similar to concentrations
required in cell lines still sensitive to cisplatin).[6]
Although other DAC compounds also lacked cross-resistance
with cisplatin in these cell lines, they were relatively
insoluble. DACCP, in contrast, is highly soluble in alkaline
solutions.

Preclinical studies by Philips and co-workers used an every two week single dosage schedule. They studied both DACCP and cisplatin. Their studies suggested that, in mice, cisplatin was 10 times more lethal than DACCP. The major histologic changes were renal tubular necrosis and bone marrow aplasia. During the Phase I trial in humans, renal toxicity was indeed seen at the higher dosage levels, but the dose-limiting factor (DLT) was thrombocytopenia. Interestingly, thrombocytopenia has also been the DLT in the Phase I trials of CBDCA (JM8) and of CHIP (JM9).[11-12]

The Phase II trials of DACCP have looked at 3 groups of solid tumors: those in which cisplatin is highly active (testicular, ovarian and bladder); diseases where cisplatin has modest activity (esophageal, gastric, lung); and disease where cisplatin is essentially inactive (colon). Almost every patient in the first group has received extensive prior therapy before entering the DACCP trial, so that the lack of activity in testicular cancer, and modest activity in ovarian and bladder tumors, is not surprising. Studying investigational agents in testicular cancer, a highly curable disease, is difficult, as one is reluctant to use these drugs as early therapy for fear of compromising responses to conventional chemotherapy. For patients with ovarian and bladder cancer, where, in advanced disease chemotherapy is far less likely to be curative, using cisplatin analogues up front is a more acceptable concept.

For those diseases where cisplatin has been of only modest activity, DACCP has not been more effective. In lung cancer, pooled data from several Phase II trials indicates that cis-platin has 15-20% activity in previously untreated patients; in those who have had prior therapy, the response rate was even lower. Thus, the preliminary data with DACCP, having a range of 0-17% (95% confidence limits), suggests similar activity. The situation applies in esophageal and gastric cancer where cisplatin also has activity in the 10-20% range. Finally, in colon cancer, where cisplatin is essentially an inactive agent, DACCP has also failed to demonstrate significant response.

As was the case in the Phase I trial, Phase II studies suggest that DACCP has less renal toxicity and is less emetogenic than cisplatin. Furthermore, the degree of myelosuppression seen in these patients, who had not received as much prior chemotherapy, was substantially less. It is possible that higher dosages of DACCP could be given, but at that point, nephrotoxicity may be more of a factor, requiring a larger fluid diuresis.

Thus, DACCP has to date demonstrated only minimal to modest activity in those tumors studied. Formulation problems have always been a major factor in the use of this agent, and they have have not been overcome. Before DACCP undergoes further Phase II trials, these formulation questions must be solved.

REFERENCES

1. Higby, D.J., Wallace, H.J., Jr., and Holland, J.F. Cisdiamminedichloroplatinum (NSC-119875): a Phase I study. Cancer Chemotherapy Rep. 57:459-463, 1973.
2. Hayes, D.M., Cvitkovic, E., Golbey, R.B., et.al. High dose cis-platinum diammine dichloride: amelioration of renal toxicity by mannitol diuresis. Cancer 39:1372-1381, 1977.
3. Wiltshaw, E., and Kroner, T. Phase II study of Cis-dichlorodiammineplatinum (II) (NSC 119875) in advanced adenocarcinoma of the ovary. Cancer Treat Rep. 60:55-60, 1976.
4. Yagoda, A., Watson, R.C., Gonzalez-Vitale, C., et.al. Cis-dichlorodiammineplatinum (II) in advanced bladder cancer. Cancer Treat Rep. 60:917-923, 1976.
5. Einhorn, L. and Donohue, J. Cis-Diammine dichloroplatinum, vinblastine and bleomycin combination chemotherapy in disseminated testicular cancer. Ann. Intern.Med. 87:293-298, 1977.
6. Burchenal, J., Kalaher, K., Dew, K., et al. Studies of cross-resistance, synergistic combination, and blocking of activity of platinum derivatives. Biochimie 60:961-965, 1978.
7. Miller, A.B., Hoogstraten, B., Staquet, M., et.al. Reporting results of cancer treatment. Cancer 47:207-214, 1981.
8. Kelsen, D.P., Ahudja, R., Hopfan, S. et.al. Combined Modality Therapy of Esophageal Cancer. Cancer 48:31-37, 1981.
9. Kelsen, D.P., Hoffman, J., Alcock, N. et.al. Pharmaco-kinetics of cisplatin regional hepatic infusions. Am. J. Clin. Oncol. 5:173-178, 1982.

10. Kelsen, D.P., Scher, H., Alcock, N. et.al. Phase I
    Clinical Trial and Pharmacokinetics of 4'Carboxyphthalato
    (1,2 diamminecyclohexane) Platinum (II). Cancer Research
    42:4831-4835, 1982.
11. Calvert, A. et.al. Early Clinical studies with cis-Diammine
    1,2 cyclobutane Dicarboxylate Platinum II. Cancer Chemo-
    therapy Pharmacol. 9:140-147, 1982.
12. Creaven, P., et.al. Phase I study of a new Antineoplastic
    Platinum Analogue Cis-dichloro-trans-dihydroxy-bis-isopro-
    pylamine Platinum (IV) (CHIP) Proceed ASCO 1:102, 1982.

High Dose Cisplatin in Hypertonic Saline: Renal Effects and Pharmacokinetics of a 40 MG/M² QD × 5 Schedule

R.F. Ozols, B.J. Corden, J. Collins and R.C. Young

1. INTRODUCTION

Cisplatin appears to have a clinically important dose-response in both testicular and ovarian cancer patients. Cisplatin at 120 mg/m^2 produced a 50% response rate in ovarian cancer patients who had failed cisplatin at a dose of 50-75 mg/m^2 (1). Similarly, a 55% response rate was reported with cisplatin at 120 mg/m^2 in testicular cancer patients who were refractory to a combination chemotherapy regimen which included cisplatin at a lower dose (2). Cisplatin, however, has not been routinely administered at doses greater than 100-120 mg/m^2 due to an unacceptable incidence of nephrotoxicity which develops even in the presence of adequate hydration and mannitol or furosemide diuresis. Nevertheless, it would be potentially clinically useful to escalate the dose of cisplatin since there remain subsets of patients with ovarian cancer and testicular cancer, primarily characterized by the presence of bulk disease, in whom standard dose cisplatin based combination therapy is not optimal (3-5).

Litterst (6) and Earhardt (7), however, have recently demonstrated in animals that cisplatin nephrotoxicity, but not the antitumor effect, is affected by the vehicle of administration of cisplatin and by the maintenance of a chloruresis. On the basis of these studies, we have administered cisplatin at 40 mg/m^2 qd x 5 (twice the standard dose) in hypertonic saline in testicular and ovarian cancer patients in whom an enhanced chloruresis was maintained using saline and KCl hydration.

2. MATERIALS AND METHODS

2.1. Patients

Two groups of patients have been treated with high dose cisplatin: (1) Twenty previously untreated poor prognosis testicular cancer patients have received high dose cisplatin as part of an intensive 4-drug regimen termed PVeBV, Table 1; (2) 7 relapsed ovarian cancer patients who had failed cisplatin-containing combination chemotherapy regimens (total dose 360-1140 mg) were treated on an ongoing Phase II trial of high dose cisplatin.

2.2. High dose cisplatin

The details of high dose cisplatin administration are summarized in Table 2. The patients were carefully observed for signs and symptoms of fluid overload. Serum electrolytes, magnesium, BUN and creatinine were measured daily during therapy. Intravenous magnesium was administered to hypomagnesemic patients. Creatinine clearances were measured prior to each cycle of high dose cisplatin. Patients with tumor-produced obstructive uropathy were treated without dose modification of cisplatin or alteration in the hydration regimen.

Table 1. PVeBV Chemotherapy[a]

Cisplatin	(P)	40 mg/m^2 i.v. qd x 5	
Vinblastine	(Ve)	0.2 mg/kg i.v. day 1	q 21 days
VP-16-213	(V)	100 mg/m^2 i.v. qd x 5	
Bleomycin	(B)	30 u i.v. q wk x 9	

[a]Ozols et al., Cancer 1983; 51: 1803-1807.

Table 2. Administration of High Dose Cisplatin

Hydration:	Normal saline with 20 meq KCl per liter at 250 ml/hour starting 12 hours prior to the first dose of cisplatin and finishing 12 hours after the last dose on day 5.
Diuretic:	Twenty mg intravenous furosemide immediately prior to each dose of cisplatin.
Cisplatin:	40 mg/m^2 dissolved in 250 ml of 3% saline and administered over 30 minutes.
Antiemetic:	Dexamethasone or metaclopramide.

2.3. Pharmacokinetic analysis

Pharmacokinetic analysis of cisplatin was performed as previously described (8). Briefly, blood was collected after the completion of the cisplatin infusion and the plasma was separated into two fractions by ultrafiltration through membrane cones with a molecular weight cut-off of 25,000 Daltons. Platinum content was then determined in the two fractions using atomic absorption spectroscopy.

3. RESULTS

3.1. Renal effects in previously untreated testicular cancer patients

The effects of high dose cisplatin in hypertonic saline upon renal function in 17 poor prognosis testicular cancer patients receiving PVeBV chemotherapy have previously been reported (8,9). There was no difference in the mean value for the serum creatinines prior to therapy and after completion of 3-4 cycles of high dose cisplatin. All the patients had serum creatinines in the normal range after completion of therapy. There were only 2 patients who developed elevated serum creatinines while on therapy and both of these patients were in septic shock at the time of renal failure. One of these patients recovered and was subsequently retreated with high dose cisplatin without further elevations in serum creatinine.

Creatinine clearances were also not significantly altered in these patients. There was no significant difference in the mean of the creatinine clearance prior to and after completion of 3-4 cycles of PVeBV. There were 8 patients who had evidence of tumor associated obstructive uropathy including one patient with a completely non-functioning kidney and a creatinine clearance of 35 ml/min. These patients were treated without modification of the dose of cisplatin or of the hydration regimen. The mean post-treatment creatinine clearance in this group of patients was 91 ml/min. The one patient with complete obstruction of a kidney had rapid improvement of renal function and resolution of the obstruction with the first cycle of PVeBV (9).

Hypomagnesemia occurred in 90% of the patients during therapy and even though the patients were asymptomatic, we administered supplemental intravenous magnesium. All patients, however, had normal magnesium levels, without oral or intravenous supplementation, within 2-4 months after the last dose of PVeBV.

3.2. Renal effects in previously treated ovarian cancer patients

Seven patients with refractory ovarian cancer who had previously received standard doses of cisplatin have been treated on an ongoing Phase II trial of high dose cisplatin in hypertonic saline (8). The pretreatment serum creatinines were normal and their creatinine clearances ranged from 35 ml/min to 90 ml/min. Four of the patients have not had any significant changes in creatinine or creatinine clearance while on high dose cisplatin. Three patients had an elevation of creatinines (↑2.0 mg/dl) with their first cycle of high dose cisplatin. Two of these patients were retreated with high dose cisplatin when their renal function had returned to pretreatment levels and did not have any elevation in creatinine with their second and subsequent cycles of high dose cisplatin. One patient with a creatinine clearance of 35 ml/min prior to high dose cisplatin developed asymptomatic transient renal failure with a peak serum creatinine of 5.5 mg/dl. Her renal function returned to pretreatment levels over a 4-week period but she has not received any further high dose cisplatin.

3.3. Volume effects of hydration

The extensive hydration (6L normal saline per day) and the 3% saline have been well tolerated by both the young men (medium age 26, range 18-34 years) with testicular cancer and the middle aged women (median age 56, range 40-62 years) with advanced ovarian cancer. There were only two instances of ovarian cancer patients developing transient trace-1+ pitting edema in the lower extremities while receiving the five days of hydration and cisplatin. However, none of the patients developed signs or symptoms of congestive heart failure.

3.4. Non-renal toxicity of high dose cisplatin

The toxicity of the PVeBV regimen in testicular cancer patients has previously been described (9,10). The major toxicity is myelosuppression. Post treatment audiograms have also demonstrated a high tone frequency loss in all patients after 3-4 cycles of high dose cisplatin. However, only 2/15 testicular cancer patients who have completed therapy have developed functional hearing impairment which has required the use of a hearing aid. In addition, 30% of the patients have had transient peripheral neuropathies associated with PVeBV.

In the heavily pre-treated refractory ovarian cancer patients receiving high dose cisplatin, the major toxicity has been myelosuppression, particularly thrombocytopenia. All patients have also received prophylactic platelet transfusions with at least one cycle of high dose cisplatin for transient platelet counts below 20,000/ul. In addition, 4/7 patients have developed numbness and tingling in the distal extremities resulting in gait disturbances. The duration of the peripheral neuropathy as well as the exact incidence of this toxicity will require more patients and further follow-up. The peripheral neuropathy is likely multifactorial as all the ovarian cancer patients had received prior therapy with other neurotoxins including misonidazole, hexamethylmelamine, and standard dose cisplatin.

3.5. Therapeutic benefit of high dose cisplatin

The preliminary results of PVeBV in poor prognosis non-seminomatous testicular cancer patients have recently been reported (9,10). The overall complete remission rate with PVeBV is 85% which is markedly superior to our previous results with a standard dose cisplatin regimen which resulted in a 43% complete remission rate in a similar group of poor prognosis patients (11).

The response rate of high dose cisplatin in refractory ovarian cancer patients awaits the completion of the ongoing Phase II trial. However, in the first 6 evaluable patients treated with high dose cisplatin, there have been 3 partial responses, and 2 patients have had stabilization of disease.

3.6. Pharmacokinetic analysis of high dose and standard dose cisplatin

The pharmacokinetic analysis of high dose cisplatin has previously been reported (8) and is summarized in Table 3. Of note is the longer half life of disappearance of ultrafilterable platinum (36 minutes) in heavily treated patients receiving high dose cisplatin compared to previously untreated patients receiving either high dose cisplatin or standard dose (20 mg/m^2 qd x 5) cisplatin (20 minutes). This difference may be due to saturation of cisplatin binding sites. While the pharmacokinetic analysis does not explain the absence of nephrotoxicity associated with the administration of high dose cisplatin in hypertonic saline, the measurement of chloride levels in the urine and plasma indicated that a brisk chloruresis was induced by the hydration regimen as well as (in some patients) a mild hyperchloremia which rapidly returned to normal after completion of the infusion.

Table 3. Pharmacokinetics of High Dose Cisplatin (40 mg/m^2 qd x 5)[a]

1. Decay of ultrafilterable platinum from serum follows first order kinetics.

 a) Half life for disappearance of ultrafilterable platinum was not different on days 1 and 5.

2. There was a significant difference in the half life for heavily pretreated patients (36.3 $\pm$ 6.3 minutes) compared to that in previously untreated patients or in patients receiving conventional doses of cisplatin (19.9 $\pm$ 3.2 minutes).

3. Total urinary chloride excretion was six times greater in patients on high dose cisplatin compared to normal patients.

4. Serum chloride concentrations were also greater in some patients on high dose cisplatin compared to patients receiving standard dose cisplatin.

[a]Corden et al. Proc. Amer. Soc. Clin. Oncol. 1983; 24: C-132.

4. DISCUSSION

These results demonstrate that high dose cisplatin administered in hypertonic saline with concomitant maintenance of a vigorous chloruresis is not nephrotoxic in previously untreated testicular cancer patients. Of particular note was the observation that even in patients with tumor associated obstructive uropathy, high dose cisplatin did not result in any nephrotoxicity. These results are in contrast to previous reports in testicular cancer patients in which it was demonstrated that the creatinine clearance after 6 cycles of PVeB (which contain the same total dose of cisplatin as 3 cycles of PVeBV) resulted in a 40% decrease in the creatinine clearance compared to pretreatment levels (12).

The exact mechanism for the protective effect on renal function of chloride ion has not been established. It has previously been postulated that a high chloride ion concentration suppresses hydrolysis of cisdichlorodiammine platinum and thereby decreases the concentration of toxic aquated species of cisplatin in the renal tubule (6,7). In contrast, intracellularly, where the chloride concentration is markedly lower than in the serum, the equilibria now favors formation of the aquated species. Alternatively, a high chloride ion concentration may suppress the direct reaction of dichlorodiammine platinum with nucleophiles. A suppression of the reaction of cisplatin with sulfhydryl containing macromolecules in the renal tubules may account for the decreased nephrotoxicity observed when a chloruresis is maintained.

The extensive chloruresis observed in our patients who have received this hydration regimen provides indirect support for both hypotheses. From our data it is not possible to determine the role of hypertonic saline, per se, compared to the vigorous hydration with normal saline in the prevention of nephrotoxicity. Additional support for the importance of the chloruresis stems from our observation that hypertonic saline does not protect from the non-renal toxicities of cisplatin, namely gastrointestinal, peripheral neuropathy, ototoxicity, and myelosuppression. While the exact mechanisms for these toxic effects of cisplatin have not been established, it seems likely that toxicity is a function of intracellular cisplatin levels in susceptible cells. The small changes in serum chloride concentration would not be likely to lower the intracellular content of reactive species of cisplatin in hematologic stem cells, for example, which would be required to decrease the myelosuppressive effects of cisplatin.

The relative frequency and severity of the non-renal toxicities of high dose cisplatin compared to standard dose cisplatin have not yet been determined and await the completion of ongoing prospective clinical trials in previously untreated patients. Thus, while we have observed a disturbing incidence of neurotoxicity in the Phase II trial of high dose cisplatin in refractory ovarian cancer patients it is possible that this may not be dose limiting in previously untreated ovarian cancer patients who have not had prior exposure to neurotoxins such as hexamethylmelamine, standard dose cisplatin, and misonidazole as have the patients in the Phase II trial. The absence of severe neurotoxicity in the previously untreated testicular cancer patients receiving high dose cisplatin as part of PVeBV provides further support for this possibility.

The clinical benefit of high dose cisplatin has not yet been established. However, the preliminary results of PVeBV in poor prognosis non-seminomatous testicular cancer patients [complete remission rate of 85% (9,10)] are markedly superior to our previous studies in which a 43% complete remission rate was obtained in a similar group of patients treated with a standard dose cisplatin combination chemotherapy regimen (11). The responses observed in the ongoing Phase II trial of high dose cisplatin in patients who had failed standard dose cisplatin regimens have led to clinical trials in the Medicine Branch, NCI of escalated cisplatin doses in previously untreated ovarian cancer patients.

REFERENCES

1. Bruckner HW, Wallach R, Cohen CJ, Deppe G, Kabakow B, Ratner L, and Holland JF. High-dose platinum for the treatment of refractory ovarian cancer. Gynecol. Oncol. 1981; 12: 61-67.

2. Hayes DM, Cvitkovic E, Golbey RB, Scheiner E, Helson L, Krakoff IH. High dose cis-platinum diamminedichloride: amelioration of renal toxicity by mannitol diuresis. Cancer 1977; 39: 1372-1381.

3. Ozols RF and Young RC. Patterns of failure of chemotherapy in gynecologic malignancies. Cancer Treat. Rep. 1983; in press.

4. Einhorn LH, Donahue JP. Cis-diamminedichloroplatinum, vinblastine, and bleomycin combination chemotherapy in disseminated testicular cancer. Ann. Int. Med. 1977; 87: 293-298.

5. Samson MR, Fisher R, Stephens RL, Rivkin S, Opipavi M, Maloney J, Groppe CW. Vinblastine, bleomycin, and cis-diamminedichloroplatinum in disseminated testicular cancer: response to treatment and prognostic correlations. Europ. J. Cancer 1981; 16: 1359-1366.

6. Litterst CL. Alterations in the toxicity of cis-dichlorodiammine-platinum and in tissue localization of platinum as a funciton of NaCl concentration in the vehicle of administration. Toxicol. Appl. Pharm. 1981; 61: 99-108.

7. Earhart RH, Martin PA, Tutsch KD, Erturk E, Wheeler RJ and Bull FE. Improvement in the therapeutic index of cisplatin (NSC-119875) by pharmacologically induced chloruresis in the rat. Cancer Res. 1983; 43: 1187-1194.

8. Corden BJ, Hill JB, Collins J, and Ozols RF. High dose cisplatin in hypertonic saline: Absence of nephrotoxicity and pharmacokinetics of 40 mg/m^2 qd x 5 schedule of administration. Proc. Amer. Soc. Clin. Oncol. 1983; 24: C-132.

9. Ozols RF, Deisseroth AB, Javadpour N, et al. Treatment of poor prognosis non-seminomatous testicular cancer with a "high dose" platinum combination chemotherapy regimen. Cancer 1983; 51: 1803-1807.

10. Ozols, RF, Javadpour N, Jacob J, and Young RC. PVeBV chemotherapy in poor prognosis non-seminomatous testicular cancer. Presented at American Urologic Association, 1983.

11. Javadpour N, Ozols RF, Barlock A, Anderson T, Wesley R, and Young, RC. A randomized trial of cytoreductive surgery followed by chemotherapy vs chemotherapy alone in bulky stage (poor prognosis non-seminomatous testicular cancer). Cancer 1982; 50: 2004-2010.

12. Vogelzang NJ and Kennedy BJ. Hypomagnesemia and renal dysfunction during cisplatin-based chemotherapy of germ cell cancer. Proc. Amer. Soc. Clin. Oncol. 1982; 1: 117.

Clinical Experience with 1,1-Diaminomethylcyclohexane (Sulphato) Platinum (II) (TNO-6)

J.B. Vermorken, W.W. ten Bokkel Huinink, J.G. McVie, W.J.F. van der Vijgh and H.M. Pinedo

1. INTRODUCTION.

Cis-diamminodichloroplatinum II (cisplatin) is the first member of a group of platinum coordination complexes, which were shown to possess antitumor activity (1). With the introduction of cisplatin into the clinic the spectrum of tumors which can be treated effectively with chemotherapy has broadened (2). This agent is increasingly utilized in first-line regimens against testicular cancer, ovarian cancer, head and neck cancer, bladder cancer, while results in squamous cell cancer of the uterine cervix and in some childhood solid tumors like neuroblastoma and osteogenic sarcoma have been most promising. However, the use of the drug is hampered by some serious side effects. Its major clinical disadvantages are intense nausea and vomiting and renal impairment (3,4). Nausea and vomiting are much more distressing than found with other cytostatic drugs and cannot be effectively prevented. Adequate hydration and attention paid to optimal urinary flow results in a decrease in the incidence and the severity of nephrotoxicity. Nevertheless, substantial decrease in glomerular filtration rate and effective renal plasma flow can be found, which may be at least partially irreversible (5,6). Other toxicities include neurotoxicity, ototoxicity, myelosuppression, diarrhea and occasional liver function test abnormalities, electrolyte imbalances and occasional anaphylactic-like reactions (7). Although nephrotoxicity is generally considered as the major dose limiting toxicity, methods to overcome this toxicity have created the possibility to administer multiple courses of the drug. With prolonged treatment other toxicities may become dose-limiting. Recognition of these limitations has stimulated a widespread search for alternative

platinum complexes with equal or greater antitumor activity
but with decreased toxicities.

A number of cisplatin analogs in which the ammonia has been
substituted by a diaminomethylcyclohexane moiety were synthesized
at the Institute of Applied Chemistry TNO, Utrecht, The Netherlands. 1,1-Diaminomethylcyclohexane sulphato platinum II (TNO-6)
underwent extensive antitumor and toxicology screening at the
Radiobiological Institute, Rijswijk, The Netherlands, in collaboration with the Free University, Amsterdam, The Netherlands
and Bristol Laboratories, Syracuse, U.S.A. The drug was chosen
as candidate for a clinical phase I trial because of its favourable toxicity profile (less nephrotoxicity compared with cisplatin), its similar experimental antitumor activity, its increased potency and its suggested lack of cross-resistance with
cisplatin.

2. DRUG INFORMATION

2.1. Chemistry

TNO-6 is a 1,1-diaminomethylcyclohexane(sulphato)platinum II
complex with a molecular weight of 442.41. Its structural
formula is shown in Fig. 1.

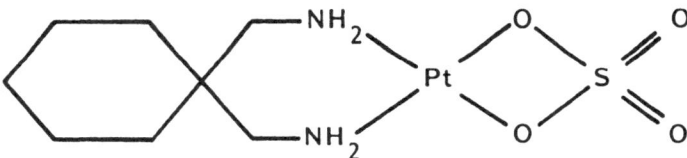

FIGURE 1.   1,1-diaminomethylcyclohexane(sulphato)platinum(II)
(TNO-6)

Chemistry data suggest that TNO-6 might react with water molecules in plasma to generate the monoaquo and/or diaquo species.
In addition, the reaction with active ligands present in plasma
is likely to generate a variety of new species which will complex
with other plasma molecules. TNO-6 is more water soluble than
cisplatin (1-20 mg-ml and 1 mg-ml respectively). In solutions
containing high concentrations of reactive ligands like chloride
(e.g. saline) TNO-6 will be rapidly converted into the poorly

soluble diaminomethylcyclohexane-dichloride-platinum(II) (TNO-1).
In 5% dextrose, TNO-6 is stable for 5 months at room temperature.

2.2. Mechanism of action

The mechanism of action of cisplatin and of other neutral
platinum coordination complexes have been ascribed to their
ability to bind to DNA. Inter- and intrastrand cross-links as
well as DNA-protein cross-links are produced (8). The main
cytotoxic lesions induced by platinum complexes appear to be
related to DNA-DNA interstrand cross-linking (9,10). Although
no specific studies on the mode of action of TNO-6 have been
performed, it is anticipated that TNO-6 acts similarly at the
molecular level (11).

2.3. Experimental antitumor activity

The anti-leukemic activity of TNO-6 in L1210 bearing mice
is comparable or marginally superior to that of cisplatin (12,
13). In cisplatin resistant L1210 leukaemia, TNO-6 shows a
therapeutic efficacy comparable to that which is observed in
cisplatin sensitive L1210 leukaemia, suggesting lack of cross-
resistance with cisplatin (13). Comparable antitumor effect to
cisplatin was found in B16 melanoma (14), while the activity
of TNO-6 in Lewis lung carcinoma, murine osteosarcoma and Madison
109 lung carcinoma is inferior to cisplatin (12,13). In preclinical screening (L1210) no schedule dependency has been
observed.

2.4. Animal toxicology

The acute LD_{50} in mice after a single intraperitoneal dose
ranges from 11 mg/kg to 20 mg/kg, while after a single intravenous dose this was 9 mg/kg (11). The LD_{10} in mice after a
single intraperitoneal injection of TNO-6 was found to be
7.9 mg/kg. The currently available toxicity data on TNO-6 in
animals show that this compound is, like cisplatin, nephrotoxic. Comparative studies however, indicate that in therapeutic doses, this toxicity is less pronounced than that of
the parent compound. Severe nephrotoxicity was observed in

two dogs after a single lethal dose of TNO-6 (2 mg/kg i.v.) (15).
In both animals major degenerative changes of the renal tubular
epithelium were observed. Bone marrow toxicity, usually mild
after cisplatin, may be more severe after TNO-6 administration.
In addition, experimental data in rats suggest that some myelo-
cardial damage may be induced after high doses of TNO-6 (11).

3. MATERIALS AND METHODS

3.1. Patient selection and evaluation

Fifty-three patients with advanced solid tumors considered
resistant to conventional treatment entered a phase I clinical
trial since 1980. The characteristics of the 53 patients are
shown in Table 1.

Table 1. Patients characteristics

Total number of patients	53
Male / female	27 / 26
Median age (range)	59 (21- 79)
Median performance status (range)	80 (50-100)
Prior chemotherapy (cisplatin)	44 (23)
Prior radiotherapy	29
Prior chemotherapy and radiotherapy	23

The tumor types included in the study were: ovarian carcinoma
(8 patients), breast cancer (7), gastrointestinal tumors (7),
non-small cell lung cancer (6), renal cell carcinoma (5),
melanoma (5), small cell lung cancer (4), soft tissue sarcoma (4)
and miscellaneous (7).

At the time of entry into the study all of the patients had
recovered from the toxic side effects of prior therapy, with
a white blood cell count (WBC) $\geq 4,0 \times 10^3/mm^3$ and a platelet
count $\geq 100 \times 10^3/mm^3$. Liver function tests and liver enzymes were
within the normal range unless abnormalities could be ascribed
clearly to liver involvement due to malignancy. Except for four
patients all others had a normal kidney function as measured
by serum creatinine and creatinine clearance (≥ 60 ml/min).
Patients with serious heart disease, brain metastases, or
evidence of an infectious disease were not eligible for the
study. An estimated life expectancy of more than 6 weeks

was required.

Patients were hospitalized for study and treated in the
Department of Oncology, Free University Hospital, Amsterdam
and in the Netherlands Cancer Institute, Amsterdam, and written
informed consent was obtained. Patients were carefully observed
for symptoms and signs of drug toxicity and anti-tumor effects.
Serial hematological, hepatic, and renal function studies were
performed. Serial 24-hour urine collections were obtained prior
to and at regular time intervals after administration of the
drug (days 1-7, 15 and 22).

3.2. Administration of drug

During the first part of the study patients received a single
intravenous dose of TNO-6 at 3 week intervals. The starting
dose was 2.5 mg/m^2 representing 1/10 of the LD_{10} in mice. Thirty-
two of the 53 patients received the drug in this manner over
the dose range of 2.5, 5, 10, 15, 25, 30 and 35 mg/m^2. TNO-6
was given in 5% dextrose-water solution (D_5W) without prior
hydration as long as there was no tumor progression and as long
as the patient's condition permitted drug administration.

During the second part of the study patients received TNO-6
by a 3-6 hour infusion at 3 week intervals, initially dissolved
in 40 ml of D_5W. At a later stage the drug was dissolved in
250-500 ml D_5W. Twenty-three patients received the drug by
this method over the dose range 30-40 mg/m^2.

Doses were not escalated in individual patients, while at
least three patients were treated at each dose level. The 53
patients received besides their initial treatment cycle 73
additional cycles, giving a total of 126 cycles. The total
number of courses per dose level varied from 1 to 38 and the
number of courses per patient varied from 1 to 15.

Antiemetics were not given at first administration of the
drug, but only after the patient has experienced nausea and
vomiting during the first cycle, or for the first time in later
cycles.

3.3. Pharmacokinetics

Pharmacokinetic studies were performed at each dose level. Concentrations of platinum in plasma, plasma ultrafiltrate and urine samples were determined by flameless atomic absorption spectrophotometry using a Perkin Elmer atomic absorption spectrophotometer Model 373 (16). Pharmacokinetic data were compared with those for cisplatin.

4. RESULTS

4.1.1. Myelosuppression.

In patients, who have received prior chemotherapy, thrombocytopenia was observed for the first time at 25 mg/m^2 during the first treatment cycle. A drop in the WBC count and platelet count was observed at the 30 mg/m^2 dose level (Table 2). In this table all evaluable patients who did not have a decreased renal function at the start of treatment are included, irrespective of the method of administration.

Table 2. WBC count and platelet count nadirs (x10^3/mm^3) during cycle I related to TNO-6 dose in pretreated patients.

	Dose (mg/m^2)		
	25	30	35
No. of patients	3	11	14
Median WBC nadir(range)	4.0(3.9-5.2)	3.0(0.9-4.5)	2.0(1.3-5.5)
Day of WBC nadir(range)	7 (7-20)	14 (10-27)	14 (8-24)
Day of recovery(range	20 (14-27)	21 (16-33)	25 (16-29)
Median platelets nadir	175 (53-182)	84 (10-247)	62 (9-270)
Day of platelets nadir	13 (8- 15)	13 (4- 22)	14 (5- 39)
Day of Recovery	21	22 (16- 36)	28 (16- 36)

The maximum tolerated dose (MTD) in these patients was 35 mg/m^2. In non-pretreated patients the MTD was 40 mg/m^2. However, all patients who received TNO-6 at the 40 mg/m^2 level received the drug by prolonged infusion. This might be of importance, because slight differences in severity of myelosuppression seemed to occur at certain dose levels, possible related to differences in infusion duration. In Table 3 the lowest counts per patient were taken into consideration.

Table 3. Myelosuppression related to the dose of TNO-6 and the method of administration in pretreated patients.

	30 mg/m^2		35 mg/m^2	
	10 min	3-6 hr	10 min	3-6 hr
No. of cycles	12	7	9	17
No. of patients	7	4	5	9
Median WBC count nadir	2.0	2.2	1.8	1.5
Range in WbC nadir	0.9-4.5	0.9-3.2	1.3-3.2	1.1-2.8
Median platelets nadir	104	43	36	44
Range in platelets nadir	10-247	27-129	31-220	9-128

In patients receiving the drug for 3 or more cycles the nadir appeared to be lower with subsequent courses. It was also reached slightly earlier, indicating that the 3 week schedule causes some cumulative toxicity. Anemia was observed in those patients who received TNO-6 at the higher dose levels (30-40 mg/m^2) for 2 or more cycles and red cell transfusions were occasionally needed.

4.1.2. Renal toxicity. No significant elevation of serum creatinine was observed during treatment at doses up to 30 mg/m^2 in patients with normal serum creatinine at start of treatment. Even long term administration did not result in a significant increase at this dose level (Table 4). However, it should be stated that only two patients received 4 or more cycles at the 30 mg/m^2 level.

Table 4. Cumulative effect on serum creatinine (mg/100 ml)

Dose mg/m^2	Values before each cycle							
	I	II	III	IV	V	VI	VII	XV
5	1.2	1.2	1.4	1.5				
10	0.9	0.9	0.8	1.0	0.9			
15	0.8	0.7	0.8	0.8				
25	0.9	0.9	1.0	1.1				
25	1.1	1.1	1.1	1.2	1.2	1.4	1.3	1.4
30	0.7	0.8	0.9	1.0	0.9	1.1	1.1	
30	1.1	1.2	1.3	1.3				
35	0.9	1.1	1.2	1.7				
35	1.1	1.1	1.2	1.5	3.5			
35	1.2	1.3	1.8					
40	0.6	0.6	0.7	0.7				

In contrast, 3 of the 20 patients, who received 35 mg/m^2 of
TNO-6 showed a 50-220% increase of the serum creatinine concentration after the second, the third and the fourth treatment
cycle, respectively (Table 4). One patient was a 59 year old
woman, in whom the left kidney had been removed 2 years earlier
because of renal cell carcinoma. A 50% transient increase in
serum creatinine was observed during the first treatment cycle
(day 4). A rise in serum creatinine to a maximum of 4.0 mg/100 ml
occurred one week after the fourth cycle. The serum creatinine
remained at this level for several months. The second patient
was a 60 year old woman with a disseminated malignant melanoma,
who received prior chemotherapy with DTIC and AZQ. One week
after the third administration of TNO-6 the serum creatinine
increased to 1.6 mg/100 ml, after which it decreased slowly to
1.4 mg/100 ml. The third patient was a 77 year old man with a
disseminated stomach cancer, who had received two courses of
a mitomycin C, adriamycin and cisplatin combination previously.
This patient had a transient 50% rise in serum creatinine after
the first administration (day 7). After the second administration of TNO-6 serum creatinine increased to a level of 3.1
mg/100 ml over a 3 week period, while it decreased very slowly
thereafter. All three patients had received TNO-6 by prolonged
infusion. Analysis of the two methods of administration at the
35 mg/m^2 dose level showed a transient increase in serum
creatinine of >25% after the first cycle in 4 of 8 patients
receiving a rapid infusion, while a similar increase was observed in 7 of 12 patients, who had received a prolonged infusion. It may therefore be concluded that at the 35 mg/m^2
dose level there is a definite risk to develop renal toxicity.

An unexpected side effect during the first part of the
study, when TNO-6 was only given by rapid infusion, was the
occurrence of proteinuria. This was observed at doses of
25 mg/m^2 or higher. This proteinuria was dose dependent and
seemed cumulative, as shown in Table 5.

338

Table 5. TNO-6 induced proteinuria* related to dose and
treatment cycle

Dose mg/m^2	Maximum proteinuria (G/24 hr):median(range)		
	Cycle I	Cycle II	Cycle III
25	1.3 (1.3- 1.4)	1.0	5.1
30	2.3 (0.9- 1.9)	4.5	3.5
35	3.2 (0.6-10.0)	5.2 (3.8-6.3)	7.7

* 10 min infusion

The median day at which the maximum proteinuria occurred was
day 5, and recovery was evident mostly within 2 weeks. Because
of the severity of the proteinuria, indicating glomerular
damage, we have searched for methods to avoid this. The use
of hydration or of corticosteroids did not seem to prevent
this side effect. However, prolongation of infusion time did
diminish the proteinuria. At 30 mg/m^2 of TNO-6 half of the
patients who were given a rapid infusion showed proteinuria,
while none of the four patients who received prolonged infusions during their first treatment cycle did.

When TNO-6 was given in a concentrated solution (dissolved
in 40 ml D_5W) over several hours phlebitis was observed in
nearly all patients. However, dilution in 250-500 ml D_5W has
greatly reduced this side effect. Using this method of administration we have not encountered serious phlebitis.

Electrolyte disturbances (especially hypophosphataemia,
but also hypomagnesaemia) and an increase in beta-2-micro-
globulin excretion in the urine (with a maximum on days 3-5)
were observed and were indicative for tubular damage. These
manifestations were already present at much lower dosages of
TNO-6, but were of no clinical importance. However, they
seemed to be cumulative as might be evident from Fig. 2,
showing serum phosphate levels in three successive cycles in
a patient, who received rapid infusions of TNO-6 at a dose of
25 mg/m^2 each time.

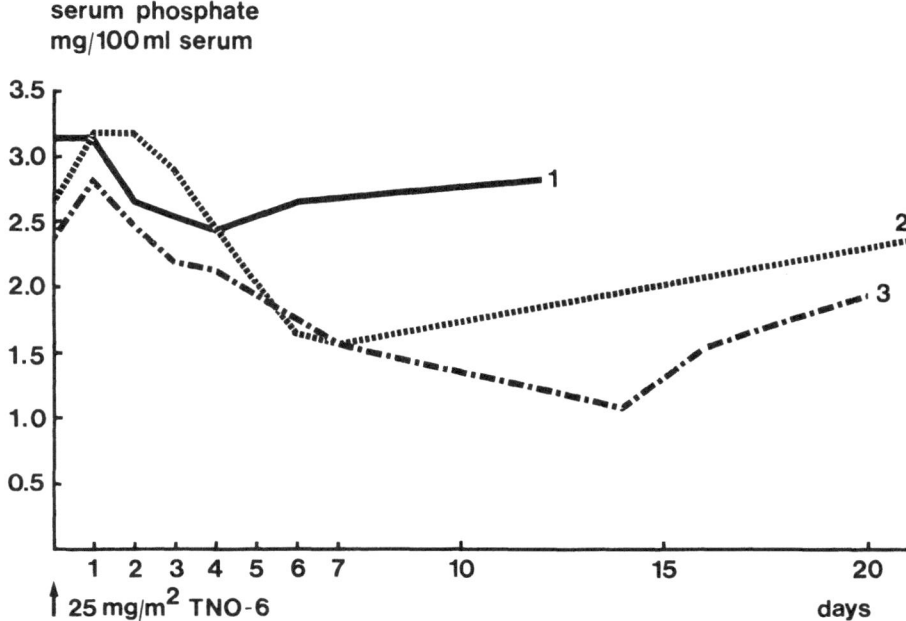

FIGURE 2. Serum phosphate levels determined during 3 successive cycles of TNO-6 in a patient who received the drug by rapid infusion at a dose of 25 mg/m^2 at 3 week intervals.

Because of the very low levels found after the third administration oral substitution was given to this patient. No specific symptoms were expressed.

4.1.3. <u>Other toxicities</u>. Table 6 summarizes other non-hematological side effects of TNO-6. Nausea and vomiting were observed in nearly all patients and seemed to be dose-related. Overall, this side effect was less severe compared to that caused by the administration of moderate or high dosages of cisplatin. There was a definite response to conventional antiemetics in some patients, but others failed to respond.

Table 6.   Non-hematological side effects
of TNO-6 observed in 53 patients

Dose related vomiting
Diarrhea (14 patients)
Dry mouth (16)
Loss of taste (10)
Tnnitus (3)
Paraesthesias (4)
Myalgia (1)
Drowsiness (3)
Anaphylactic-like reactions (1)

We have seen severe cellulitis and necrosis as result of such
extravasation of the drug in one patient.

4.2. Pharmacokinetics

Data on the pharmacokinetics of TNO-6 following a rapid infusion of the drug have been reported earlier (17). Table 7
summarizes these data.

Table 7.   Pharmacokinetic parameters of TNO-6 compared to
cisplatin in blood and urine after bolus injection

Parameter*	TNO-6 (n=8)	Cisplatin (n=7)
$t_{\frac{1}{2}\alpha}$ (min)	6.2 + 2.9	15.9 + 5.2
$t_{\frac{1}{2}\beta}$ (day)	3.4 + 1.4	5.4 + 1.0
V_c (liter)	5.8 + 1.1	13.2 + 3.0
V_d^{ss} (liter)	18.4 + 4.6	62.7 + 16.1
AUC^∞/mg Pt/m^2	729 + 209	332 + 66
B/mg Pt/m^2	0.094 + 0.014	0.029 + 0.005

*
    Total platinum kinetics

Mean cumulative excretion of platinum in the urine after 3
days is 27.9% + 7.5%(SD) in 6 patients compared with 35.6 +
4.5% for cisplatin.

In short the following observations have been made for bolus
injections of TNO-6:

-Total and unbound platinum have a shorter half-life of distribution than with cisplatin. Mean platinum half-life in plasma
ultra-filtrate (free platinum) was 4.6 + 0.7 min in three
patients.

-Half-life of elimination is only slightly shorter with TNO-6
as compared to the values obtained after cisplatin.

-The area under the total platinum concentration curve in plasma
for TNO-6 is about twice that of cisplatin, and duration of
distribution time is shorter for TNO-6.
-Cumulative urinary platinum excretion for TNO-6 is similar to
that of cisplatin.

Preliminary results of data on the pharmacokinetics of TNO-6
after prolonged infusion showed that, with the exception of
peak levels and half-life of the initial phase, pharmacokinetic
parameters did not differ from those found with rapid infusions.
In Fig. 3 an example of the concentration-time curves of total
and free platinum, and the cumulative urinary excretion during
and after a 6-hour infusion of TNO-6 is depicted.

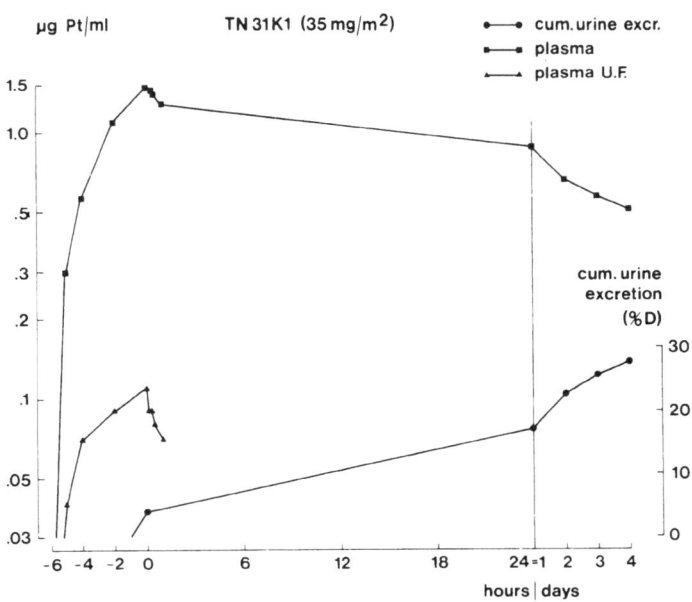

FIGURE 3. Semilogarithmic plot of platinum concentrations in
plasma and plasma ultrafiltrate, and linear plot of the
cumulative urinary excretion of platinum versus time in a
patient receiving TNO-6 by 6-hour infusion.

4.3. Antitumor effect

One complete remission has been observed in a patient with
breast cancer (lung metastases). One partial response has been
achieved in a patient with adenocarcinoma of the lung, while

minor responses were observed in patients with ovarian cancer, small cell lung cancer and testicular cancer (each tumor type one patient). Except for the patient with breast cancer all patients had shown to be resistant to cisplatin.

5. CONCLUSIONS

TNO-6 is an interesting analog which can be given without hydration on an outpatient basis. Dose-limiting toxicity was observed at 35 mg/m^2 for pretreated patients and 40 mg/m^2 for non-pretreated patients. Toxicity at these dose levels consisted of myelosuppression and renal failure. At the dose level of 30 mg/m^2, given at 3 week intervals, which is recommended for phase II trials, proteinuria was observed when the drug was given by rapid infusion. This latter side effect could be limited by extending the duration of infusion to 4-6 hours, which is an additional suggestion for phase II studies.

REFERENCES
1. Rosenberg B, Van Camp L, Trosko JE, et al. 1969. Platinum compounds: a new class of potent antitumour agents. Nature 222, 385-386.
2. Einhorn LH and Williams SD. 1979. The role of cis-platinum in solid-tumor therapy. N.Eng.J.Med. 300, 289-291.
3. Vermorken JB and Pinedo HM. 1982. Gastrointestinal toxicity of cis-diammine-dichloro-platinum(II): a personal experience. Neth.J.Medicine 25, 270-274.
4. Krakoff IH. 1979. Nephrotoxicity of cis-dichlorodiammine-platinum(II). Cancer Treat.Rep. 63, 1523-1525.
5. Dentino M, Luft FC, Yum MN, Williams SD, Einhorn H. 1978. Long term effect of cis-diamminedichlorideplatinum (CDDP) on renal function and structure in man. Cancer 41, 1274-1281.
6. Meyer S. 1982. Cis-platinum and the kidney. Ph.D. thesis. Groningen.
7. Von Hoff DD, Schilsky R, Reichert CM, et al. 1979. Toxic effects of cis-dichlorodiammineplatinum(II) in man. Cancer Treat.Rep. 63, 1527-1532.
8. Zwelling LA and Kohn KW. 1979. Mechanism of action of cis-dichloro-diammine-platinum(II). Cancer Treat.Rep. 63, 1439-1444.
9. Zwelling LA, Michael S, Schwartz H, Dobson PP, Kohn KW. 1981. DNA cross-linking as an indicator of sensitivity and resistance of mouse L1210 leukaemia to cis-diammine-dichloroplatinum(II) and L-phenylalanine mustard. Cancer Res. 41, 640-649.
10. Erickson LC, Zwelling LA, Ducore JM, Sharkey NA, Kohn KW. 1981. Differential cytotoxicity and DNA cross-linking in

normal and transformed human fibroblasts treated with cis-diamminedichloroplatinum(II). Cancer Res. 41, 2791-2794.

11. Lee FH, Canetta R, Issell SF, Lenaz L. 1983. New platinum complexes in clinical trials. Cancer Treat.Rev. 10, 39-51.

12. Lelieveld P, Atassi A, Van Putten LM. 1981. Preclinical toxicity studies of cisplatin and three currently developed analogs. Abstracts of Proceedings Int.Cong.Chemother. Florence, Italy.

13. Rose WC, Schurig JE, Bradner WT, Huftalen JB. 1982. Anti-tumor activity and toxicity of cis-diamminedichloroplatinum (II) analogs. Cancer Treat.Rep. 66, 135-146.

14. Lelieveld P. Personal communication.

15. Lelieveld P, Van Putten LM. 1981. Preclinical investigations with the new PT compound TNO-6. Proceeding 12th Int'l Cong.Chemother. 12, 60.

16. Vermorken JB, van der Vijgh WJF, Klein I, Gall HE, Pinedo HM. 1982. Pharmacokinetics of free platinum species following rapid 3-hr and 24-hr infusions of cis-diammine-dichloro-platinum(II) and its therapeutic implications. Eur.J.Cancer Clin.Oncol. 18, 1069-1974.

17. Pinedo H, Ten Bokkel Huinink W, Simonetti G, et al. 1982. Phase I study and pharmacokinetics of cis-1,1-di(amino-methyl)-cyclohexane Pt II sulphate (TNO-6). Proc.Am.Soc. Clin.Oncol. 1, 32.

POSTER PRESENTATIONS

VI-1   SYNERGISTIC LETHAL EFFECTS OF CISPLATIN IN COMBINATION WITH NUCLEOSIDES.
B. Drewinko, M.A. Dipasquale and L.Y. Yang.

VI-2   CATALYTIC ACTIVITY OF METAL ANTITUMOR AGENTS.
J. Turkevich, Z. Xu and R.S. Miner.

VI-3   FURTHER ADVANCES IN THE MANAGEMENT OF MALIGNANT TERATOMAS OF THE TESTIS AND OTHER SITES.
E.S. Newlands, R.H.J. Begent, G.J.S. Rustin, D. Parker and K.D. Bagshawe.

VI-4   STEROIDAL-CISPLATIN (II) COMPLEXES: NEW ANTICANCER AGENTS WITH POTENTIAL SELECTIVITY.
O. Gandolfi, J. Blum and F.M. Shavit.

VI-5   A PILOT STUDY OF THE CONCOMITANT USE OF *cis*-PLATINUM CHEMOTHERAPY AND RADIATION THERAPY IN PATIENTS WITH ADVANCED HEAD AND NECK CANCER.
M.D. Green, J.S. Cooper, N. Cohen and F. Muggia.

VI-6   PHASE II TRIAL OF 1,2-DIAMINOCYCLOHEXANE (4-CARBOXYPHTHALATO) PLATINUM (II) (DACCP) IN NON-SMALL CELL LUNG CANCER.
H. Scher, D. Kelsen, L. Kalman and R. Gralla.

VI-7   INTRA-ARTERIAL *cis*-PLATINUM (IACP) ADMINISTRATION IN PATIENTS WITH ADVANCED SOLID TUMORS.
D. Lehane, R. Sessions, G. Ehni, N. Bryan, L. DeSantos, B. Horrowitz, M.A. Zubler, W. Grose, F. Smith and M. Lane.

VI-8   *cis* AND *trans-bis* (NITROMIDAZOLO) PLATINUM (II) COMPLEXES: PREPARATION, CHARACTERIZATION AND RADIOSENSITIZATION PROPERTIES.
J.R. Bales, C.J. Coulson, D.W. Gilmour, R. Kuroda, M. Laverick, M.A. Mazid, S. Neidle, A.H.W. Nias, B.J. Peart, C.A. Ramsden and P.J. Sadler.

VI-9   COMBINED MODALITIES MANAGEMENT FOR UNRESECTABLE NON-OAT CELL CARCINOMA OF THE LUNG: A PILOT STUDY OF HIGH DOSE EXTENDED FRACTIONATION THORACIC IRRADIATION PLUS CONCOMITANT *cis*-PLATINUM AND 5-FU.
D.J. Moylan, M. Mohiuddin, H. Brodovsky and K. Aceto.

VI-10   FLUOROURACIL (5FU) AND CISPLATIN (DDP) AS SALVAGE CHEMOTHERAPY IN OVARIAN CANCER (OC).
M.V. Fiorentino, F. Tredese, O. Nicoletto, G. Nardelli, P. Biondetti, T. Maggino, D. Marchesoni, S. Bolzonella, O. Daniele and A. Onnis.

VI-11   CISPLATIN (DDP) PLUS VINDESINE (VDS) VERSUS DDP PLUS VP 16-213 VERSUS DOXORUBICYN (DOXO) PLUS CYTOXAN (CY): A RANDOMIZED STUDY IN ADVANCED NON-SMALL CELL CANCER OF THE LUNG (NSCCL).
M.V. Fiorentino, A. Paccagnella, L. Salvagno, V. Chiarion Sileni, A. Brandes, O. Vinante, L. Endrizzi, S. Bolzonella and V. Fosser.

VI-12   EFFECTIVE RADIATION SENSITIZATION OF HYPOXIC *S. TYPHIMURIUM* CELLS BY SLIGHTLY TOXIC Pt(II)-COMPLEXES.
R.C. Richmond and E.B. Douple.

VI-13   *cis*-PLATINUM IN RECURRENT BRAIN TUMORS.
A.B. Khan, B .J. D'Souza, M.D. Wharam, L.F. Sinks, S. Woo, D. McCullough and B.G. Leventhal.

VI-14   MECHANISM OF ACTION OF FREE OR INCORPORATED INTO LIPOSOMES *cis*-DICHLORODIAMMINOPLATINUM II: A COMPARATIVE STUDY IN EHRLICH TUMOR CELLS.
M.C. De Pauw-Gillet, C. Houssier, G. Weber and R. Bassleer.

VI-15   PHASE II TRIAL OF *cis*-DIAMMINE-1,1-CYCLOBUTANE DICARBOXYLATE PLATINUM II (CBDCA, JM8) IN PATIENTS WITH CARCINOMA OF THE OVARY NOT PREVIOUSLY TREATED WITH CISPLATIN.
A.H. Calvert, J.W. Baker, V.M. Dalley, S.J. Harland, A.C. Jones and J. Staffurth.

VI-16   PHASE II STUDY OF *cis*-DIAMMINE-1,1-CYCLOBUTANE DICARBOXYLATE PLATINUM II (CBDCA, JM8) IN CARCINOMA OF BRONCHUS.
S.J. Harland, I.E. Smith, N. Smith, D.L. Alison and A.H. Calvert.

VI-17   BINDING SITES FOR CYTOTOXIC METAL IONS AND COMPLEXES WITHIN EHRLICH CELLS.
A. Kraker, S. Krezoski, J. Schneider, J. Schmidt and D. Petering.

VI-18   PLATINUM-RADIATION BASED COMBINED MODALITY APPROACH FOR LOCALLY-ADVANCED CANCER OF THE HEAD AND NECK.
C.T. Coughlin and E.B. Douple.

VI-19   POTENTIATION OF CELL KILL BY COMBINING NITROIMIDAZOLE-PLATINUM COMPLEXES WITH RADIATION.
E. Douple and B.A. Teicher.

VI-20   COMBINATION CHEMOTHERAPY INCLUDING *cis*-PLATINUM (DDP), METHOTREXATE AND 5-FLUOROURACIL (PMF) IN ADVANCED OVARIAN CANCER.
P.F. Conte, M. Bruzzone, M.R. Sertoli, R. Rosso, A. Rubagotti and G. Pescetto.

VI-21   CHEMOPOTENTIATION OF MITOMYCIN C CYTOTOXICITY *IN VITRO* BY *cis*-DIAMMINEDICHLOROPLATINUM (II) AND THREE NEWLY SYNTHESIZED PLATINUM COMPLEXES.
B.A. Teicher.

VI-1 SYNERGISTIC LETHAL EFFECTS OF CISPLATIN IN COMBINATION
WITH NUCLEOSIDES. Benjamin Drewinko, Maria A. Dipasquale
and Li Y. Yang. Dept. Lab. Med., M.D. Anderson Hospital and Tumor
Inst., Houston, Tx 77030

We have previously reported that combinations of cisplatin and
ara-C exhibited a potentiated cytotoxic effect on human tumor cells
and that this synergistic effect was related to increased DNA interstrand crosslinks (Cancer Res.; 41:25, 1981). To ascertain whether
this phenomenon was common to other, natural nucleosides we treated
an established human colorectal carcinoma cell line (LoVo cells)
for 1 hr with combinations of cisplatin (5 µg/ml) and increasing
concentrations (100 to 1000 µg/ml) of the deoxynucleosides of
thymine, cytidine, uracil and adenine. Cytotoxicity was measured
by inhibition of colony-formation, and DNA interstrand crosslinking
was evaluated on proteinase K-treated samples (0.5 mg/ml) by the
alkaline elution method. With the exception of high concentrations
(>500 µg/ml) of dThd, treatment with deoxynucleoside alone failed
to exert any significant lethal effect. Simultaneous treatment with
cisplatin and every deoxynucleoside showed a linear, dose-dependent,
synergistic increment in cytotoxicity reaching, at concentrations
of 1000 µg/ml, a greater than 10-fold increase over the calculated
additive effects. For every deoxynucleoside, degree of cytotoxicity
correlated linearly with increments in the DNA crosslinking factor.
Thus, it appears that natural nucleosides interact with cisplatin
to increase its bifunctional binding to DNA that leads to cell death.
Such results support the previously advanced rationale for clinical
trials employing cisplatin with high doses of natural nucleosides
in a effort to further expand the cytotoxic efficacy of this
platinum derivative without a concomitant increase in toxicity to
normal tissues. (Supported by Grant CA-23272 from the NCI, USPHS.)

VI-2 CATALYTIC ACTIVITY OF METAL ANTITUMOR AGENTS. John
Turkevich, Zhusheng Xu, Robert S. Miner, Chemistry Department, Princeton University, Princeton, NJ 08544 USA

We have found that certain therapeutically active metal coordination compounds react at 40°C with DNA, RNA and their constituents to
produce soluble complexes which are active catalysts for the decomposition of hydrogen peroxide. This activity is most marked with
cytosine and less so with thymine, guanine, hypoxanthine and uracil.
Adenine and alpha pyridone complexes showed negligible activity. The
therapeutically active compounds studied were diammino Pt(II) and
1,3 diamino cyclohexane Pt(II) derivatives and Rhodium (II) diace-
tate. Therapeutically inactive but chemically related compounds
trans diammino Pt(II) and 1,2 diaminocyclohexane Pd(II) compounds
did not form a catalytically active complex with cytosine. The
platinum (IV) analogue of cis diammino Pt(II) did not produce a catalytically active complex with cytosine but it enhanced the activity
of the Pt(II) compound. Adenine is not only inactive with cis
platinum but is antagonistic to cytosine. The kinetics of formation
of catalytically active species was studied as function of temperature and ratio of reactants and different reactants. Thus similar
results were obtained with different cytidine, guanosine, adenosine
complexes of cis platinum with cytidine derivatives showing high activity. Poly C showed high activity when reacted in ratio of one
mole of platinum to one base. Poly G showed unusual behavior of
first developing high catalytic activity and then dramatically losing
it. Poly A, Poly I and Poly U showed low catalytic activity with
cis platinum. Transdihydroxy diammino Pt(II) produced with Poly C
a complex with negligible catalytic activity.

DNA from salmon sperm and from calf thymus on reaction with cis
platinum at 40°C did not produce any catalytic activity in 72 hours,
however heating to 90°C developed catalytic activity consistent with
its cytosine content.

A possible mechanism for the therapeutic action of cis platinum
drugs is the formation of catalytically active species on runs of
cytosine in single stranded DNA. These runs transcribe as proline
which may distort the nucleosome sufficiently to weaken its binding
to DNA and lead to formation of single stranded DNA. This will
favor uncontrolled transcription and replication.

Helpful discussions with Dr. Joseph H. Burchenal and Dr. Leyland-
Jones of the Memorial Sloan Kettering Cancer Center are gratefully
acknowledged. This work was supported by Research Corporation.

VI-3 FURTHER ADVANCES IN THE MANAGEMENT OF MALIGNANT TERATOMAS OF THE TESTIS AND OTHER SITES.

E.S. Newlands, R.H.J. Begent, G.J.S. Rustin, D. Parker and K.D. Bagshawe, Dept. of Medical Oncology, Charing Cross Hospital, Fulham Palace Road, London W6 8RF, United Kingdom

We have developed sequential combination chemotherapy for the management of large volume metastatic malignant teratomas. The chemotherapy consists of cis-platinum (120 mg/m), vincristine, methotrexate and bleomycin (POMB) alternating with VP 16-213 (etoposide), cyclophosphamide and actinomycin D (ACE) (Newlands et al, Brit. J. of Cancer 1980, 42, 378). Since we increased the number of courses of POMB given to each patient, 69 male patients have completed treatment (1 Nov. 1982). 67% of these had advanced and bulky metastatic disease and life table analysis projects a survival of 83%. Complete remissions have been obtained in 15/18 (83%) with advanced abdominal disease; 15/16 (94%) with advanced lung disease; 8/11 (73%) with advanced abdominal and lung disease. Liver and brain involvement is not an adverse prognostic factor and 6/8 (75%) patients with widespread liver metastases and 3/4 (75%) of patients with brain metastases are in complete remission. Multivariate analysis indicates that clinical staging and the size of metastases have little influence on survival. The strongest determinant of survival is the initial serum concentration of human chorionic gonadotrophin and/or alpha-foetoprotein. Prior radiotherapy is also an adverse prognostic factor.

The toxicity with this sequential chemotherapy is manageable and less than our experience with high-dose vinblastine regimens. The haematological toxicity has been reported (Newlands et al, Brit. J. Cancer 1980, 42, 378). 24% of patients required antibiotics for neutropaenic fever. Multiple courses of high-dose cis-platinum induce a renal leak of magnesium which can become symptomatic, presenting with tetany in epileptic fits. Routine supplementation with 4 g of magnesium sulphate with each course of cis-platinum has eliminated this problem (Macaulay et al, Cancer Chemotherapy and Pharmacology - in press).

VI-4 STEROIDAL-CIS-PLATINUM (II) COMPLEXES: NEW ANTICANCER AGENTS WITH POTENTIAL SELECTIVITY.

O. Gandolfi*, J. Blum*, F.M. Shavit. *Dept. Organic Chemistry, The Hebrew University, Jerusalem, Israel and Dept. Bacteriology of the Hebrew University-Hadassah Medical School, Jerusalem, Israel.

The severe limitation encountered in the application of Pt complexes in cancer chemotherapy is their high level of toxicity. Non specific recognition between tumor cells and normal cells prevents an increase in concentration of the current Pt drugs in neoplastic tissue rather than in normal tissue. A number of tumors are now known to be hormone dependent (e.g. breast and renal cancer, human meningiomas, several forms of lymphatic leukemia, etc.). The presence in tumor cells of cytosol receptors, which recognize specific steroids, has suggested the possibility of utilizing antitumor drugs bound to hormonally active lipophilic carriers, in order to achieve an increased selectivity and, consequently, a decrease in toxicity.

In accordance with these ideas, we have prepared a number of cis-platinum (II) complexes with functionalized o-catechol ligands, of general formula: $[Pt(1,2-O_2C_6H_3-R)(PPh_3)_2]$ where $1,2-O_2C_6H_3-R$ is the catecholate form of 3,4-dihydroxybenzoic acid, 3,4-dihydroxyphenylacetic acid, 3,4-dihydroxycinnamic acid, dopamine, L-dopa, α-methyl-dopa, D,L-dopa, isoprotenerol, L-norepinephrine, L-epinephrine, adrenalone. Derivatives of catecholamines have recently been discovered also as antitumor agents.

Some of the new platinum-o-catecholate complexes, which by themselves inhibit the growth of L1210 mouse leukemic cells, could be anchored via carboxyl or amine function, to a variety of steroids: $[Pt(1,2-O_2C_6H_3-CH_2CH_2-X-S)(PPh_3)_2]$, where X=CO or NH and S=derivative of estrogens, androgen, progesterone, colic acids.

The activity of some of the steroidal-platinum complexes in breast cancer cell line, MCF-7, has been determined, in a first effort to seek a recognition by the progesterone and estradiol receptors within these cells.

VI-5 A PILOT STUDY OF THE CONCOMITANT USE OF CIS-PLATINUM CHEMO-
THERAPY AND RADIATION THERAPY IN PATIENTS WITH ADVANCED

HEAD AND NECK CANCER. Michael D. Green*, Jay S. Cooper+, Noel Coher°,
Franco Muggia*. New York University Medical Center, 550 First Ave.,
New York, NY 10016. Divisions of Medical Oncology*, and Radiation
Oncology+ and Department of Otoloryngology°.

A considerable amount of preclinical data suggests that cis-
Platinum (CDDP) given concomitantly with radiation (RT) causes a
synergistic effect on tumor cell kill. In an attempt to test this
in the clinic we have designed a study in which CDDP is administered
concurrently with a conventional dose and schedule of RT in patients
(pts) with advanced head and neck cancers not suitable for surgery.
The primary aim of the study was to test treatment tolerance so that
pts who were treated for palliative purposes as well as those who
were treated for cure were included.

CDDP was administered as an intravenous infusion at dose of
$20mg/m^2$ for 5 days every 3 weeks concurrent with RT (180-200cGy per
day 5 times per week). 26 pts have been entered with a median follow
up of 8 months (2-15). 25 are evaluable for toxicity (1 is currently
on treatment) and 22 are evaluable for response. Two pts have been
lost to follow up and one had no evaluable disease. One pt had stage
III, 18 stage IV and 5 had recurrent disease following surgery. Six
pts had a total RT dose <6000cGy and 18 had a total RT dose >6000cGy.
Two pts received 1 course of CDDP (both refused further treatment)
12 pts received 2 courses and 11 pts received 3 courses of CDDP.

Toxicity was evaluated in 25 pts and was mainly hematologic with
9 (36%) developing thrombocytopenia (<100,000), 4 (17%) neutropenia
(<2000 WBC), and 3 (12%) anemia (Hgb <10%). Mucositis ($\geq$ Gr 2)
occurred in 6 (24%), a moderate to severe peripheral neuropathy in 2
(8%) and an elevated serum creatinine in 3 (13%) precluding additional cisplatin. Nausea and vomiting were generally tolerable, and
severe only in 3. There were no episodes of sepsis or treatment
related deaths. Disease cleared completely in 9 pts (43%) and partially ($\geq$50%) in 8 (38%).

This pilot experience is highly encouraging since minimal
interference with the contemplated dose of radiation and considerable
efficacy was observed in a population consisting mostly of bulky
tumors. The simultaneous use of cisplatin and radiation must be
explored further in prospective trials to determine both the optimal
dose schedules and the efficacy relative to radiation alone or
sequential regimens.

Supported in part by Lila Motley Fund and Cancer Center Grant
#CA16087.

VI-6 PHASE II TRIAL OF 1,2-DIAMINOCYCLOHEXANE (4-CARBOXY-
PHTHALATO) PLATINUM (II) (DACCP) IN NON-SMALL CELL LUNG

CANCER. Howard Scher, David Kelsen, Leonard Kalman and Richard
Gralla. Memorial Sloan-Kettering Cancer Center, 1275 York Avenue,
New York, New York 10021, U.S.A.

DACCP is a second generation platinum analog that demonstrated
in-vitro actitivy against L1210 and P388 cell lines resistant to
cisplatin. In Phase I evaluation at MSKCC, thrombocytopenia was
the dose limiting toxicity. Nephrotoxicity (creatinine $\geq$1.5mg% was
uncommon. A Phase II evaluation in non-small cell lung cancer was
performed. 33 patients (pts) (28 males and 5 females) were entered.
Patient characteristics included a median age of 55 (range 34-74)
and PS (Karnofsky) 70 (range 50-100). 12 pts had received no prior
chemotherapy (CT); 18 had received prior cisplatin. 20 pts had
adenocarcinoma and 11 epidermoid cancer. Indicator lesions included
pulmonary nodules in 22, soft tissue and nodal masses in 9 and liver
metastases in 2. The starting dose was 640 mg/m^2 administered IV
every 3 weeks. Escalations to 720 mg/m^2 were performed if no myelosuppression (WBC <3000 cells/mm^3, platelets <125,000 cells/mm^3) or
nephrotoxicity was noted. Hydration consisted of 500 cc D$_5$½NS pre
and post therapy. 30 pts were entered at 640 mg/m^2 and 4 escalated
to the 720 mg/m^2 dose level; 3 were entered at 720 mg/m^2. Myelosuppression was uncommon at all levels as only 2/29 (7%) evaluable pts
had WBC nadirs below 3000 cells/mm^3 and 3/29 (11%) had platelet
nadirs below 125,000 cells/mm^3. Nephrotoxicity was mild Of pts
who had received no prior CT, a creatinine $\geq$ 1.5mg% was noted in 1/11
(9%) evaluable pts and 5/21 (22%) of pts who received prior CT.
Acute toxicities included mild nausea and vomiting in 90%, diarrhea
in 30% and fever in 10%. Allergic reactions, manifested as hives
and urticaria, were observed in 4 pts (2 of whom had not received
prior platinum based chemotherapy). A sensorimotor peripheral
neuropathy was noted in 3 pts, which required discontinuation of
therapy in one. 29/33 pts were evaluable for response, including
11 who had received no prior CT. Of the inevaluable pts, 2 developed allergic reactions and did not complete the drug infusion and 2
were lost to follow up. One partial remission of 3 months duration
was noted in a pt who had previously responded to cisplatin but
then developed progressive disease. One pt remained stable over
4 months but was removed for toxicity. No other responses were
seen. We conclude that DACCP has limited therapeutic activity in
non-small cell lung cancer (95% confidence limits 0-10%).

VI-7 INTRA-ARTERIAL CIS-PLATINUM (IACP) ADMINISTRATION IN PATIENTS WITH ADVANCED SOLID TUMORS. Daniel Lehane, Roy Sessions, George Ehni, Nick Bryan, Luis DeSantos, Barry Horrowitz, MaryAnne Zubler, William Grose, Frank Smith and Montague Lane. Baylor College of Medicine, 1200 Moursund Ave., Houston, TX 77030.USA

The effectiveness of IACP is unique since little pharmacologic advantage can be demonstrated for the intra-arterial administration of most other chemotherapeutic agents. This report presents the results of IACP in 192 patients with 133 complete and partial responders (69%) including 50 patients with squamous cell carcinoma of head and neck region (H&N), 36 adenocarcinoma of the colon (C) and 30 primary high grade malignant gliomas (MG). Patients were selected for this study if they had a creatinine clearance of at least 70cc/min. Cis-platinum (CP) was diluted in 0.9% NaCl at a final concentration of 1 mg/ml and infused at a dose of 100 mg/m^2. CP solutions were prefiltered using a 0.5 mμ filter. Patients with H&N tumors were divided into 3 subgroups: 21 patients previously treated, including prior radiation therapy (XRT), 7 CR, 12 PR (90%) with a median survival of 7 months, 21 patients with unresectable stage 3 and 4 disease receiving IACP + XRT, 6 CR, 14 PR (95%) with a median survival of 11 months, and 8 patients with resectable stage 3 disease receiving preop IACP 8 of 8 CR + PR, median survival 13+ months. There are 36 patients with advanced, metastatic C with an overall response rate of 75% and a median survival of 11 months for responders and 2 months for non responders p = .002. In 26 patients with liver metastases, pretreatment performance status was 3 or worse in 62%, 70% had prior chemotherapy and 44% had abnormal liver function yet had a 65% response rate and a median survival of 6 months for responders and 1.5 months for non responders p=.004. Ten patients with recurrent MG, all of whom had previously received XRT and nitrosourea chemotherapy received internal carotid IACP. 7 patients achieved an objective response, but with a median survival of only 3 months. Of 20 patients with grade 3 and 4 MG receiving postop adjuvant IACP + XRT and CCNU, the median survival was increased to 83.5 + weeks with less than a 5% incidence of neurotoxicity. We conclude that there are increased response rates and improved survival in patients treated with IACP. The 2 to 10-fold increase in response rates suggests that IACP is the optimum route of administration for CP.

VI-8 CIS AND TRANS-BIS(NITROIMIDAZOLO)PLATINUM(II) COMPLEXES : PREPARATION, CHARACTERIZATION AND RADIOSENSITIZATION PROPERTIES. John R. Bales*, Christoper J. Coulson†, David W. Gilmour†, Reiko Kuroda‡, Margaret Laverick, Muhammad A. Mazid*, Stephen Neidle‡, Anthony H.W. Nias, Barry J. Peart†, Christoper A. Ramsden† and Peter J. Sadler*,*Chemistry Department, Birkbeck College, Malet Street, London WC1E 7HX, U.K.,†The Research Laboratories, May and Baker Ltd., Dagenham, Essex,RM10 7XS, ‡Cancer Research Campaign Biomolecular Structure Research Group, Department of Biophysics, King's College, Drury Lane, London, WC2B 5RL, and Richard Dimbleby Department of Cancer Research, St Thomas's Medical School, London, SE1, U.K.

The preparation and properties of bis(nitro-imidazolo)Pt(II) dihalides and dicarboxylates have been investigated. The product from direct reaction of the 5-NO$_2$ imidazole metronidazole with K$_2$PtCl$_4$ is the cis complex, FLAP, whereas that from the 2-NO$_2$ imidazole misonidazole is the trans complex, I. Simple preparative routes to trans-FLAP have been devised. Structures were confirmed by X-ray crystallography and the contrasting properties and reactivities of these complexes will be discussed.

FLAP has a low toxicity, and good hypoxic cell radiosensitization properties. A 1 hour pretreatment of CHO cells at a non-toxic dose of 50μM gave an enhancement ratio of 2.4. FLAP is orally absorbed and is currently undergoing further evaluation.

FLAP

I

VI-9 COMBINED MODALITIES MANAGEMENT FOR UNRESECTABLE NON-OAT CELL CARCINOMA OF THE LUNG: A PILOT STUDY OF HIGH DOSE EXTENDED FRACTIONATION THORACIC IRRADIATION PLUS CONCOMITANT CIS-PLATINUM AND 5-FU. David J. Moylan, M.D., Mohammed Mohiuddin, M.D., *Harvey Brodovsky, M.D. and Kathleen Aceto, B.S.N. Jefferson Medical College, Thomas Jefferson University, Dept. of Radiation Therapy and Nuclear Medicine and *Dept. of Medicine, Eleventh & Walnut Streets, Philadelphia, Pennsylvania 19107, U.S.A.

At Thomas Jefferson University Hospital, we have an ongoing program for the treatment of patients with localized, unresectable non-oat cell carcinoma of the lung to high tumor doses in the range of 6600-6800 rads using large priming tumor doses followed by extended fractionation radiotherapy. In an attempt to improve local control and survival, we have undertaken a phase I-II study combining this regimen with Cis-platinum 100 mg/M^2 on day 1 and 5-FU infusion 1 gm/M^2 for 24 hours on days 2-6. Chemotherapy was administered concomitantly with high-dose, small-volume tumor irradiation (600 rads on day 2 and 400 rads on day 4). This is followed by large field irradiation to a dose of 3500 rads. At this point the patient is given a 4 to 10 day rest. The entire cycle is then repeated for a total tumor dose of 7000 rads with the mediastinal dose limited to 5500-6000 rads, supraclavicular dose in the range of 4400-4800 rads and the spinal cord dose under 4600 rads. To date, 10 patients have been entered onto this treatment regimen. Two patients died before completing treatment and are unevaluable for response. One of these whose initial performance status was poor died of respiratory arrest; a second patient, who had an exploratory thoracotomy, developed pleural dissemination halfway through the treatment. Local tumor response and normal tissue reaction are assessed. The acute toxicity of this regimen has been limited to mild to moderate dysphagia and moderate leukopenia. There have been no fatalities related to treatment. Six of 8 patients evaluable for response have had a rapid and significant reduction (greater than 75%) in their tumor volume, with 4 of these being complete responses. Two patients developed clinically significant radiation pneumonitis requiring steroids.

The complete response rate seen in this pilot study is encouraging. Nevertheless, local recurrence and distant metastases remain a problem.

VI-10 FLUOROURACYL (5Fu) AND CISPLATIN (DDP) AS SALVAGE CHEMOTHERAPY IN OVARIAN CANCER (OC). M.V. Fiorentino*, F. Tredese*, O. Nicoletto*, G. Nardelli, P. Biondetti, T. Maggino, D. Marchesoni, S. Bolzonella*, O. Daniele*, A. Onnis. Divisions of *Medical Oncology and of Gynecology, Padova Medical Center, 35100 Padova, Italy.

From June '82 to April '83, 23 advanced OC patients (pts) entered a DDP-5Fu chemotherapy program, mainly after failure to Adriamycin (ADM) and alkilating agents. One patient with stage IV° for liver was lost for follow up and could not be evaluated; two further pts underwent early death. 20 Pts are now evaluable after 2 or more courses.
Cycles were given every 4 weeks: 5Fu at the dosage of 500 mg/M2.days 1 to 5 and DDP 100 mg/M2 in day 7. 14/20 evaluable pts had tumor residues >5 cm, assessed by surgery or CT Scan or Ultrasonography. Mean performance status was 70 (range 50 to 90).
Dose reductions were adopted for DDP, in case of renal function impairment: 75% of planned dose being administered when serum creatinine (SC) was between 1,5 and 2 mg/liter (14/85 administered courses) and 50% when SC was between 2 and 3 mg (18 courses).
5Fu was reduced to 75% in 9 courses, and 50% in 3 other cycles for hematological problems (out of 85 cycles given).
No nadir of WBC under 2300/cmm and of platelets under 80.000/cmm occurred. 7/20 evaluable pts obtained partial remission. 3/20 pts had been platinum pretreated and one responded for less than 2 months.
Duration of remission up to now have been 8+, 6+, 6, 4, 4+, 2+, 1+ months.

VI-11 CIS-PLATIN (DDP) PLUS VINDESINE (VDS) VERSUS DDP PLUS VP 16-213 VERSUS DOXORUBICYN (DOXO) PLUS CYTOXAN (CY): A RANDOMIZED STUDY IN ADVANCED NON SMALL CELL CANCER OF THE LUNG (NSSCL). M.V. Fiorentino, A. Paccagnella, L. Salvagno, V. Chiarion Sileni, A. Brandes, O. Vinante, L. Endrizzi, S. Bolzonella, V. Fosser. Divisione di Oncologia Medica - USL 21 - 35100 Padova (Italy).

Between March 1981 and March 1983, 98 patients (pts) with disseminated or inoperable histologically cnfirmed NSCCL entered into a randomized study with three arm: arm A: DDP (100 mg/M2 i.v. with a two hour infusion) every 4 weeks plus VDS (3 mg/M2 i.v.) weekly for 6 doses then every 2 weeks: arm B: DDP (as above) plus VP 16-213 (125 mg/M2 i.v.) on day 1,3,5 every 4 weeks; arm C: DOXO (40 mg/M2 i.v.) on day 1 plus CY (700 mg/M2 i.v.) on day 4; recycle every 3 weeks. Before randomization pts were stratified by histology (epidermoid/adeno/large cell type) and by diffusion of disease (limited/extensive according to VALG' criteria). Evaluation was after the third course. 3 further courses were given to responsive pts; 25% of pts had received prior radiotherapy or surgery. Up to now 76 pts are evaluable, with the following results:

	PTS	CR	PR	CR+PR	NR	
Arm A	25	3(12%)	11(44%)	14(56%)	11(45%)	A vs B: NS
Arm B	26	1(4%)	8(30%)	9(35%)	17(65%)	A vs C:P 0.001
Arm C	25	-(0%)	2(4%)	2(4%)	23(96%)	B vs C:P 0.05

Median duration of response is 4 mo.; no difference in responce duration among A-B-C. Toxicity: DDP-related gastrointestinal toxicity was noted in 100% of pts; treatment related death after DDP-VDS: haematological toxicity was minimal in all the 3 arms. Conclusions: containing regimens give a higher response rate than DOXO+CY; duration of response is similar in the 3 arms so that on increase in survival is not apparent for the moment.

VI-12 EFFECTIVE RADIATION SENSITIZATION OF HYPOXIC S. typhimurium CELLS BY SLIGHTLY TOXIC Pt(II)-COMPLEXES.
Robert C. Richmond and Evan B. Douple. Norris Cotton Cancer Center, Dartmouth-Hitchcock Medical Center, Hanover, NH 03755,U.S.A.
Barton L. Bergquist and James C. Chang. University of Northern Iowa, Cedar Falls, IA 50614,U.S.A.
Abdul R. Khokhar. University of Vermont, Burlington, VT 05405,U.S.A.
Beverly A. Teicher. Sidney Farber Cancer Institute, Boston, MA 02115,U.S.A.

The antitumor drug cis-dichlorodiammine Pt(II) (cis-DDP) is known to sensitize radiation-induced inactivation of hypoxic bact- erial cells. Analagous experiments in tissue culture with mammalian cells have shown only marginal hypoxic cell radiation sensitization by cis-DDP (i.e., synergistic inactivation caused by drug presence only during irradiation). In tissue culture the limiting cis-DDP concentration is low (ca. 10 micromolar) due to toxicity. This limiting concentration likely does not produce sufficient free radical interactions needed for radiation sensitization. This assumption requires that cis-DDP radiation sensitization operates through a compartment of free solution.

There are available a number of proven or potential Pt(II) antitumor drugs that are less toxic on a molar basis than cis-DDP. Lowered toxicity allows for the exposure of cells to higher concen- tration of platinum drug, and thus a more likely effective free solution compartment of radiation sensitization. Five Pt(II) com- plexes have been tested for radiation sensitization in order to begin examination of the free solution compartment of Pt(II)-induced radiation sensitization. Hypoxic stationary phase S. typhimurium cells were irradiated in PBS, pH 7, in the presence and absence of these Pt(II)-complexes. All complexes are essentially non-toxic at the concentrations used, and all are effective radiation sensitizers of these hypoxic cells. Cis-dichlorobis(fluoresceinamine) Pt(II) (synthesized by J. Chang and B. Bergquist) at 100 micromolar con- centration gives an ehnancement ratio of 1.7 (ratio of slopes of survival curves). Cis-bis(ascorbate)(1,2-diaminocyclohexane) Pt(II) (synthesized by A. Khokhar) at 200 micromolar gives an enhancement ratio of 1.4, as do 200 micromolar of cis-(1,1-cyclobutanedicarbox- ylato)(diammine) Pt(II) (JM-8 from Johnson-Matthey) and 200 micro- molar of cis-(2-ethylmalonato)(diammine) Pt(II) (JM-10 from Johnson- Matthey). An enhancement ratio of 1.6 is obtained from 200 micro- molar of the 2-nitroimidazole complex cis-dichlorobis(azomycin) Pt(II) (synthesized by B. Teicher). For reference, an oxygen en- hancement ratio of 2.6 is obtained from this system.
(Work supported by NIH grant CA26045).

VI-13 CISPLATINUM IN RECURRENT BRAIN TUMORS. Ativa B. Khan*, Bernard J. D'Souza*, Moody D. Wharam*, Lucius F. Sinks+, Shiao Woo+, David McCullough+ and Brigid G. Leventhal*. Johns Hopkins Oncology Center*, 600 N. Wolfe Street, Baltimore, Maryland 21205, U.S.A., Georgetown University+, 3800 Reservoir Road, Washington, D.C. 20006, U.S.A.

Twenty-two patients with brain tumors were treated initially with surgery, radiotherapy and/or adjuvant chemotherapy. At recurrence, demonstrated by CT scan, they were given cisplatinum 60 mg/m^2 i.v./d x 2 days every 3 weeks. Five patients received only 1 course and are not evaluable for response. Responses are graded as clinical improvement $\pm$ CT scan improvement as follows:

Tumor Type	# Evaluable Response	Response CT & Clin.	Clin.	NR	Response Duration (Mos.)
Glioma	7	2	1	4	(7+ - 34+)
Ependymoma	6	1	3	2	(1+ - 34+)
Others	4	4			(2 - 5)
Total	17	7	4	6	

"Others" included 1 dysgerminoma, 1 teratocarcinoma, 1 pinealoma and 1 small cell tumor. Toxicity was graded by CALGB criteria. The number of patients showing grade 3-4 toxicity were: platelets 7; white count 4; renal 3; GI 9. Nine out of eleven patients tested showed high frequency hearing loss. Acute fluid retention with low serum electrolytes and some serious, but reversible changes in mental status were seen in 13 patients. In summary, platinum appears active in a spectrum of brain tumors and should be further studied for therapeutic efficacy. Toxicity is manageable. Severe fluid and electrolyte problems are more common in patients with brain tumors.

VI-14 MECHANISM OF ACTION OF FREE OR INCORPORATED INTO LIPOSOMES CIS-DICHLORODIAMMINOPLATINUM II : A COMPARATIVE STUDY IN EHRLICH TUMOR CELLS. Marie-Claire De Pauw-Gillet[a], Claude Houssier[b], Georges Weber[c] and Roger Bassleer[a]. Institutes of Histology[a], Chemistry[b] and Nuclear Physics[c]. University of Liège, Belgium.

A better survival of animals bearing tumor cells has been obtained with cis-dichlorodiamminoplatinum II (or cis-DDPt) incorporated into liposomes; this is probably due to the local increase of cis-DDPt inside the tumor (1, 2). In the case of Ehrlich tumor cells (ELT) transplanted into the mouse peritoneal cavity we observed that a better survival of the animals was not obtained when cis-DDPt was given in association with fluid or solid negatively charged liposomes. An inflammatory reaction was noted in the peritoneal cavity.

On the contrary, cis-DDPt loaded liposomes were generally more cytotoxic than free cis-DDPt in ELT cells cultivated in vitro. An ultrastructural analysis of ELT cells cultivated and treated in vitro with cis-DDPt either free or incorporated into negatively charged fluid liposomes was performed. Free cis-DDPt provoked chromatin dispersion or condensation and formation of ribosomal aggregates in helicoïdal conformation. When incorporated into liposomes, cis-DDPt produced dense material accumulation inside small cytoplasmic vacuoles. However, ribosomal aggregation or chromatin modifications were not noted.

From in vitro experiments, we conclude that free cis-DDPt penetrates into the cell by permeation and reacts with nucleic acid in the cytoplasm and the nucleus, in which it induces similar modifications as those we had observed before in vegetal cells (3). When incorporated into liposomes, the agent essentially enters the cell by phagocytose and reaches the lysosomial apparatus, where lipids are degraded, liberating a part of cis-DDPt as a free drug; the latter could be activated inside the vacuoles by acidic pH and react with lysosomial enzymes or leave the vacuoles. Fusion of liposomes with plasma membrane could also liberate cis-DDPt in a free state, but these two mechanisms are very limited as judged by the nucleic acids ultrastructural modifications.

The lack of activity of cis-DDPt loaded liposomes in ELT bearing mice is probably due to several factors : macrophage and lymphatic absorption (4); heterogeneity of degree of endocytosis in ELT cells population; eventually lack of fusion with plasma membrane in vivo (4)

VI-15 PHASE II TRIAL OF CIS-DIAMMINE-1,1-CYCLOBUTANE DICARBOXYLATE PLATINUM II (CBDCA, JM8) IN PATIENTS WITH CARCINOMA OF THE OVARY NOT PREVIOUSLY TREATED WITH CISPLATIN
A Hilary Calvert, Joan W Baker, Vera M Dalley, Stephen J Harland, Adrian C Jones, Jean Staffurth
Royal Marsden Hospital, Surrey and London, England

CBDCA is an analogue of cisplatin shown to be virtually without nephrotoxicity and ototoxicity in phase I studies, while neurotoxicity and emesis were considerably less than would be expected from cisplatin treatment (Cancer Chemother. Pharmacol. $\underline{9}$ 140-147, 1982). In an early phase II study clinical responses were seen in patients with ovarian cancer, most of whom had previously been treated with cisplatin. In the present study thirty four patients not previously treated with cisplatin have been treated with CBDCA. A dose of 400 mg/m2 was given 4 weekly without hydration. Dose reductions were made for patients with previous myelosuppressive therapy or impaired renal function. Eight patients had received prior alkylating agent therapy. Six are currently not assessed, and of the remaining 28 there are 8 complete remissions (4 confirmed by laparotomy), 11 partial remissions, and 9 with no response. Toxicities seen were myelosuppression (median WBC nadir 3.4, range 1.9-7.0, median platelet nadir 98, range 58-531) and vomiting. Vomiting seldom persisted beyond 24 hours, and half the patients were treated as outpatients. JM8 given in this dose and schedule has activity comparable to that of cisplatin, but the toxicity to the patient is markedly reduced.

VI-16 PHASE II STUDY OF CIS-DIAMMINE-1,1-CYCLOBUTANE DICARBOXYLATE PLATINUM II (CBDCA, JM8) IN CARCINOMA OF BRONCHUS. Stephen J Harland, Ian E Smith, Neil Smith, Dawn I. Alison and A Hilary Calvert. The Lung Unit,Royal Marsden Hospital Downs Road, Sutton, Surrey, England.

CBDCA an analogue of cisplatin, which showed less nephrotoxicity and emesis in phase I studies has been used as a single agent for the treatment of patients with carcinoma of bronchus. The drug was given as a 1 hour infusion every 4 weeks at a dosage of 400 mg/m' with reductions being made for advanced age previous radiotherapy and poor renal function. 18 patients with small cell anaplastic histology have been treated. Nine of these had relapsed on other treatment and none of them responded to CBDCA. Four out of six who had relapsed following a good remission from previous combination chemotherapy responded to CBDCA. Three previously untreated patients all responded to CBDCA overall response rate = 39%. Of nine untreated patients with non small cell carcinoma two have shown a response to the drug. The only side effects noted were nausea and myelosuppression. Nausea was easily controlled in these patients and myelosuppression was never more severe than grade 1. The results suggest that CBDCA is an active drug in small cell anaplastic carcinoma of bronchus when patients are not resistant to previous chemotherapy. The lack of alopecia makes this form of treatment particularly attractive to female patients with poor prognosis. If the single agent activity is maintained in a larger series the drug deserves consideration for use in combination regimens in bronchial carcinoma.

VI-17 BINDING SITES FOR CYTOTOXIC METAL IONS AND COMPLEXES WITHIN EHRLICH CELLS. A. Kraker, S. Krezoski, J. Schneider, J. Schmidt, and D. Petering, Department of Chemistry, University of Wisconsin-Milwaukee, Milwaukee, Wisconsin 53201.

Ehrlich ascites tumor cells contain a Zn binding protein with the chemical and immunological properties of metallothionein (Mt). Mt plays a central part in Zn, Cu, and Cd metabolism in normal tissues. In the present study the interactions of cytotoxic forms of Cu, Cd, and Pt have been investigated. When 3-ethoxy-2-oxobutyraldehyde bis-(thiosemicarbazonato) Cu(II) (CuKTS) is reacted with Ehrlich cells in vitro, in culture, or in vivo, Cu(II) is reduced, dissociated from the complex, and bound to Mt as zinc is displaced. Titration of Ehrlich cells with CuKTS shows that Mt is the principal site of binding of Cu until it is saturated; subsequently Cu binds to other protein sites. In this same concentration range, DNA synthesis is inhibited and cell proliferation is inhibited as well. After a pulse of CuKTS to Ehrlich cells in culture, Mt-Cu is stable over a 24 hr period. Other protein-bound Cu is lost with a first order rate constant of 0.06 hr^{-1}, and new ZnMt is slowly made. Within hours after ZnMt appears, proliferation begins. A similar relationship exists between the binding of Cd to Mt, displacement of zinc, and inhibition of proliferation of Ehrlich cells in culture. Finally, at concentrations of cis-diaminedichloro Pt(II) which inhibit cell proliferation by 50%, 30% of the cellular Pt is bound to Mt. In zinc-deficient mice, there is a correlation between the loss of Zn from Mt and the suppression of cell proliferation. Thus, in several different systems there is an empirical relationship between Mt-zinc and Ehrlich cell proliferation. Whether this is a causal association has yet to be determined. However, the finding that Mt exists in at least 6 transplantable tumor lines indicates that this protein may be a major binding site for metals in a variety of tumors.
(Supported by GM 29583-01).

VI-18 PLATINUM-RADIATION BASED COMBINED MODALITY APPROACH FOR LO-CALLY-ADVANCED CANCER OF THE HEAD AND NECK. *Christopher T. Coughlin and Evan B. Douple. *Norris Cotton Cancer Center, Dartmouth-Hitchcock Medical Center, Hanover, New Hampshire 03755, U.S.A.

Twenty-five patients with locally-advanced carcinoma of the head and neck (stage III and IV) have been treated with a regimen utilizing induction chemotherapy. Cis-dichlorodiammineplatinum (II) (cis-DDP) at 100 mg/m2 was given day 1 followed by a Bleomycin infusion of 15 u/m2 over 24 hours-days 2-5. Day 21, a second dose of cis-DDP at 100 mg/m2 was delivered I.V. over ½ hour. Day 22, radiotherapy was initiated at 2 Gy/day tumor dose to the primary site and both sides of the neck. This was administered in standard fashion to 48 Gy in 5 weeks. During the radiation sequence, the platinum was administered weekly on an outpatient basis at 20 mg/m2 I.V. one hour prior to irradiation. Response after 48 Gy was assessed and patients were consolidated either with surgery or with a boost of 20 Gy to the primary site and areas of previous clinically involved nodal disease with no further platinum. This protocol is designed to exploit cis-DDP in a dual role of active tumoricidal agent and radiation potentiator. Twenty-one out of 24 patients evaluable for response were in complete clinical response at the end of all therapy; 17 maintained good local control, and 13 are still alive and well at an average of 15 months post therapy. Six patients had biopsies obtained after cis-DDP infusion. These were assayed for tumor tissue platinum concentration using atomic absorption spectroscopy. Only two samples contained detectable amounts of platinum. This most likely represents inadequate sample size as well as inconsistent timing of the biopsy post cis-DDP infusion. The levels obtained were in the 1 micromolar range, which is consistent with the concentrations necessary to show sensitization in vitro.

VI-19 POTENTIATION OF CELL KILL BY COMBINING NITROIMIDAZOLE-
PLATINUM COMPLEXES WITH RADIATION. Evan B. Douple and
Beverly A. Teicher. Norris Cotton Cancer Center, Dartmouth-
Hitchcock Medical Center, Hanover, New Hampshire 03756, U.S.A. and
Sidney Farber Cancer Institute, Boston, Massachusetts 02115, U.S.A.

Studies are now employing radiation sensitizers in attempts to
overcome the radioresistance afforded by hypoxia in solid tumors.
Results of clinical trials using the two electron affinic drugs
metronidazole and misonidazole are discouraging because of toxicity.
Potentiation of radiation-induced cell kill in hypoxic cells by cis-
dichlorodiammineplatinum(II) has also been reported previously, but
this effect is achieved in vitro at levels of drug concentration
which are quite toxic, presumably due to the platinum complex
binding to DNA. We report here results of experiments designed to
test interaction between radiation and two platinum complexes which
include potential radiosensitizers as ligands in their structure.
It is hypothesized that the potentiation by classic radiosensitizers may be enhanced by delivering the active ligand to the DNA
using the platinum complex as a carrier. The first complex tested
was A6431 [cis-dichlorodi-1-(2-hydroxyethyl)2-methyl-5-nitro-3-
imidazole platinum(II)], obtained courtesy of C. Coulson (May &
Baker Ltd). The second complex was 2NIPt[cis-dichlorobis(azomycin)-
platinum(II)],synthesized by one of us (B. Teicher). Unfed
plateauphase (6 day) confluent monolayer cultures of V79 cells were
rendered hypoxic and exposed 100-400 μm concentrations of platinum
complex in complete medium for 90 min before irradiation.
Surviving fractions were determined by CFU analysis of trypsinized
and subcultured cells. Cells which received the combined
2NIPt-radiation treatment revealed a potentiation of cell kill
which was enhanced with increasing dose. The effect was not
apparent when the radiation dose was delivered under ambient
conditions. When A6431 or 2NIPt were added to cells immediately
after irradiation in air and present during a post-irradiation
incubation, cellular recovery, defined operationally as repair of
potentially lethal damage (PLD), was totally inhibited. Both of
these effects were observed using essentially nontoxic doses of
A6431 (SF=0.90) and 2NIPt (SF=0.98). These results suggest a
rationale for the design of platinum complexes which incorporate
radiosensitizer ligands. The design of therapy protocols should
consider coordination of the irradiation with the platinum complex
as as to exploit radiosensitization and/or modulation of PLD
recovery. The radiosensitizer-platinum complexes might be
administered with conventional radiosensitizers to produce further
potentiation of hypoxic cell kill with less normal tissue toxicity.

VI-20 COMBINATION CHEMOTHERAPY INCLUDING CIS-PLATINUM(DDP),METHO-
TREXATE AND 5-FLUOROURACIL(PMF) IN ADVANCED OVARIAN CANCER.
PierF. Conte[*] Milena Bruzzone[*] Mario R. Sertoli[*][+] Riccardo Rosso[*]
Alessandra Rubagotti[*] Giuseppe Pescetto[.]Istituto Scientifico Tumori[*]
Istituto Oncologia Università[*][+]Clinica Ginecologica Università[.]16132
Genova, Italy.

The usual therapeutic approach for advanced ovarian cancer is based
on maximal debulking surgery followed by aggressive combination chemo
therapy (CT) containing DDP,alkylating agents or adriamycin.Gastro
intestinal and renal toxicity of platinum and the cardiotoxicity of
adriamycin reduce the number of patients who can be submitted to
these regimens.In order to minimize side effects related to treatment,we used the following chemotherapeutic regimen:DDP 25mg/M^2d.1,8;
MTX 25mg/M^2d.1; 5-FU 600mg./M^2d.1 q.28 d(PMF).The aims of the study
were:1)to assess the effectiveness of a combination CT with DDP and
antimetabolites; 2)to evaluate the possibility to reduce DDP gastro-
intestinal-renal toxicity by administrating DDP in divided doses.
Starting from June 1981 38 pts (28untreated,10 pretreated) were
submitted to PMF. Clinical response was evaluated after 6 courses
of CT: 2 pts(pretreated) who died after the 1st cycle were considered
for survival,not for response.Of the 26 stage III-IV untreated pts,
7underwent optimal surgery(residual disease < 2cm),19 suboptimal
surgery before CT.Only 2/10 pretreated pts underwent cytoreductive
surgery(residual disease < 2cm) before CT.13 pts(8 untreated,5pretreg
ted)progressed(36.1%).7pts (1 pretreated,6untreated) had a clinical
partial response(CPR) after 6 cycles(19.4%);5/7 were submitted to
surgical 2nd look and 4/7 underwent further cytoreductive surgery;in
1 case a pathological complete remission(PCR)and in 3 cases residual
disease < 2cm were obtained.16 pts(4 pretreated,12 untreated) had a
clinical complete response(CCR) (44.5%)and underwent surgical 2nd look
7(2 pretreated,5untreated)proved to be PCR;2 untreated pts revealed
persistent microscopic disease(positive washing only)and 7(2 pretreated,5 untreated)persistent nodular widespread disease surgically resectable in 2 cases.Pts achieving CPR or having persistent disease at
the 2nd look were submitted to further 6 courses of PMF.The overall
survival at 12 and 24 mo. is 55% and 19.2% respectively.The overall
relapse free survival at 12 and 24 mo. is 42% and 10.2% respectively.
Analysis of data in relation to the extent of residual disease after
surgery and prior chemotherapy shows that the most important prognostic factor in our series seems to be the extent of postsurgical residual disease:of the 9pts with < 2cm disease,8 achieved CCR,4 of
which pathologically confirmed.No renal toxicity was observed and
gastrointestinal side effects of treatment were very moderate.

VI-21 CHEMOPOTENTIATION OF MITOMYCIN C CYTOTOXICITY IN VITRO BY CIS-DIAMMINEDICHLOROPLATINUM(II) AND THREE NEWLY SYNTHE-SIZED PLATINUM COMPLEXES. Beverly A. Teicher, Sidney Farber Cancer Institute, 44 Binney Street, Boston, MA 02115, U.S.A.

The potential of cis-diamminedichloroplatinum(II) (CDDP), cis-di(2-amino-5-nitrothiazole)dichloroplatinum(II) (Plant), cis-(1,2-diamino-4-nitrobenzene)dichloroplatinum(II) (Plato), and cis-dipyridinedichloroplatinum(II) (PyPt) to act as chemosensitizers of mitomycin C toward EMT6 cells under oxygenated and hypoxic conditions has been assessed. For a 2 hr. exposure, CDDP had an ED_{50} of 0.006 uM (oxygenated) and an ED_{50} of 0.0089 uM (hypoxic). The ratio of ED_{50}'s oxygenated/hypoxic for CDDP was 0.67 indicating that this drug is almost equally cytotoxic toward oxygenated and hypoxic cells. Plant had an ED_{50} of 9.42 uM (oxygenated) and an ED_{50} of 0.008 uM (hypoxic); the ratio of ED_{50}'s was 1,000 showing that Plant is more cytotoxic toward hypoxic cells. In oxygenated cells, Plato had an ED_{50} of 25,000 uM, while the ED_{50} (hypoxic) was 0.25 uM. The ratio of ED_{50}'s was 100,000 indicating that Plato was significantly more cytotoxic toward hypoxic cells. For PyPt the ED_{50} (oxygenated) was 0.011 uM and the ED_{50} (hypoxic) was 3.75 uM giving a ratio of oxygenated to hypoxic cell killing of 0.003. Therefore, PyPt is more cytotoxic toward oxygenated cells than hypoxic cells. Two concentrations of each platinum complex, 0.1 and 0.01 uM, were tested in combination with mitomycin C at 1, 0.1 and 0.01 uM. The results were analyzed via isobolograms. Under oxygenated conditions the combination of CDDP and mitomycin C produced a 2-3-fold enhancement in cell killing. Under hypoxic conditions enhancements of 5-fold, 20-fold and 60-fold were obtained with 1, 0.1 and 0.01 uM mitomycin C, respectively. The Plant-mitomycin C combination produced a 2-3-fold enhancement in cell killing under oxygenated conditions, and a 5-14-fold enhancement in cell killing under hypoxic conditions. Under hypoxic conditions the combinations of 0.1 and 0.01 uM Plato and mitomycin C were 30-60-fold more cytotoxic than expected. At 0.01 uM Plato an 8-16-fold enhancement in cytotoxicity was observed under hypoxic conditions. Plato plus mitomycin showed a 3-fold enhancement over additivity under oxygenated conditions. PyPt and mitomycin C were strictly additive under oxygenated conditions and the combination produced an 8-14-fold enhancement in cytotoxicity under hypoxic conditions. Overall, the two most effective chemopotentiators or mitomycin C cytotoxicity toward hypoxic cells were CDDP and Plato. PyPt and Plant were only slightly less effective.

DAVID B. BROWN
MEMORIAL LECTURE

Cisplatin — Past, Present and Future
S.K. Carter

Cisplatin is a triumph which elucidates many aspects of clinical cancer research in general and drug development research in particular. As is well known cisplatin was discovered initially by a brilliantly intuitive serendipitous observation by Dr. Barrett Rosenberg.[1] The critical step in bringing the drug to clinical trial was the observation by the NCI drug development program that the compound was highly effective in its experimental tumor systems. It was this experimental activity which led the NCI to develop the drug for clinical study and ultimately file an Investigational New Drug application (IND) with the Food and Drug Administration.[2] It is worth noting that the first patient treated with the drug was at the Wadley Institute in Dallas, without an IND, and at initially very high doses. In the NCI sponsored trials it was initially observed that the drug was active and toxic to the kidney. Some early views were that the renal toxicity would obviate general widespread use of the drug. The potential value of the drug was so obvious however that experimentation eventually found, through hydration, a mechanism to significantly ameliorate the renal toxicity. With the ability to circumvent renal toxicity, higher doses of the drug could be administered and a wide range of solid tumor activity was uncovered. This activity brought the drug into the disease-oriented strategies of the national cancer programs clinical research thrust. For example the activity in testicular cancer, first observed at Roswell-Park Memorial Institute,[3-4] by the group under James Hollands leadership, had significant impact on the development of curative chemotherapy for this disease in its metastatic phase (Figure 1). Golbey and associates first combined cisplatin with vinblastine, bleomycin and actinomycin D after the important observation by Samuels[6] of the great activity of high dose vinblastine combined with bleomycin. Einhorn[7] achieved the most successful, and widely accepted results, combining cisplatin with high dose vinblastine and bleomycin, initially with BCG.

The license for marketing cisplatin was obtained by the Bristol-Myers Company and they prepared the new drug application (NDA) which enabled the drug to be approved by the FDA for sale in the indications of testicular cancer and ovarian cancer. Subsequently Bristol-Myers also obtained NDA approval for the additional indication of bladder cancer.

The history of cisplatin is therefore a mixture of academic, government and industrial input and collaboration which is representative of what has occurred with the great majority of successful cancer drugs since the beginning of the modern era of cancer chemotherapy.

Figure 1

CISPLATIN HISTORY IN TESTICULAR CANCER

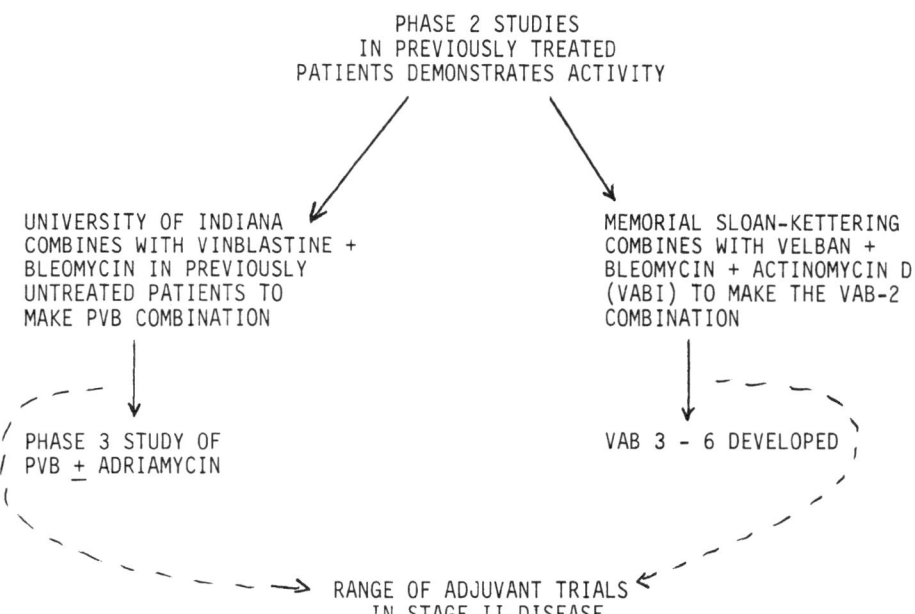

PHASE 2 STUDIES
IN PREVIOUSLY TREATED
PATIENTS DEMONSTRATES ACTIVITY

UNIVERSITY OF INDIANA
COMBINES WITH VINBLASTINE +
BLEOMYCIN IN PREVIOUSLY
UNTREATED PATIENTS TO
MAKE PVB COMBINATION

MEMORIAL SLOAN-KETTERING
COMBINES WITH VELBAN +
BLEOMYCIN + ACTINOMYCIN D
(VABI) TO MAKE THE VAB-2
COMBINATION

PHASE 3 STUDY OF
PVB $\pm$ ADRIAMYCIN

VAB 3 - 6 DEVELOPED

RANGE OF ADJUVANT TRIALS
IN STAGE II DISEASE

STUDY NEVER PERFORMED

R
— VINBLASTINE + BLEOMYCIN
— VINBLASTINE + BLEOMYCIN + CISPLATIN

Cisplatin is one of the most effective anti-cancer drugs ever discovered. Despite the fact that it is only commercially approved for use in 3 tumor types (testicular, ovarian and bladder cancer) it has demonstrated evidence of activity against a wide range of other malignancies (Table 1). Despite the fact that clinical investigation with cisplatin began in 1971 the clinical research which still remains to be undertaken is enormous. While a great deal of clinical research with cisplatin has been undertaken, the majority of this research has been disease-oriented in nature ignoring the drug oriented question of elucidating the exact role of cisplatin in the disease under study. The research has involved platinum in combinations with other drugs and/or modalities in an approach geared exclusively to improve the therapeutic results within the disease. This approach does not concern itself with attempts to dissect out the value or role of the individual component parts of the regimen under study. In this disease-oriented strategy, the lowest priority study is the pivotal Phase 3 study demanded by the FDA for clearly establishing the approvability of a given drug for marketing in that disease. These studies must be stimulated, supported and analyzed by the pharmaceutical industry if an NDA is to be filed. The needed cisplatin research can be viewed in both disease-oriented (Table 2) and modality oriented (Table 3) terms. In disease-oriented terms this research involves:

1. elucidating the single agent activity;

2. probing the multiple potentials for combination regimens with other active drugs;

3. probing the potentials for combining cisplatin alone or in combination with radiation therapy;

4. probing the potential as surgical adjuvant treatment;

5. clearly elucidating the role of the drug in the optimal therapy of the disease within its various stages, and obtaining approval from the FDA for marketing the indication.

This disease oriented approach needs to be undertaken for every disease in Table 3 and for every other disease in which appropriate Phase 2 studies still remain to be undertaken if they should turn out to be positive.

In drug oriented terms this research involves:

1. exploring new dosage schedules;

2. exploring alternate routes of administration e.g., intra-arterial and intraperitoneal;

3. exploring various high dose level approaches with either hypertonic saline or renal toxicity protectors e.g. sodium thiosulfate;

4. explore approach to blocking or ameliorating the renal toxicity;

5. explore approach to blocking or ameliorating the nausea and vomiting caused by the drugs;

6. explore the role of the drug as a radiosensitizer and how to optimally combine it with radiation therapy;

7. explore the interaction of the drug with the immune system and the body's host defenses against neoplastic disease;

8. exploring the mechanisms of tumor cell resistance to the drug with goal of developing ameliorative strategies to overcome resistance.

TABLE 1

Tumor types for which cisplatin has shown evidence of
anti-tumor activity which indicates the need for further
clinical research to establish the true indication
(exclusive of ovary, testes, and bladder)

1. Squamous cell carcinoma of the head .and neck.

2. Squamous cell carcinoma of the cervix.

3. Oat cell or small cell anaplastic lung cancer.

4. Non small cell lung cancer (in combination with VP-16 or
    vinca alkaloids).

5. Adenocarcinoma of the stomach.

6. Carcinoma of the esophagus.

7. Adenocarcinoma of the prostate.

8. Osteogenic sarcoma.

9. Soft tissue and bone sarcomas.

10. Non Hodgkins lymphoma.

11. Adenocarcinoma of the breast.

12. Brain tumors.

13. Thyroid cancer.

14. Endometrial cancer.

TABLE 2

DISEASE-ORIENTED[*]
STRATEGIES FOR CISPLATIN

1. Combine with other active drugs:

    A.   Begin with Phase 1-2 pilot or exploratory study.

    B.   Phase 3 study to elucidate actual role.

2. Where appropriate combine with surgery:

    A.   As adjuvant after surgical resection.

    B.   As neoadjuvant prior to surgery resection
         (example: head and neck).

    C.   With cytoreductive surgery
         (example: ovary, oat-cell, lung).

    D.   With surgical resection of metastases
         (example: sarcoma).

3. When appropriate combine with radiation therapy:

    A.   As adjuvant therapy after radiation.

    B.   As a sensitizer given just prior to and/or
         simultaneously with x-ray.

    C.   A combination of the above.

4. Determine role(s) for drug within the various stages of disease
    therapeutic situations and therapeutic sequences.

[*]All options potentially exist after Phase 2 studies indicate a
meaningful level of activity.

TABLE 3

DRUG-ORIENTED OPTIONS*
FOR IMPROVING THE THERAPEUTIC INDEX OF CISPLATIN

I. DRUG MANIPULATIONS

1. Increase dose:

A. with hypertonic saline;

B. with toxicity protectors such as sodium thiosulfate, WR-2721 etc;

2. Change schedule:

A. continuous infusion;

B. more chronic schedules;

3. Change route:

A. intraperitoneal;

B. intra-arterial;

C. intravesical;

4. Toxicity blocking:

A. anti-renal;

B. anti-emetic.

II. ANALOGUE DEVELOPMENT

1. Improve activity in responsive tumors.

2. Broaden spectrum of activity.

3. Diminish acute or chronic toxicity.

4. Lack of cross-resistance with cisplatin:

A. use sequentially with cisplatin;

B. combine with cisplatin.**

*All of these at Phase 2 level interact with disease-oriented study.
**Starts a new drug-oriented flow.

The complexity of the disease-oriented research potential with cisplatin can be demonstrated in head and neck cancer. In this tumor there is ample Phase 2 evidence demonstrating that cisplatin as a single agent gives response rates in the 30 to 40% range when effectively delivered to advanced disease patients without prior exposure to cytotoxic drugs.[8] Therefore, platinum appears to be equally effective, or potentially superior to methotrexate and bleomycin which are considered to be the two established effective agents against the disease.[9] Other drugs with evidence of activity include mitomycin C, 5-fluorouracil and vinblastine.[9]

One strategy of research would be to clearly define the single agent activity of cisplatin in comparison to the other active single agents. A clinical trial design to accomplish that is shown below:

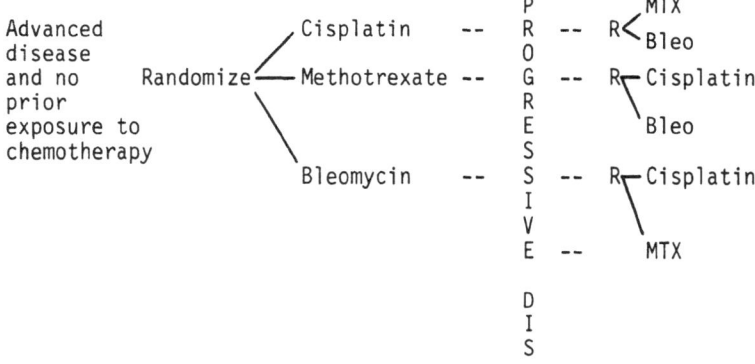

Combination chemotherapy brings forth a tremendous number in potential clinical research. Within the three active agents the following combination potentials exist:

- Cisplatin + MTX
- Cispaltin + Bleo
- Bleo + MTX
- Cisplatin + Bleo + MTX

All of these combinations have been looked at in a Phase 1-2 sense and there is evidence that all of the cisplatin containing combinations might be superior to single agent uses. Only a small percentage of the Phase 3 studies which potentially could be undertaken have actually been performed. The Northern California Oncology Group has compared in a randomized fashion cisplatin + MTX to cisplatin alone. While the combination resulted in a higher partial response rate, no survival gain has been demonstrated.

The combination of cisplatin + Bleomycin has been demonstrated to be active in several studies by the group at Memorial Sloan-Kettering in New York.[10] Its true role however still remains to be elucidated by Phase 3 studies. The potential Phase 3 studies which could be undertaken include the following:

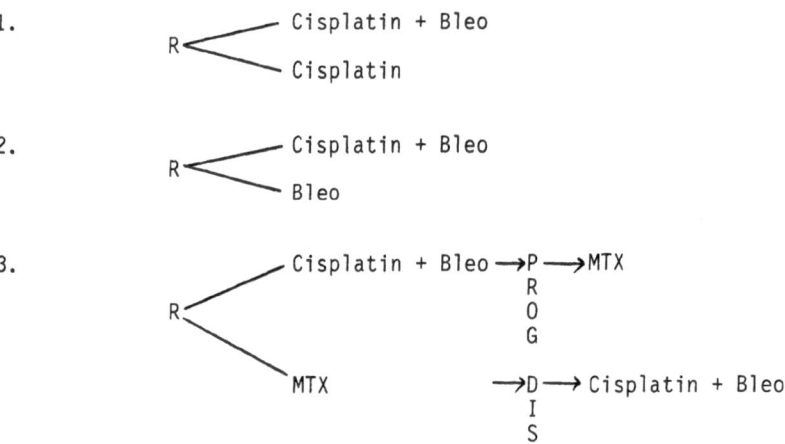

The disease oriented combination chemotherapy becomes even more complex when three additional drugs are added to the potential constituents for combination chemotherapy. The number of two, three and four drug regimens which can be derived from six drugs utilizing cisplatin become quite large and only a few of these have in actuality been given Phase 1-2 clinical trials to date.

Still another level of complexity is brought to bear when combined modality approach with cisplatin, either alone, or in combination, are considered for the treatments of stage 3-4 disease. These broad options include the following:

1. Radiation + chemotherapy for inoperable stage 3-4 disease.

2. For operable stage 3-4 disease:

*Chemotherapy $\longrightarrow$ Surgery

*Chemotherapy $\longrightarrow$ Surgery $\longrightarrow$ x-ray

*Chemotherapy $\longrightarrow$ Surgery $\longrightarrow$ chemotherapy$^+$

Surgery $\longrightarrow$ x-ray $\longrightarrow$ chemotherapy$^+$

X-ray $\longrightarrow$ surgery $\longrightarrow$ chemotherapy$^+$

* = neoadjuvant chemotherapy.

+ = adjuvant chemotherapy.

Currently there has been some investigation of cisplatin + Bleo as neoadjuvant chemotherapy and cisplatin alone as adjuvant chemotherapy. One actual trial which has been on-going for several years is evaluating the following options:

Operable
Stage 3-4   R
Disease

Cisplatin + Bleo $\longrightarrow$ surgery $\longrightarrow$ x-ray

Cisplatin + Bleo $\longrightarrow$ surgery $\longrightarrow$ x-ray $\longrightarrow$ cisplatin

Surgery $\longrightarrow$ x-ray

The seven options just discussed offer seven potential arms of a randomized Phase 3 study which the chemotherapy could be cisplatin alone or cisplatin + Bleo to focus on just two chemotherapy options. All of this ignores the added variables of number of drug courses, schedule and intensity of treatment delivery.

The options for inoperable stage 3-4 disease with x-ray include the following:

1. Chemotherapy $\longrightarrow$ x-ray
2. X-ray + chemotherapy
3. X-ray $\longrightarrow$ chemotherapy
4. 1 + 2
5. 2 + 3
6. 1 + 2 + 3

This offers six potential arms for a randomized Phase 3 study which the chemotherapy could be cisplatin alone or cisplatin + Bleomycin.

In summary, the various options for the role of cisplatin chemotherapy within the context of advanced (stage 3-4) head and neck are the following:

1. Drug treatment of recurrent disease after surgery and/or x-ray and metastatic disease beyond the scope of local control;

2. Neoadjuvant surgical therapy for operable disease.

3. Adjuvant surgical therapy for operable disease.

4. Radiation sensitizer and/or adjuvant therapy for locally inoperable disease.

Within each option there exist the further option of cisplatin alone or in combination with other drugs and the potential control groups for pivotal studies designed to satisfy the FDA requirements.

Each of the other 13 diseases listed in Table 1 need to be approached in a way similar to the ones just discussed for head and neck cancer. This would involve an initial panoply of exploratory research studies to focus on the potential optimal area within the diseases, to utilize cisplatin, either alone or in combination. This would be followed by the design and execution of the required controlled clinical trials to establish the efficacy and safety of the drug for this indication.

The drug oriented research strictly would follow a Phase 1   2   3 flow with an intergration into the disease oriented strategy.

One example would be intraperitoneal administration of cisplatin. After a Phase 1 study to establish the highest safe dose by this route there would occur a Phase 2 study in ovarian cancer to evaluate whether a response rate is observed which gives a reasonable hope of being superior to standardly administered parenteral cisplatin. If the Phase 2 study was positive then intraperitoneal cisplatin would be integrated into a series of disease oriented ovarian cancer trials to clearly demonstrate the efficacy of this approach.

A second example includes intra-arterial cisplatin administered into the hepatic artery. There is early exploratory data (Phase 1-2) indicating that this regional delivery methodology might increase the response rate in hepatic metastasis from gastrointestinal adenocarcinomas, including colorectal cancer, as well as in primary hepatomas. What will be needed are large scale prospectively randomized trials to demonstrate that i.a. cisplatin, alone or in combination is safe, efficacious and superior to the same parenterally administered drugs. This i.a. route opens up the potential for cisplatin to be studied in tumors such as colorectal cancer, pancreatic cancer and hepatomas.

CISPLATIN ANALOGS

The essence of evaluating an analog is the comparison with the parent compound. The comparison is made in terms of efficacy, as well as acute and chronic toxicity. The clinical trial of an analog must take place within the context of the role that has been established for the parent compound. This context determines where the analog can be studied, and in the case of a highly effective compound e.g. cisplatin, can put significant limitations on the clinical trial strategy.

A new analog of platinum could improve the therapeutic index by either diminishing the toxicity or increasing the efficacy. The diminished toxicity could be either of the acute kind (nausea and vomiting and/or myelosuppression) or the chronic (renal, ototoxicity, or neuro-toxicity). The increased efficacy could be either a higher response rate in the responsive tumors or a broadening of the spectrum of clinical activity. A third possibility for an analog would be lack of cross-resistance with cisplatin in tumors responsive to the parent compound.

A toxic modification in an analog of cisplatin could be of significant value. The renal toxicity impacts on cisplatin usage in a variety of ways. It limits chronic dosing and therefore hinders effective maintenance regimens. Since the drug is part of highly effective regimens, this is an important consideration. In addition, high doses of cisplatin can only be given with vigorous hydration, which makes it one of the more complex drugs to administer successfully. If renal toxicity could be reduced then an "MTD" could be established based on myelosuppression, which theoretically might be more efficacious.

Another problem is the nausea and vomiting that is ubiquitous with cisplatin and that is a great discomfort to many patients. This too limits chronic dosing to some degree. An improvement in this toxicity could also be an important benefit in an analog.

In the selection of patients for Phase 2 studies, with cisplatin analogs, the prior therapy choices can be manifold and can impact upon the end-result which is felt to indicate positivity. In a cisplatin sensitive tumor e.g. ovarian cancer the variables can be as follows:

1. no prior chemotherapy;

2. prior chemotherapy but no exposure to cisplatin;

3. prior exposure to cisplatin without evidence of resistance;

4. prior exposure to cisplatin with evidence of resistance.

At the Royal Marsden Hospital it is felt to be acceptable that ovarian cancer patients be treated with CBCDA, as a single agent, in patients without prior chemotherapy exposure. In the United States, where combination chemotherapy, usually including cisplatin, is considered the regular first line drug approach. This single agent design would be more difficult to use.

The minimal level of activity in a Phase 2 study, which would warrant Phase 3 studies being undertaken, would have to depend on the prior treatment characteristics of the patients chosen. The difference in potential responsiveness between a women with ovarian cancer and no prior chemotherapy exposure vs one failing on a cisplatin containing combination is obvious (Table 4). Ideally trials, and end-points, should be individually designed for each of the critical pre-therapeutic subsets.

TABLE 4

PLATINUM ANALOGUES
PHASE II STRATEGY OPTION
OVARIAN CANCER

I.	NO PREVIOUS CHEMOTHERAPY	30-40%
II.	PREVIOUS CHEMOTHERAPY (No Cisplatin)	20-30%
III.	PREVIOUS CHEMOTHERAPY (Including Cisplatin)	15-25%

With a drug as active as cisplatin, with its multiple analogs already in clinical trial, a myriad of research opportunities exist (Table 5). It is obvious that only a portion of this research can be undertaken and that it must be complete in the marketplace of research ideas, for its proper priority. The value of scientific meetings, such as this one, is that it enables a flow of ideas to occur among the researchers interested in the platinum area, so that hopefully the optimal research ideas can be pursued with minimal overlapped duplication.

375

TABLE 5

A LIFETIME OF CLINICAL RESEARCH
OPPORTUNITIES WITH 3 CISPLATIN ANALOGS

I. Single Agent Approaches

    1. Compare with cisplatin   Previously untreated

    2. Compare with each other   Previously treated
                                                   A. no cisplatin
    3. Compare with other single agents   B. cisplatin

II. Combination Approaches

    1. Combine with other drugs   Phase I-II
                                              pilot studies
    2. Combine with cisplatin   ↓
        A. CBCDA + cisplatin   Phase II disease
        B. Chip + cisplatin   specific studies
        C. TNO-6 + cisplatin   ↓
        D. Three 3-drug combinations   Phase III studies
        E. Four drug combination

    3. Combine with each other

                    All of the above

                    ± irradiation

                    ± biologic response modifiers

REFERENCES

1. Rosenberg B: Cisplatin: its history and possible mechanisms of
    action in, Prestayko AW, Crooke ST and Carter SK (eds): Cisplatin:
    Current Status and New Developments; Academic Press, NYC, pp 9-21,
    1980.

2. Carter SK and Goldsmith M: The development and clinical testing of
    new anti-cancer drugs at the National Cancer Institute - example
    cis-platinum (II) diamminedichloride (NSC 119875) in, Connors TA and
    Roberts JJ (eds): Platinum Coordination Complexes in Cancer
    Chemotherapy; Springer-Verlag, Heidelberg, pp 137-145, 1974.

3. Wallace HJ and Higby DJ: Phase 1 evaluation of cis-platinum (II)
    diamminedichloride (PDD) and a combination of PDD plus Adriamycin.
    Ibid 2, pp 167-177

4. Higby DJ, Wallace HJ, Albert DJ, et al: Diamminedichloride-
    platinum: a Phase 1 study showing responses in testicular and other
    tumors. Cancer 33:1219, 1974.

5. Wittes RE, Yagoda A, Silvay O, et al: Chemotherapy of germ cell
    tumors of the testing. Cancer 37:637, 1976.

6. Samuels ML, Johnson DE, Holoye PY: Continuous intravenous bleomycin
    therapy with vinblastin in stage III testicular neoplasium. Cancer
    Chemother Rep 59:563, 1975.

7. Einhorn LH and Williams SD: The management of disseminated
    testicular cancer in, Carter SK, Livingston RB and Glatstein E:
    Principles of Cancer Treatment; McGraw-Hill, NYC, pp 605-612, 1982.

8. Jacobs C: The role of cisplatin in the treatment of recurrent head
    and neck cancer. Ibid 1, pp 423-431.

9. Carter SK and Livingston RB: The chemotherapy of head and neck
    cancer. Ibid 7, pp 644-652.

10. Wittes R, et al: Cis-dichlorodiammineplatinum (II) based
    chemotherapy as initial treatment of advanced head and neck cancer.
    Cancer Treat Rep 63:1533, 1979.

AUTHOR INDEX

SUBJECT INDEX